Pandemic, States and Societies in the Asia-Pacific, 2020–2021

Hawksley and Georgeou bring together scholars and practitioners from across the region to analyse the main effects of the first two years of the COVID pandemic in a range of case studies from Southeast Asia, East Asia, South Asia, and Oceania.

The book provides a broad survey of how Indonesia, Bangladesh, Japan, the Philippines, Vietnam, Nepal, Australia, Cambodia, Taiwan, and New Zealand attempted to manage the COVID pandemic; the challenges they faced; and how they fared. Drawing on insights from politics, economics, sociology, law, public health, education, and geography, most authors are nationals of the cases they discuss. Written in non-specialist language, ten case studies are examined, providing a useful analysis of the first two years of COVID in the Asia-Pacific from the emergence of COVID in January 2020 to the lifting of restrictions in December 2021. Chapters focus on different issues according to the scholar's academic expertise, and a wide diversity of national pandemic experiences, challenges, and responses are showcased.

An essential read for scholars and students interested in the areas of Asia-Pacific politics, sociology, and public health.

Charles Hawksley is Senior Lecturer in Politics and International Studies at the University of Wollongong (UOW), Australia. Charles holds a PhD in politics from UOW. His research on the politics of the Asia-Pacific has appeared in *Third World Quarterly*, *Rethinking Marxism*, and *Global Change Peace and Security*.

Nichole Georgeou is Associate Professor in Humanitarian and Development Studies at Western Sydney University, Australia. Nichole holds a PhD and an MA (Research) from UOW in development sociology. She is the author of *Neoliberalism, Development and Aid Volunteering* (Routledge) among many other publications.

Routledge Studies on the Asia-Pacific Region

Local Political Participation in Japan
A Case Study of Oita
Dani Daigle Kida

The US-Japan Security Community
Theoretical Understanding of Transpacific Relationships
Hidekazu Sakai

Opportunities and Challenges for the Greater Mekong Subregion
Building a Shared Vision of Our River
Edited by Charles Samuel Johnston and Xin Chen

Diversity and Inclusion in Japan
Issues in Business and Higher Education
Edited by Lailani Alcantara and Yoshiki Shinohara

Pandemic, States and Societies in the Asia-Pacific, 2020–2021
Responding to COVID
Edited by Charles Hawksley and Nichole Georgeou

For more information about this series, please visit: https://www.routledge.com/Routledge-Studies-on-the-Asia-Pacific-Region/book-series/RSAPR

Pandemic, States and Societies in the Asia-Pacific, 2020–2021

Responding to COVID

Edited by Charles Hawksley and Nichole Georgeou

Routledge
Taylor & Francis Group

LONDON AND NEW YORK

First published 2024
by Routledge
4 Park Square, Milton Park, Abingdon, Oxon OX14 4RN

and by Routledge
605 Third Avenue, New York, NY 10158

Routledge is an imprint of the Taylor & Francis Group, an informa business

© 2024 selection and editorial matter, Charles Hawksley and Nichole Georgeou; individual chapters, the contributors

The right of Charles Hawksley and Nichole Georgeou to be identified as the authors of the editorial material, and of the authors for their individual chapters, has been asserted in accordance with sections 77 and 78 of the Copyright, Designs and Patents Act 1988.

All rights reserved. No part of this book may be reprinted or reproduced or utilised in any form or by any electronic, mechanical, or other means, now known or hereafter invented, including photocopying and recording, or in any information storage or retrieval system, without permission in writing from the publishers.

Trademark notice: Product or corporate names may be trademarks or registered trademarks, and are used only for identification and explanation without intent to infringe.

British Library Cataloguing-in-Publication Data
A catalogue record for this book is available from the British Library

ISBN: 978-1-032-31821-9 (hbk)
ISBN: 978-1-032-31822-6 (pbk)
ISBN: 978-1-003-31152-2 (ebk)

DOI: 10.4324/9781003311522

Typeset in Galliard
by SPi Technologies India Pvt Ltd (Straive)

Contents

List of Figures   *vii*
List of Tables   *ix*
List of Editors   *x*
List of Contributors   *xi*
Preface   *xiv*

1 Pandemic, States and Societies in the Asia-Pacific 2020–2021:
  Responding to COVID   1
  CHARLES HAWKSLEY AND NICHOLE GEORGEOU

2 Indonesia's response to the COVID-19 pandemic:
  from herbal cure-alls to a science-based response   12
  YOHANA SUSANA YEMBISE AND ROB GOODFELLOW

3 Pandemic, migrant workers, and the economy of Bangladesh   34
  MAMTA B. CHOWDHURY

4 Japan: Moralised politics in countering COVID-19   55
  YUKIKO NISHIKAWA

5 Making sense of behavioural restrictions and institutional
  controls: the Philippine COVID-19 experience   82
  LESLIE A. LOPEZ, JESSICA SANDRA R. CLAUDIO, DENNIS B. BATANGAN,
  JOSELITO T. SESCON AND HARAYA MARIKIT C. MENDOZA

6 Vietnam: COVID-19 in Vietnam   107
  TOAN DANG

7 Nepal: pandemic and unusual state response 122
UDDHAB PYAKUREL AND SUPRIYA GURUNG

8 Australia and COVID-19: Cracks in the Commonwealth 136
CHARLES HAWKSLEY AND NICHOLE GEORGEOU

9 Taiwan: how COVID-19 sharpens Taiwanese identity 162
TSE-MIN HUNG

10 Cambodia: the thin line between development and human
rights during COVID-19 182
NATALIA SZABLEWSKA, MUY SEO NGOUV AND RATANA LY

11 Aotearoa New Zealand: is the grass really greener here?
Social, political, and cultural implications of COVID-19
in New Zealand 201
CHRISTINA ERGLER, NICHOLE GEORGEOU, SARAH LOVELL AND
ROBERT HUISH

Conclusion 217
CHARLES HAWKSLEY AND NICHOLE GEORGEOU

Index 222

Figures

1.1	Daily COVID deaths (global) on 10 April 2023	3
1.2	World Health Organization COVID deaths by WHO region	5
2.1	HIV infections Indonesia 2005–2018	16
2.2	Economic growth and official unemployment rates in Indonesia 2014–2018	19
2.3	Dates and severity of restricted internal movement by country	21
2.4	Confirmed COVID-19 cases from March 2020 to September 2021	22
2.5	Daily confirmed COVID-19 cases, Indonesia, March 2020–November 2021	24
3.1	Overseas recruitments and remittances flow to Bangladesh 1976–2021	39
3.2	Overseas recruitment of migrant workers, 2021 (major country-wise)	40
4.1	Graph showing COVID-19 cases per one million population 22 December 2021	56
4.2	Graph showing number of COVID-19-infected persons (January 2020–February 2022)	57
4.3	Graph showing number of deaths per day (January 2020–February 2022)	57
4.4	Organisational chart for novel coronavirus response in Japan	61
5.1	Quarantine classification system (March 2020–September 2021)	84
5.2	COVID-19 alert level and granular lockdown system	85
5.3	Cumulative confirmed COVID-19 cases (Philippines)	87
5.4	Cumulative confirmed COVID-19 cases (Southeast Asia) March 2020–April 2022	89
5.5	Cumulative confirmed COVID-19 deaths (Southeast Asia)	90
5.6	COVID-19 vaccination status (initial and booster doses)	91
5.7	Quarterly GDP growth rate (2020–2021, in percentages)	94
8.1	Australia—COVID deaths per million March 2020–December 2022	138
8.2	Daily COVID cases Australia February 2020–March 2023	139

8.3 Timeline of Australian states and territories in and out of
lockdown 2020–2021 (by quarters) 144
8.4 COVID deaths to 31 December 2021 by age cohort (Australia) 150
9.1 Full-page ad in the *New York Times* 15 April 2020 170
9.2 Enlarged text of Figure 9.1 171
9.3 Text of the UNGA Resolution 2758 of 1971 expelling
Taiwan from the United Nations 174
11.1 Clear and simple visual communication of six easy steps to
keep people safe after the move to alert level 1 in 2020 202
11.2 New Zealand's pandemic timeline 206

Tables

1.1	COVID deaths in Asia-Pacific case studies	6
3.1	Socio-economic indicators of South Asia and Bangladesh (selected years)	36
4.1	Total expenses of emergency measures (20 April 2020)	58
4.2	Economic stimulus package (8 December 2020)	58
4.3	Partial amendments made in the Special Measures Acts (before and after)	64
5.1	Allotment and utilisation of funding sources for the Philippine COVID-19 response (in billions, as of 31 December 2021)	97
5.2	Selected schemes under the SAP implementation of the DSWD	98
8.1	National, state and territory populations, government leaders, total COVID cases and COVID deaths to 31 December 2021	149
9.1	Taiwan's COVID alert levels	166

Editors

Charles Hawksley is a senior lecturer in Politics and International Studies at the University of Wollongong (UOW), Australia. Charles holds a PhD in Politics from UOW and a first class Honours (History) from University of New South Wales, Sydney, Australia. His research on the politics of the Asia-Pacific has been published in journals such as *Third World Quarterly*, *Rethinking Marxism*, and *Global Change Peace and Security*.

Nichole Georgeou is an associate professor in Humanitarian and Development Studies at Western Sydney University (WSU), Australia, and Director of the Humanitarian and Development Research Initiative (HADRI) at WSU. Nichole holds a PhD and an MA (Research) from UOW in Development Sociology. Among many other publications, Nichole is the author of the 2012 study *Neoliberalism, Development and Aid Volunteering* (Routledge).

Contributors

Dennis B. Batangan conducts research at the Institute of the Philippine Culture (IPC), Ateneo de Manila University, the Philippines. He is a member of the faculty of the Ateneo School of Government (ASoG) Master in Public Management (MPM) Health Governance Track.

Mamta B. Chowdhury holds a PhD in Economics and a Master of Economics (Development) degree from the Australian National University (ANU) in Canberra, Australia. She is a senior lecturer in Economics, Finance and Property at Western Sydney University and has authored some significant publications in the area of worker's remittances, especially their effects on economic and financial growth and development, and stock markets of developing countries.

Jessica Sandra R. Claudio is a lecturer at the Department of Sociology and Anthropology and a research associate at the Institute of Philippine Culture, Ateneo de Manila, the Philippines, where she manages an ASEAN-level project on health technologies (or eHealth). She obtained her Masters in Sociology in 2018 from Ateneo de Manila University.

Toan Dang is the CEO and Founder of the Central Highlands Center for Community Development and Climate Change Adaptation (CHCC), Vietnam. He holds a Master's degree in Social Planning and Development from the University of Queensland and a PhD from Western Sydney University (WSU). He is a consultant, researcher, and development practitioner in Development Studies.

Christina Ergler is a senior lecturer in the School of Geography/Te Iho Whenua at University of Otago, New Zealand. She holds a PhD from University of Auckland, New Zealand. Her research lies at the cross-roads of geography, sociology, and public health in the minority and majority world with a focus on the relationships between well-being, place, and lived everyday experiences.

Rob Goodfellow holds a PhD in History from UOW and often works as a cultural consultant in Indonesia. He is an adjunct fellow and researcher with the Humanitarian and Development Research Initiative (HADRI) at Western Sydney University, Australia.

Robert Huish is an associate professor in the Department of International Development Studies Faculty of Arts and Social Sciences at Dalhousie University, Canada. His research explores global health inequity, and the role of social activism in bringing about improved health outcomes in resource-poor settings. He recently completed an international research project looking at comparative stigma emerging from the COVID-19 pandemic.

Tse-Min Hung holds a Master's degree in Social Work from Western Sydney University, Australia. She is a journalist, interpreter, and social researcher.

Leslie A. Lopez is a lecturer and the Director of the Development Studies Program at Ateneo de Manila, the Philippines. With a background in sociology with extensive experience in monitoring and evaluation, she received her PhD in Sociology at the University of the Philippines, Diliman, in 2019.

Sarah Lovell is an associate professor in the School of Health Sciences at University of Canterbury, New Zealand. She holds a PhD from Queen's University, Canada. She is a qualitative health researcher concerned with access and delivery of care in the community, with a particular focus on sexual and reproductive health.

Ratana Ly is completing her PhD in Law at the University of Victoria. Her research interests lie in the fields of human rights, international criminal law, labour law, and the environment. Ratana is also a senior research fellow at the Center for the Study of Humanitarian Law, Cambodia.

Haraya Marikit C. Mendoza is a fellowship coordinator at the Institute of Philippine Culture at Ateneo de Manila, the Philippines.

Yukiko Nishikawa in a professor (Doctoral Program) at the Doshisha University Graduate School of Global Studies where she researches Peace and Development Studies. Among many other works, she has authored *Political Sociology of Japanese Pacifism* (Routledge 2018) and *Human Security in Southeast Asia* (Routledge 2010).

Muy Seo Ngouv is a researcher and lecturer at the Center for the Study of Humanitarian Law at the Royal University of Law and Economics, Cambodia, where she researches and writes on topics including human rights law, humanitarian law, and public international law.

Uddhab Pyakurel is Global Associate Director, Engagement Division at Kathmandu University, Nepal and a lecturer in Development Studies at the School of Arts. He holds a PhD from the Centre for the Study of Social Systems at the Jawaharlal Nehru University, New Delhi. He researched extensively on poverty, development, state restructuring, Indo-Nepal relations and other socio-political issues.

Joselito T. Sescon is an assistant professor in the Department of Economics at Ateneo de Manila, the Philippines. Joselito holds a Master of Arts and a Master of Development Economics degrees from the University of the Philippines, Diliman. He works on economic policy, poverty, and the rural sector.

Natalia Szablewska is a professor in Law and Society at the Open University, United Kingdom and a fellow of the Center for the Study of Humanitarian Law at the Royal University of Law and Economics, Cambodia. She is a legal and social scholar whose research and practice focus has been predominantly on modern slavery and the wider business and human rights agenda. Among other degrees, Natalia holds a PhD in Law and Legal Studies from the University of Aberystwyth (Wales).

Professor Yohana Susana Yembise is an Indonesian academic at the Faculty of Education, Cenderawasih University, Jayapura, Papua Province. She is a former politician who served as Indonesia's Minister of Women's Empowerment and Child Protection in President Joko Widodo's first Working Cabinet (2014–2019).

Preface

In early 2020, a new disease began sweeping the globe. Severe Acute Respiratory Syndrome-Coronavirus Disease 2019 (SARS-COVID-19, or just 'COVID-19' or 'COVID' for short) quickly affected the lives of everyone on earth. As the virus spread and people became infected and began to die, states took a range of actions. One of them was restricting movement so that the virus did not spread.

In early May 2020, the editors of this book conceived of a quick survey publication while under lockdown regulations in Wollongong, Australia. In discussions during our one-hour maximum morning walks, we decided we wanted to pull together as many people as we could to deliver short 'snapshots' of how states had handled the first months of the COVID-19 pandemic. Our focus was to provide a comparative study to explore the diverse responses in what was then fast emerging as a major public health crisis. As a 'pre-vaccine document', it tried to capture the emerging severity of the pandemic problem and how states were attempting to control transmission.

That book, *State Responses to COVID-19: A Global Snapshot at 1 June 2020*, was published by the Humanitarian and Development Research Initiative (HADRI) at Western Sydney University. Free and online *State Responses to COVID-19* was creative commons and has been shared in multiple downloads, with over 10,000 downloads that we have been able to track. It was purposely created as open access to increase comparative knowledge of what was happening around the world and how different states and territories were handling, and often mishandling, the outbreak of COVID.

Our brief to those authors was to cover in less than 1,500 words what they thought was most important about the first six months of COVID in their case study. We tried to get a level of similarity about a state's focus on health, economic, and (as academics) educational responses of many different societies as COVID settled over the globe. We succeeded in bringing together—in a ridiculously short deadline of six weeks from conception to publication—70 contributors writing on 43 state/territory/region case studies across 4 continents. We also included ten issue papers on diverse matters such as undocumented migrants, the activities of non-governmental organisations during the pandemic, or the health of healthcare workers. These various contributions provide glimpses as to how the COVID pandemic had affected specific states or specific concerns within states.

Back in June 2020, there was no COVID vaccine, although there was a massive global effort invested in finding one. There was (and still is) a lack of knowledge about where COVID had come from—although there were numerous unproven theories—and how it could be best resisted. By this time most governments had adopted the time-proven tactics of isolation, masks, and lockdowns, but there was great variation in approach. There was still a genuine fear that COVID really would overwhelm many state health systems. Pictures from hospitals and mortuaries in New York and in the north of Italy confirmed the desperation of the situation and the utter exhaustion of medical staff battling the virus. Written at a time before terms like 'Delta' and 'Omicron' entered common parlance, the 137 pages of *State Responses to COVID-19* still make for interesting reading three years later, and the book remains an important historical source, as it showcases what might be seen as denial on behalf of some states' governments, while others acted early and attempted to keep the virus out. The states that could afford to do so offered financial support, and the book attempted to capture how the pandemic was being handled across the world, with contributions from the Americas, Europe, Africa, the Middle East, South Asia, East Asia, and Oceania.

The success of that project developed into a vision to provide a longer and deeper assessment of fewer states in the Asia-Pacific region. Wherever possible, we wanted scholars from this region as authors.

We pitched the idea over Zoom to Simon Bates of Routledge in Singapore in late 2021 and emailed and organised authors during the first half of 2022. As editors, we pushed them to finish, as we wanted to get it out quickly, and they complied. All chapters were submitted by October of 2022, but of course, we then contracted COVID ourselves. The delay in getting the book out is partly due to our own illness, as well as family matters. We thank all of the chapter contributors for their patience while we got better and got back to work, and we acknowledge that this publication has emerged later than we all would have liked.

Despite the delays, the case studies in this book cover the first two crucial years of COVID in the Asia-Pacific, a time that for most states was the most damaging. We hope that readers will find the diversity of the contributions as interesting as we have.

At Routledge, we thank commissioning editor Simon Bates for backing the project from the beginning, and we wish him well for his return to the United Kingdom.

Finally, a huge thanks to our Routledge Singapore editor Chelsea Low for her speed and professionalism in bringing this book to completion, and to copy editor Melissa Brown Levine for her keen editorial eye. Any remaining mistakes are owned by the editors.

Charles Hawksley
Nichole Georgeou
Wollongong, Australia, August 2023

1 Pandemic, States and Societies in the Asia-Pacific 2020–2021

Responding to COVID

Charles Hawksley and Nichole Georgeou

Introduction

A survey of COVID in the Asia-Pacific

We are not medical doctors. The editors and contributors to this volume cannot inform you why there are so many variants of the Severe Acute Respiratory Syndrome-Coronavirus 2 2019 (SARS-CoV-2 virus) (or hereinafter 'COVID' or COVID-19)—Alpha, Beta, Gamma, Delta, Omicron, or those yet to come are outside of our area of expertise. We do not know anything about spike proteins, except that they exist, and we are unable to tell readers with any certainty from whence the COVID virus originated, whether it crossed into humans from a pangolin, a raccoon dog, a bat, some other animal, or any number of other theories.

What we can do is write about what the pandemic meant for people, and how states reacted in the form of political, social, economic, and health measures. We are approaching these issues from the point of view of how national governments ('states') dealt with the COVID pandemic and what lessons can be drawn from the case studies should a similar event occur in the future. We are academics, or to be more precise, one of the editors is a researcher across political science/history/development studies, and the other is a researcher across political sociology/humanitarian studies/development studies. The combination gives us a broad license to work with our authors of case studies who span a range of disciplines including sociology, education, law, politics, international relations, history, social work, geography, and health sciences.

This introduction has two sections. The first places the Asia-Pacific COVID experience into a global context. The second tells readers what to expect in the book, its structure, and some of the key findings.

COVID-19: the global context

During 2020–2021, the COVID pandemic was a global public health problem of a type not experienced since the 1918 influenza epidemic. Some might dispute if COVID was even a 'global pandemic', but we take the word

DOI: 10.4324/9781003311522-1

pandemic to mean the widespread occurrence of an infectious disease across states and across the world at the same time, which for our purposes is the calendar years of 2020–2021. COVID was certainly that, spreading rapidly from Asia into Europe and the Americas, and more slowly into Africa and Oceania. It showed the fragility of the interconnected world, a world that for some had previously involved travel and work opportunities in other states.

The COVID-19 pandemic has had a substantial human cost. By 10 March 2023, COVID deaths worldwide were over 6.8 million people, representing around 1% of those who contracted COVID (some 676 million people). The 6.8 million lives lost represent 0.00085% (less than one-thousandth of a percent) of the estimated global population of over 8 billion people. Statistically, this is a much smaller number of dead than those killed by the 1918 influenza—which infected around 500 million people, thought to be one-third of the world's population of 1.5 billion at that point, and killed one in ten of those (50 million) (CDC, 2023)—but still, 6.8 million people have died—grandfathers, grandmothers, mothers, fathers, daughters, sons, wives, husbands, partners, lovers, and children.

At the time of writing (March of 2023), the COVID pandemic is not over, but states and societies are learning to live with the likelihood of widespread COVID infection, and a collective amnesia appears to have settled over the past several years. The idea of eliminating COVID has passed; no state was able to do this. The year 2022 was when societies attempted to go back to how things used to be. In our post-restrictions world, mask wearing is no longer enforced on public transport, vaccination is not required to enter restaurants, and air travel has resumed. Hong Kong dropped its mask mandate on 1 March 2023, one of the last places in the world to do so (Master, 2023), but most other states had ended their mask mandates or restrictions back in late 2021. In another sign of the times, the remarkable Johns Hopkins COVID Tracking Centre—which for three years complied a daily account of infections and deaths for all jurisdictions on the planet, and which relied on official statistics from governments, some of which did not always pass on accurate information—stopped collecting data on 10 March 2023 (Johns Hopkins 2023).

There are various ways to measure the effects of the pandemic, including the decline in gross domestic product, total infections, length of lockdowns, numbers vaccinated, and of course deaths from COVID or associated medical conditions. The first two years of COVID were deadly for most societies across the globe. The graph in Figure 1.1 shows that December 2020 to January 2021 and the months on either side of March 2021 were the worst two periods globally for COVID fatalities so far (to March 2023). The global peak appears to have been reached on 21 January 2021 when 16,878 COVID deaths were recorded. These peaks are followed by July–August 2021 and then November–December 2021. The global COVID death rate looked to be falling in late 2021, but it increased in early 2022 as states relaxed their policies.

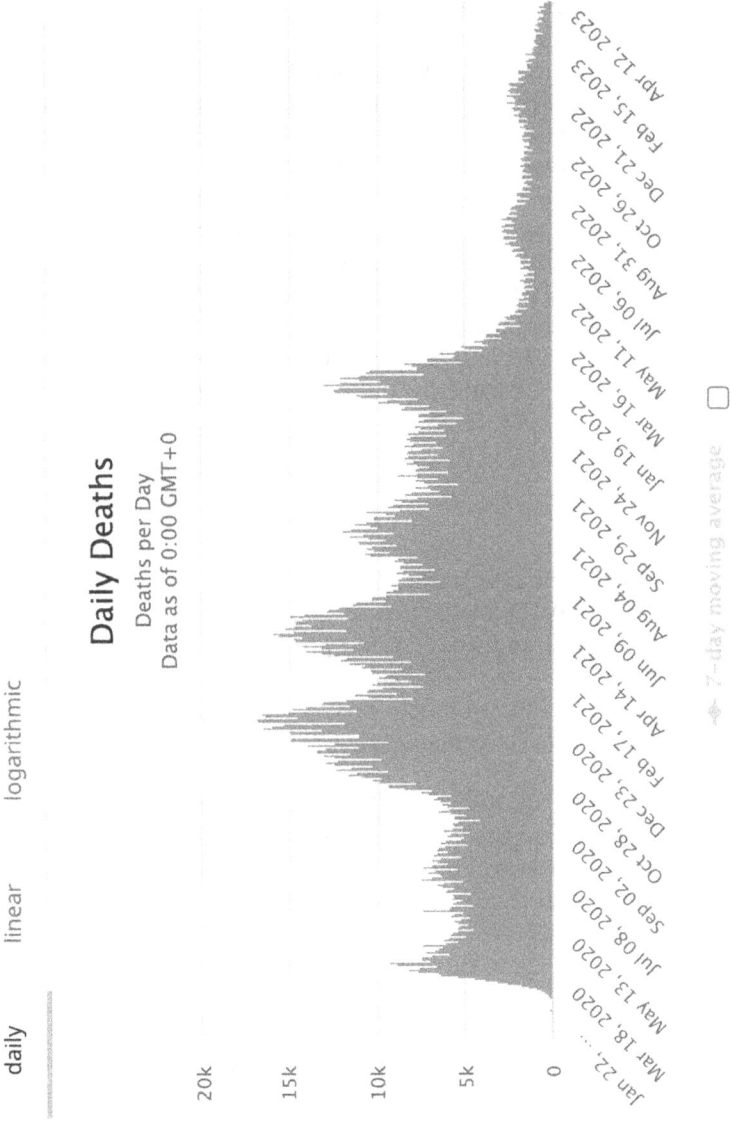

Figure 1.1 Daily COVID deaths (global) on 10 April 2023.

Source: Worldometers 2023: https://www.worldometers.info/coronavirus/

In mid-March 2023, total COVID deaths were highest in the United States (1,123,836), Brazil (699,310), India (530,779) Russia (388,521), Mexico (333,188) the United Kingdom (220,721), Peru (219,539), Italy (188,322), France (166,176), Iran (144,933), although several other states had COVID fatalities of over 100,000 in the period from 2020 to early 2023 (Poland, Spain, Ukraine, South Africa, Argentina, Columbia, China, and Turkey) (ARCGIS 2023).

The World Health Organization figures support the contention that CO-VID deaths globally have fallen markedly since the end of 2021 (Figure 1.2). Broken down regionally, World Health Organization (WHO) data indicates the Americas and Europe were the most affected by COVID deaths, followed by Southeast Asia. It should be noted however that there is no 'Asia-Pacific' for the WHO. The region of South-East Asia includes India, which has suffered two-thirds of the over 800,000 regional deaths, while the WHO's 'Western Pacific' region also includes China, which has suffered over 120,000 of the 406,000 COVID dead in that region (WHO 2023).

As both charts show, since around April of 2022, the number of people dying from COVID has fallen substantially, but in March 2023 it was still measuring in the hundreds per day (540 on 10 March 2023) (Worldometers 2023).

COVID-19 in the Asia-Pacific

In the Asia-Pacific region, the case studies included in this book have all witnessed loss of life from COVID for the period 2020–2021, and have continued to do so through 2022 and 2023. While there has been a decrease in COVID deaths worldwide, some Asia-Pacific states have gone against the global trend with respect to the numbers of COVID deaths and infections from the start of 2022 and have seen a far greater loss of life since the lifting of restrictions.

Table 1.1 shows the case studies in this book with COVID deaths on 31 December 2021 (a table that represents the first two years of COVID), and on 30 March 2023, a further 15 months, or three and a quarter years into the pandemic. The figures are worth exploring as in some states there is not much of a rise from the end of 2021 to March of 2023, which is consistent with global trends; however, in others, there is a dramatic increase. For Australia, Cambodia, New Zealand, and Taiwan, the period 2020–2021 looks like a job well done. Add another 15 months, and Australia's COVID deaths are over eight times what they were on 31 December 2021. The trend is evident for New Zealand also, which until the end of 2021 had double-digit COVID fatalities and is now over 4,000, and for Japan. Taiwan moved from 850 to 19,005 in the same period. Evidently, mass vaccination coupled with a relaxation in restrictions did not protect everyone.

Of the case studies in this book, in terms of COVID deaths, Indonesia has been the most severely affected, followed by Japan and the Philippines. At the

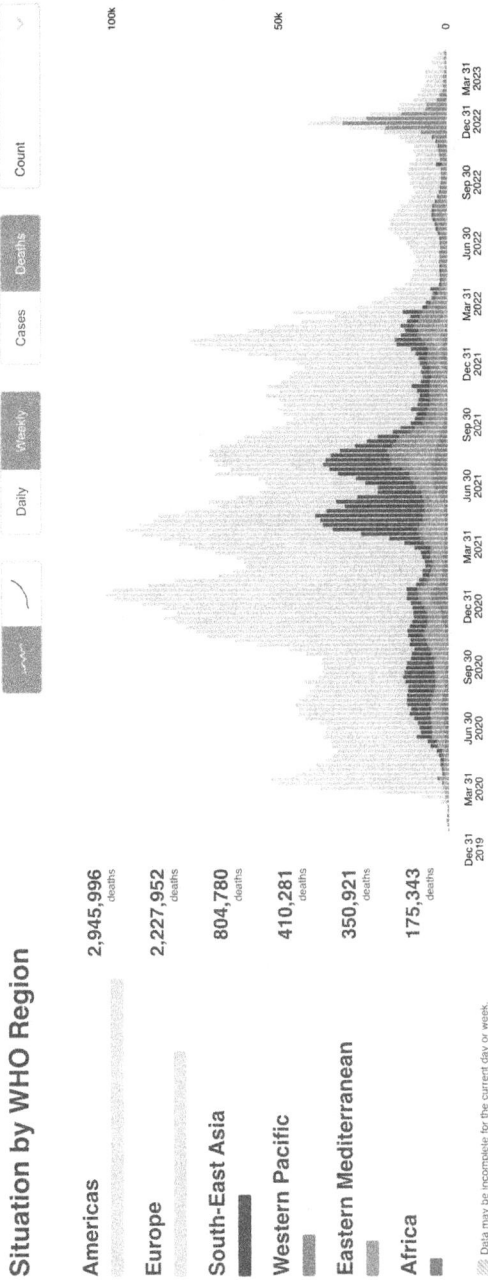

Situation by WHO Region

Americas	2,945,996	deaths
Europe	2,227,952	deaths
South-East Asia	804,780	deaths
Western Pacific	410,281	deaths
Eastern Mediterranean	350,921	deaths
Africa	175,343	deaths

Data may be incomplete for the current day or week.

Figure 1.2 World Health Organization COVID deaths by WHO region.

Source: World Health Organization.

Table 1.1 COVID deaths in Asia-Pacific case studies

Cast study	COVID deaths by 31 December 2021	COVID deaths by 30 March 2023
Australia	2,353	19,576
Bangladesh	28,072	29,446
Cambodia	3,012	3,056
Indonesia	144,094	161,092
Japan	18,393	73,865
Nepal	11,590	12,020
New Zealand	59	4,008
Philippines	51,502	66,364
Taiwan	850	19,005
Vietnam	32,610	43,186

(Compiled by authors from Worldometers data).

time of writing (13 April 2023) the figures from Cambodia would indicate its last COVID death was in April of 2022, while Vietnam has not recorded a death in 2023. The figures for Cambodia and Vietnam may well be accurate, but it may also indicate that there is less effort going into ensuring statistical accuracy. The figures for these case studies would appear to say that even those states that were initially lauded for their effectiveness in 2020, such as Australia, New Zealand, Taiwan, and Vietnam (Georgeou and Hawksley 2020) have all recorded much higher numbers of COVID deaths than would have been expected given their first two years of the COVID pandemic.

Globally, mass vaccination has reduced the chances of people dying from COVID infection. States tell us some **668** million people (about 8.5% of the world's population) have been infected with COVID and survived, but the virus has left millions of people across the world with feelings of ongoing lethargy and lacking energy, concentration, or motivation for months (dubbed 'long COVID'). Workplaces across the world reported declines in productivity due to COVID during 2020–2021 (World Bank 2021), even though working from home (via Zoom or a similar technology) has enabled greater flexibility.

Book structure

As noted, the editors are academics within the field of development studies, which is a broad field, and it is not only restricted to the so-called developing world. What we have attempted in this book is to provide some 'deep dives' into the management of the pandemic by several states in the Asia-Pacific region. We use the words 'states' to refer to governments of effectively independent polities who claim to control a given territory, regardless of the level of international acceptance. We prefer the word state to country as the former is closer to the notion of governmental apparatus—i.e. 'the machinery of *state*'.

The different chapters in this volume have sought to provide case studies, and as editors, we have not sought to impose a framework on how to understand the specific circumstances of any state or territory. Readers will observe there is no case study of COVID in India or COVID in China. This is not for lack of interest, nor due to the complexity of pulling together the experiences of over a billion people within a 5,000–6,500 words limit. Indeed, the same argument of complexity could be made for writing a chapter on Indonesia and its population of over 273 million, or for New Zealand and its 5 million people.

Wherever in the world, even for very small populations, the effects of the COVID pandemic are complex. In the 22 Pacific Islands Countries and Territories (PICTs), the populations are, with the exception of Papua New Guinea, under one million but the effects of COVID have been widely varied depending on factors such as the level of urbanisation, political status, aid relationships, proximity to sea lanes and access to medical assistance. The populations of Micronesia are highly urbanised—68.7% on average and up to 95% in Guam—however the much larger Melanesian states are predominantly rural, for example around 86% of PNG's 8.4 million people are rural. The overall PICT average urbanisation is thus just over 23%, even if over half of Fiji's population and some 70% of New Caledonia's lives in towns and cities (Georgeou et al., 2022). Providing an overall assessment of the effects of COVID on the Pacific Islands is arguably just as complex as it would be for China or India and would have as many qualifications and exceptions.

As editors, we made decisions as to which states to include and what to exclude. The specific logic to this book then is that many of the authors had worked with us on previous projects and said yes when we asked them to write a chapter. Other authors were approached to write specific chapters, and we were very pleased they could help out. Our interest was in the diversity of the different societies and governments of the Asia-Pacific, and our authors focussed on aspects of the 'national' experience that they thought were unique. Given the constraints of lockdowns, we did not ask for original research. The case studies are more what might be called general survey pieces that are based on freely available secondary data.

The results show that all states broadly adopted similar policies of attempted suppression, then containment, and all eventually were defeated by COVID and have had to learn to live with the virus. Some were faster to react than others, and by late 2021, when vaccines had become widely available, it became a political choice to 'open up' again. In some states, this led to disastrous consequences. For example, by the end of 2021, Australia had experienced 395,504 cases of COVID-19 with 2,239 deaths. By March 2023, there were over 10,000 new cases a week, and the number of COVID infections had blown out to over 11 million. The entire Australian population is only 25.9 million, so over 42% of the Australian population has now had COVID, some more than once. Most alarmingly, from the relatively strong containment of 2020–2021, and 2,239 deaths, by mid-March 2023, over 19,000 people had died from COVID in Australia (Worldometers, 2023). If learning to live with COVID has involved a sort of collective amnesia or even denial, then perhaps things are just as serious now as they were in 2020 and 2021.

There are many possible ways of organising chapters: alphabetically by case study, ranked by Human Development Index, ranked by gross domestic product per capita, geographically from East to West or West to East. We have opted to present the chapters starting with the most populous case study to the least populous. This provides something of an organising principle, largest populations to smallest, that cuts across indicators of development that might tend to group like (advanced industrial/developing) with like. Our intention was to view the pandemic as a global and regional issue, and so the responses of varied states adds to the sense of pandemic chaos that engulfed the world.

We commence in Indonesia where Yohana Susana Yembise (Universitas Cenderawasih) and Rob Goodfellow (Humanitarian and Development Research Initiative (HADRI) at Western Sydney University (WSU)) argue the Indonesian response to COVID was characterised by a fundamental shift in state policy from initial denial to more decisive national leadership. This in turn brought coordinated science-based action centred on a nationwide mass vaccination programme largely modelled on a previous experience with HIV AIDS. The chapter explains the context in which this transition in thinking and practice occurred, and notes some of the difficulties, limitations, and restrictions facing the Indonesian government. It also concentrates on the impacts of the pandemic felt by Indonesian civil society.

For Bangladesh, Mamta B. Chowdhury (WSU) has provided an assessment of the overall economic response to COVID. While there was initial criticism of a slow start, by 2021, the support packages appear to have worked well. The chapter focuses on the impact of COVID-19 on the Bangladesh economy, with a particular focus on the migrant workers and the flow of remittances to the country, which is the second-largest source of foreign exchange earnings for Bangladesh after ready-made garment (RMG) export income.

For Japan, Yukiko Nishikawa (Doshisha University) writes there were several puzzling mysteries about COVID in Japan, in particular, a low number of cases; a lack of strict measures, as well as the remarkable speed of vaccination; and the high percentage of the population that was inoculated by late 2021. She argues that law and politics helped shape a pragmatic rule-of-law system, as well as a 'moralised politics' in Japan that has functioned both to enforce the state's policies and to contain state power during the coronavirus emergency situation. In the absence of emergency powers, Japanese society evolved social responses to curb COVID transmission. These included behaviours that bordered on vigilantism, and which were locally organised. This local and regional policing was voluntary and has at its essence a desire to protect local communities from 'outsiders'.

Heading south to the Philippines, Leslie A. Lopez, Jessica Sandra R. Claudio, Dennis B. Batangan, Joselito T. Sescon, and Haraya Marikit C. Mendoza (Ateneo de Manila) explore the political, economic, and health actions of the administration of President Rodrigo Duterte, specifically focusing on the emergence of the uniformed sector as a dominant state functionary to combat COVID. They argue that the political leaders of the Philippines looked to history to militarise what was a complex public health emergency, with predictable results. The securitisation of a broad public concern such as COVID-19 was a natural extension of the administration's attempts to securitise populist issues, such as the War on Drugs.

Across the South China Sea in Vietnam, Toan Dang (Central Highlands Center for Community Development and Climate Change Adaptation) shows how the pandemic was politicised by the government to encourage people to move to a 'war footing' and defeat the virus. Certain features of Vietnam's COVID response hark back to its recent war history; however, its attitude to Chinese-produced vaccines is related to its longer and more complex relationship with China. Toan argues the Vietnamese government sought to develop a set of principles that were entirely appropriate for the population it serves. The various groups and levels of community were enlisted in non-pharmaceutical measures through unifying discourses which emphasised nationalistic duty, community well-being, and citizen responsibility. The Vietnamese population was thus not entirely without agency in how the pandemic was addressed, a claim illustrated in the way that strong cultural and historical values provoked many to avoid vaccines that were made in China.

In the Nepal chapter, Uddhab Pyakurel (Kathmandu University) and Supriya Gurung (HADRI/WSU) chronicle the government's delayed response to the surge of COVID-19 cases, and its use of measures such as travel restrictions, snap lockdowns, and a national vaccine rollout to then attempt to control the virus. It addresses how thousands of Nepali and Indian migrant workers, many of whom were carrying the COVID virus, moved through the porous border between India and Nepal after the normally open border was declared closed. The chapter also analyses some unusual government activities that occurred during the pandemic, some of which raised questions of corruption, and notes how on several occasions the Nepali state failed to capitalise on measures that would have aided in its fight against the spread of COVID-19.

Back in Australia Charles Hawksley (University of Wollongong) and Nichole Georgeou (WSU) have concentrated on the problems that eventuated in a wealthy developed state when the federal government did not actually have the emergency powers to manage the pandemic and where individual state and territory governments of Australia led the response to COVID. The Commonwealth government sought to project an image that it was indeed managing events; however, it mismanaged key aspects of the response, in particular the vaccine rollout and the administration of elder care in nursing homes. The result was that nationally agreed federal 'plans' on vaccination were delayed by months. The chapter also explores the economic response and the unequal enforcement of restrictions in lower-socio-economic status suburbs that were policed more rigorously than in wealthier suburbs.

For Taiwan Tse-Min Hung (HADRI/WSU) describes how the pandemic led to calls for a more independent voice in global affairs and for a greater definition of a Taiwanese identity. While Taiwan's early success in combatting CO-VID was in many ways due to its international exclusion, its international COVID charm offensive can be seen as a quest to re-engage with international organisations and to prosecute a case for the abandonment of China-led restrictions on its own claims for statehood. The new assertive Taiwanese identity was evidenced both internationally and domestically, and it combined through differing aspects such as effective border control, a new national passport, the protection of the public health system, and general support for the government's efficient management of the pandemic.

In the chapter on Cambodia, Natalia Szablewska (the Open University, United Kingdom/Center for the Study of Humanitarian Law at the Royal University of Law and Economics, Cambodia), Muy Seo Ngouv (the Center for the Study of Humanitarian Law at the Royal University of Law and Economics, Cambodia), and Ratana Ly, (University of Victoria, Canada/Center for the Study of Humanitarian Law at the Royal University of Law and Economics, Cambodia), argue the Cambodian government's success in combatting COVID needs unpacking. Cambodia's relatively small population (16.7 million) and the majority of Cambodian society being under the age of 30 made it less likely to have medical pre-existing conditions that could increase the risk of poor outcomes from COVID-19. Cultural restraint and following general hygiene measures avoided the infection spreading. This success was however marked by the introduction of legislation, ostensibly to combat COVID transmission, which in practice limits a number of fundamental freedoms, including freedom of expression, that further restricts critiques of government in its development-orientated policies. As such, COVID provided the government with an opportunity to silence dissent.

Finally, in the chapter on New Zealand, Christina Ergler (University of Otago), Nichole Georgeou (WSU), Sarah Lovell (University of Canterbury), and Robert Huish (Dalhousie University, Canada), argue the pandemic in New Zealand was a form of slow violence that affected specific communities and professions. They also argue that while Jacinda Arden's government was respected internationally and domestically for its COVID-19 strategy, certain domestic challenges were neglected during the pandemic. This violence of delayed destruction affected the shattered tourism industry, led to rising inflation, and to increased costs in housing and energy, which all impact the daily lives of New Zealanders, and which can ultimately exacerbate existing social and economic inequalities.

In the conclusion to this book Charles Hawksley and Nichole Georgeou offer some short observations on commonalities and differences between these case studies. Noting that none of these contributions is intended to be a final word on the subject of how states and societies experienced COVID, they argue that a lens of biopolitics may be a useful way to understand pandemic management, but suggest there are four specific areas of analysis that warrant further investigation. These are attributes that emerge at a national level when reviewing the effectiveness of the response in the region as a whole: comparative levels of development, effective implementation, unitary or federal state structure, and the quality of political leadership. We hope that you find these contributions as interesting as we found them to edit.

References

ARCGIS. (2023). 'COVID-19 Dashboard', https://www.arcgis.com/apps/dashboards/bda7594740fd40299423467b48e9ecf6.

CDC (Centre for Disease Control). (2023). '1918 Pandemic (H1N1 virus)', https://www.cdc.gov/flu/pandemic-resources/1918-pandemic-h1n1.html.

Georgeou, N. and Hawksley, C. (eds) 2020. 'State Responses to COVID-19: A Global Snapshot at 1 June 2020, HADRI/Western Sydney University,' https://doi.org/10.26183/5ed5a2079cabd

Georgeou N, Hawksley C, Wali N, Lountain S, Rowe E, West C, et al. (2022). 'Food security and small holder farming in Pacific Island countries and territories: A scoping review', *PLOS Sustain Transform* 1(4): e0000009. https://doi.org/10.1371/journal.pstr.0000009Johns, Hopkins. (2023). 'What Is the JHU CRC Now?' https://coronavirus.jhu.edu/.

Master, F. (2023, February 28). 'Hong Kong to Scrap COVID Mask Mandate,' from March 1, *Reuters*, https://www.reuters.com/world/china/hong-kong-scrap-covid-mask-mandate-march-1-2023-02-28/.

WHO (World Health Organization). (2023). 'COVID-19 Situation in WHO – Western Pacific Region', https://who.maps.arcgis.com/apps/dashboards/345dfdc82b5c4f6a815f1d54a05d18ec.

World Bank. (2021). 'Global Productivity: Trends, Drivers, and Policies', https://www.worldbank.org/en/research/publication/global-productivity.

Worldometers. (2023). 'COVID-19 Coronavirus Pandemic', https://www.worldometers.info/coronavirus/.

2 Indonesia's response to the COVID-19 pandemic

From herbal cure-alls to a science-based response

Yohana Susana Yembise and Rob Goodfellow

The Indonesian government's response to the COVID-19 pandemic was, and continues to be, characterised by a fundamental shift in state policy from initial denial to more decisive national leadership and, in turn, broad coordinated science-based action centred on a nationwide mass vaccination programme. This chapter will explain the context in which this transition in thinking and practice occurred, including some of the difficulties, limitations, and restrictions facing the Indonesian government. Finally, this chapter will outline some of the negative impacts of the pandemic felt by civil society in the world's largest archipelagic state.

Background

Since the Indonesian Declaration of Independence on 17 August 1945 and the formal transfer of sovereignty from the Dutch on 27 December 1949, Indonesia has been considered by the international community to be a geopolitically important country. Under President Sukarno (1951–1965), Indonesia was an inspiration to other post-colonial states and a leading member of the Non-Aligned Movement. Under Indonesia's second President, Suharto (1965–1998), the country experienced high levels of sustained economic growth and relative social stability. Today, under Indonesia's seventh President, Joko Widodo (2014 –), also known as 'Jokowi,' Indonesia has established a high-growth domestic economy in transition to a leading value-added export economy (World Bank Report, 2021). Indeed, with over 270 million people (Lindsey & Man 2020), Indonesia is the most populous country in the southern hemisphere and the fourth most populous in the world. It is also the largest Muslim-majority nation and, after the Suharto period has been a functioning liberal democracy. Economically, and geopolitically, what happens in Indonesia matters to the region and to the rest of the world, and this extends to Indonesia's response to the COVID-19 pandemic.

The first months of 2020 were fertile ground for populist leaders around the world—Donald Trump in the United States, Jair Bolsonaro in Brazil, Narendra Modi in India, Mahinda Rajapaksa in Sri Lanka, Jacob Zuma in South Africa, Vladimir Putin in Russia, Rodrigo Duterte in the Philippines, and Boris

DOI: 10.4324/9781003311522-2

Johnson in the United Kingdom—all of whom advanced a broadly anti-political ideology that constructed a practical appeal to ordinary people who otherwise felt that their concerns were deliberately disregarded by elites and "special interest groups" (Osuna, 2020).

Jokowi, like US President Donald Trump, made numerous public statements deliberately downplaying the known dangers of the virus in favour of 'talking up' the economy (Wolfe & Dale, 2020). Like other populists, Jokowi's initial response to the pandemic can be characterised as a form of 'pandemic populism' (Vieten, 2020) based on the idea of the "popular common good" (Kyle et al., 2018); however, it should be noted there is a significant body of literature that challenges this view (A'yun & Mudhoffir, 2022).

COVID in Indonesia

In the Indonesian context, pandemic populism is best defined as "livelihoods versus lives" (Islamaj et al., 2021). To this end, populism as an ideology was and, continues to be, exemplified in Indonesia by the promise of small but incremental improvements in the living standards of ordinary people. In *Bahasa Indonesia* (the national language) this idea is often expressed by the emotive word *rakyat* or 'the people'. In Indonesia, as elsewhere, the 'anti-ideology' of populism ostensibly reports to benefit the '*rakyat*'.

To protect livelihoods (read 'the Indonesian economy' and, in reality, the business interests of domestic oligarchs), Jokowi and at least one of his key cabinet ministers were conspicuous for initially denying the seriousness of COVID-19. In late February 2020, for example, the Indonesian health minister, Terawan Agus Putranto, suggested to journalists that 'prayers' and 'equatorial humidity' would keep Indonesians safe from coronavirus while at the same time presenting complimentary packets of powered *jamu* (a popular traditional Javanese cure-all) on behalf of the president (Lindsey & Wilson, 2020). Putranto's comments, however, also reflected a poor understanding of epidemiology by religious leaders, which had to be taken into consideration by the government. Poor communication about the *halal* status of Chinese-manufactured vaccines, combined with a largely unchecked social media misinformation campaign, also contributed to this 'dysfunction' (Jaffrey, 2021).

In April 2020, President Trump was saying something similar to Putranto, however, neither leader was offering a medical or scientific explanation to support their respective non-science-based beliefs and theories. Serious questions were, however, being raised about the Indonesian government's response. For example, the *Jakarta Post's* Ary Hermawan wrote in late February 2020,

> It appears that the problem lies with the fact that the government is worried more about the social and economic impact of a mass hysteria created by the virus outbreak than the outbreak itself, which poses an extremely serious threat to public health.
>
> (Hermawan, 2020)

During the Suharto period (1968–1998), the Javanese word '*rukun*' was widely used to describe the concept of 'social harmony', which was to be defended and preserved at all costs. If viewed in the context of this preoccupation with both the economy and national security, Jokowi's initial approach to COVID-19 begins to make more sense. This is even more so if one considers the pervasive Indonesian social value of avoiding anything that engenders social conflict or disturbs "order and stability". In short, in early 2020, the Indonesian government viewed the looming pandemic as less of a threat to public health than to the actual legitimacy of the central administration itself (Lindsey & Wilson, 2020). Indeed, a preoccupation with "*rust en orde*" (a Dutch expression meaning "peace and order") is not a new thing in Indonesia; rather, from Dutch colonial times to the present day, it has informed the worldview of both Javanese elites and now national indigenous oligarchs.

Accordingly, in March 2020, Jokowi publicly admitted that his government was withholding information about the spread of the disease because, "he didn't want to stir panic" (or rather, to disturb *rukun*). As an avowed 'economy-oriented' leader (Parker, 2019) the Indonesian President was understandably concerned about what impact a hard COVID lockdown would have on the material conditions of ordinary people (Bland, 2020). However, it is also possible that he was more concerned about the *rakyat's* reaction to such a lockdown and the resulting national security consequences.

Interestingly, the absence of reliable COVID-19 mortality figures in Indonesia during 2020 meant crude extrapolations were quickly being made in lieu of hard data. This correlation showed that COVID-19 was already well established in Indonesia by the time the first two cases were officially acknowledged. For instance, Indonesian public graveyards, such as Jakarta's sprawling Rorotan cemetery, were recording significantly increased and largely unexplained burials throughout early 2020 (Cahya, 2021). This reflected the day-to-day experiences of the president's key political constituencies—namely, the urban and rural poor—who quickly found themselves at odds with the official position on how best to protect themselves from the virus.

The Indonesian government's initial public denial of the seriousness of COVID-19 was, in fact, typified by the public health maxim, "You only find what you test for".[1] This discourse mirrored a common practice in the early 2000s of deliberately *not* testing for HIV, especially amongst sex workers and their clients in Bali, with the implicit aim of protecting the island's 'image' or, more precisely, its booming economy (Riono & Jazant, 2004). At that time, the official logic was that, if you do not test for HIV, you will not find it, so *ipso facto*, it does not exist. The counter-argument was that how can something that ostensibly "does not exist" in Bali, like HIV, damage the island's commercial interests?

In contrast to two decades of official denial dating back to President Suharto, President Widodo's policy position on HIV represented a fresh concern or, perhaps, a political recalibration. Instead of prevarication, his new policy position appeared to reflect the "popular common good". This development was immediately welcomed by public health professionals in Indonesia, as well as at the July 2014 International AIDS Conference held in Australia, where the eyes of the world were on the Indonesian HIV-AIDS response. This represented good diplomatic news for Indonesia. More importantly, however, was that the change in rhetoric resulted in the Indonesian government immediately funding widespread free testing and antiretroviral treatment in combination with a lively public education programme that squarely addressed the stigma of HIV, namely, "Hey! Let's talk about HIV/AIDS" (Bone, 2016).

By the time the first cases of novel coronavirus were detected in Wuhan, China, in late 2019 and then in north Italy from January 2020, sections of the Indonesian government had already experienced a minor public health epiphany with the president becoming increasingly responsive to rapidly rising HIV case numbers (and AIDS deaths) (Boonto & Julliand, 2021). Part of this realisation may have had to do with the fact that Bali is a critical base of support for the Indonesian President's ruling party, *Partai Demokrasi Indonesia Perjuangan* (PDI-P) [The Indonesian Democratic Party of Struggle].

When applied to COVID, the question became, how could a virus that originated in China, and which (officially) "did not exist" in Indonesia, harm the Indonesian national economy? Or, for that matter, the reputation of the president? As Javier (2021) explains, this way of thinking unfortunately permeated down to the local political level.

> Part of the problem [was] flawed policy design. Indonesia allocated $US400 million for coronavirus testing. But local governments have used only 3.8 percent of this budget, in order to keep their case counts low and evade zone-based restrictions mandated by the micro-measures. The bigger issue with health data is political. Public health experts warn that national-level data are routinely manipulated by officials to justify the government's pro-business policies. This was apparent in the recent decision to ease restrictions on business activities, based on a slight decline in new cases, which was in fact driven by a drastic reduction in tests and data entry backlogs.
>
> (Javier, 2021)

In a sense, the HIV/AIDS epidemic (Figure 2.1) gave Indonesia a *sort of* public health template for dealing with future public health challenges, like the COVID pandemic. More importantly, however, a new way of thinking about how best to address COVID-19 in Indonesia was already partially embedded within the Indonesian public health apparatus and even in the consciousness of some senior bureaucrats.

Counting COVID cases

COVID-19 was officially confirmed in Indonesia on 2 March 2020, after a dance instructor and her daughter tested positive for the virus. Contact tracers

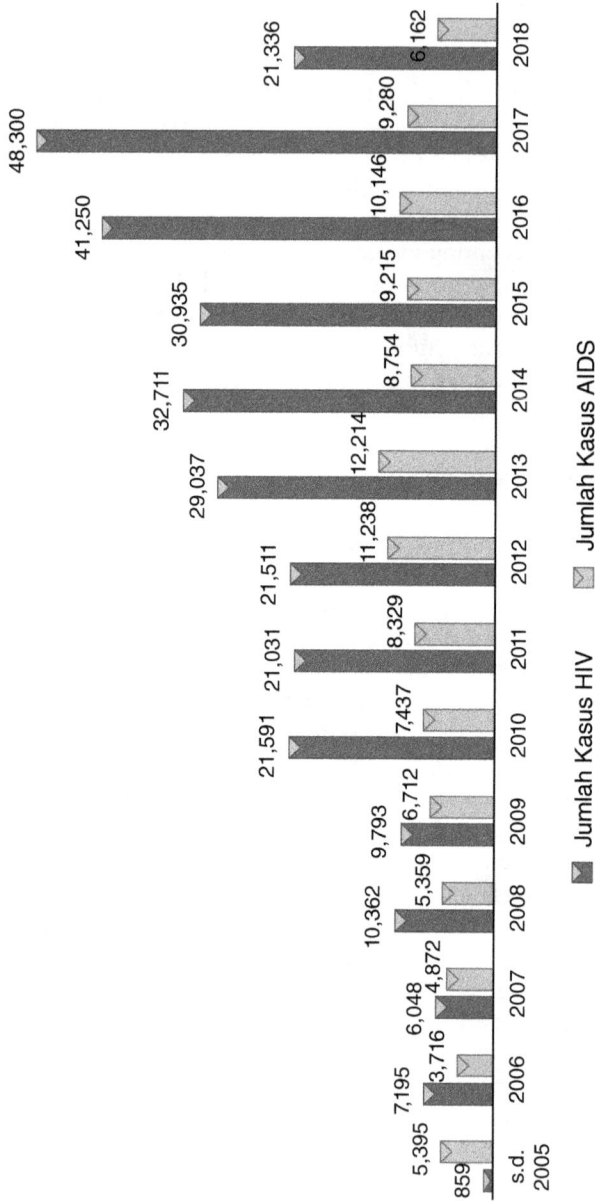

Figure 2.1 HIV infections Indonesia 2005–2018.

Source: Indonesian Ministry of Health (2018).

were able to determine that both mother and daughter were infected by a Japanese (and not a Chinese) national (Ratcliffe, 2020). This was politically very convenient, as it avoided playing into deeply entrenched anti-Chinese sentiment among Indonesians.

Despite Jokowi's initial populist rhetoric, like many other states across the world, by April 2020, the official Indonesian position was slowly beginning to conform to "the Public Health Approach"—namely, "[d]efine the problem, identify risks and any pre-existing protective factors, develop, and test prevention strategies and ensure widespread adoption of effective injury prevention strategies". For Indonesia, this was almost exclusively focused on the roll out of a mass vaccination programme (Satcher & Higginbotham, 2008: 400–403).

The shift to the Public Health Approach, at least in theory, was largely due to sustained pressure from both health professionals and medical scientists, as well as the media and the public. In fact, critics of the government had argued for three months that COVID-19's reported absence in the world's fourth most populous nation was totally implausible, especially given the large number of visitors from China, both for business and for tourism. A modelling study based on the number of travellers from Wuhan, China, for example, published by a team at the Harvard T. H. Chan School of Public Health on 11 February 2020 concluded that "even by that early period, it was highly unlikely (statistically impossible) that Indonesia did not have a single COVID-19 case", as was maintained at the time by the Indonesian government (Rochmyaningsih, 2021).

Unfortunately, early indications were that this promising acknowledgement continued to be hampered by extremely low testing rates, generally poor data management, fragmented application systems, data entry duplication, and a lack of suitably skilled human resources. Indeed, even a presidential decree mandating the integration of multiple data sources to improve decision-making was poorly implemented (Karunia, 2020). This shortcoming was acknowledged by the president's newly appointed 'COVID tsar', General (retired) Luhut Binsar Pandjaitan, the serving coordinating minister of maritime and investment affairs of Indonesia (Kurnia et al., 2021; Witoelar & Utomo, 2021), in the magazine *Kompas* on 11 May 2020. However, as Javier comments, "It is hard to think of a country other than Indonesia where the Minister for Economic Affairs is in charge of fighting an infectious disease" (Javier, 2021).

What Presidential Degree No. 7/2020 (and its amendment No. 9/-2020) did do was to effectively 'securitise' the Indonesian government's response. This was a feature shared with other regional Southeast Asian states, especially the Philippines. The new Indonesian laws mandated that rather than qualified health authorities managing the national COVID response (which would have been consistent with international best practice) instead the responsibility fell to military generals in the National Disaster Mitigation Agency (BNPB) (Hidayana & Larasati, 2021).

Again, this placed "order and stability" ahead of all other considerations, especially public health contingencies like hard lockdowns.

As an illustration of the deficiencies found in the state 'securitisation' approach, the COVID positive rate in Indonesia quickly emerged as a differentiating factor between different reporting sources.[2] For example, according to *Tempo.co*, as of 30 September 2020, the daily number of COVID-19 cases in Indonesia (as reported by the National Disaster Mitigation Agency) was 4,284 out of 30,940 people tested; therefore, the official positive rate was 13.85%. Significantly, the World Health Organization (WHO) suggests that if the positive rate is over 5%, this is likely "too high" (Javier, 2021), and a state should have a positive test rate of below 5% for two weeks before it considers reopening. Indonesia's official testing was too limited to detect that the real rate of COVID infection was likely under 1%, far below the official rate of 13.85%.

To further illustrate this point, the Indonesian Ministry of Health noted that as of 3 October 2021 (following the July 2021 historical peak in positive cases), there had been 4.2 million COVID-19 cases in Indonesia, while the local government KawalCovid-19 data set reported that the total number of cases since the beginning of the pandemic had reached 4.36 million. Discrepancies between versions of official numbers were also found in mortality data reported by both the central government and local government authorities (Javier, 2021). The media, however, bravely put a human face on these raw statistics by widely reporting on Indonesian healthcare workers who had died of COVID. According to the Risk Mitigation Team of the Indonesian Medical Association, by August 2021, mortality rates in this cohort included over 1,200 health professionals, including 598 doctors, at least 24 of whom were reported to be fully vaccinated (Tarigan, 2021; Rochmyaningsih, 2021).

However, in March 2020, the most pressing political issue for the President himself was not the COVID virus, adherence to public health orthodoxy, or even security (which is largely a military-oligarchy preoccupation), but rather the need to protect the rapidly flagging Indonesian economy. This is because "jobs and growth" were the centrepiece of Jokowi's campaign promises in both the 2014 and 2019 general elections. Clearly, the economic health of Indonesia was critical to the President's political legitimacy as "the Father of Infrastructure Development".

Figure 2.2 illustrates the context of the Indonesian President's initial pandemic preoccupation with "livelihoods over lives". The year after President Widodo was first elected in 2014, the Indonesian economy sharply contracted, with the unemployment rate rising to 6.18%. By the end of 2018, unemployment was down to 5.34%, largely through a policy of capping most commodity prices, (while at the same time, reducing ballooning energy subsidies), controlling and reducing the state deficit, and funding nationally significant infrastructure projects (like airports, railways, and roads), and by an aggressive programme of tax collection combined with reductions in unproductive state enterprises (Parker, 2019).

ECONOMIC GROWTH (%)

Indonesia's economy has accelerated since 2015, despite the country feeling the brunt of global economic slowdown.

UNEMPLOYMENT RATE (%)

Unemployment rate has also fallen since 2015.

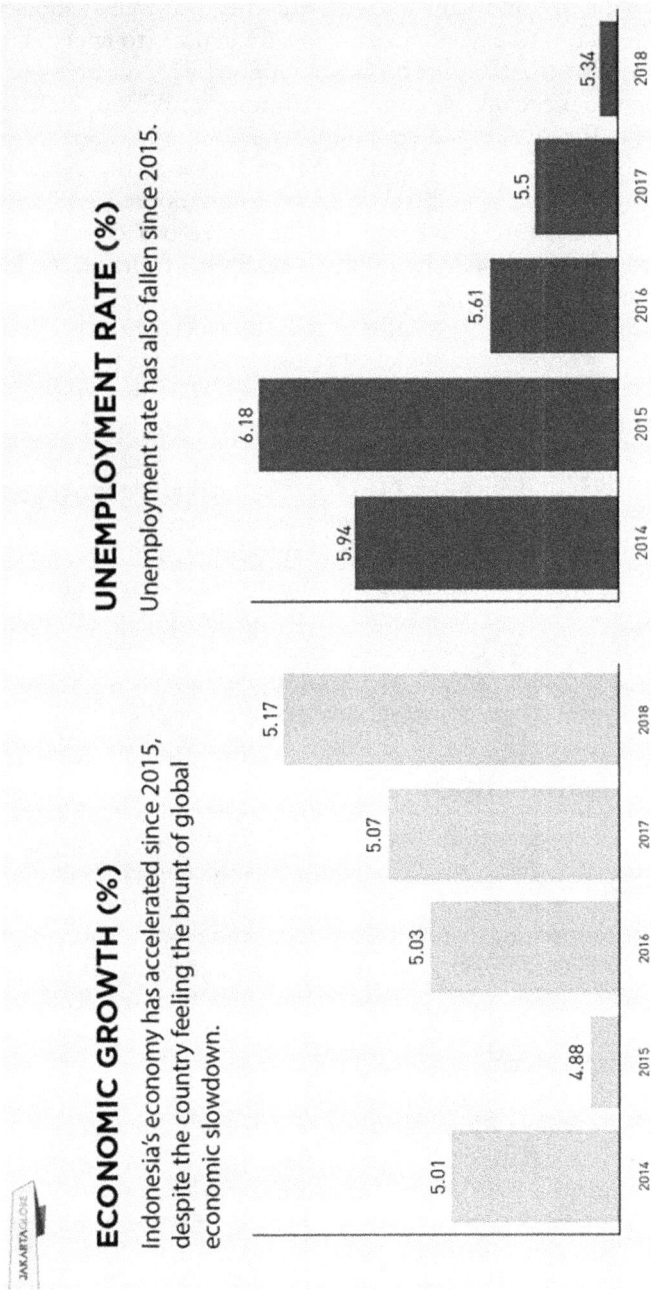

Figure 2.2 Economic growth and official unemployment rates in Indonesia 2014–2018.

Source: Javier (2021).

An indication of the President's preoccupation with matters economic at the start of the pandemic was that in March 2020, his government offered hotel discounts of up to 30% to anyone who visited Bali, as well as allocating a budget of $US8 million to engage social media influencers to encourage domestic tourists to visit the island. This was combined with a range of 'crisis packages' to support affected local businesses (Lindsey & Wilson, 2020). This was all occurring at the same time as Indonesia's neighbours were closing their borders and locking down due to COVID. Figure 2.3 shows that while Indonesia lagged many of its regional neighbours in closing borders and enacting lockdowns, the response time frame between the first recorded local case and then coordinated action was well ahead of, for example, Australia, the Philippines, India, Pakistan, and New Zealand.

Throughout early 2020, there continued to be an official focus on forestalling damage to the economy and thereby ostensibly reducing the risk of provoking the disquiet of over 25 million Indonesians who continue to live below the poverty line, or on less than $US1.90 a day per person (Asian Development Bank, 2022).

In April 2020, something new began to concern the Widodo government—unilateral localised and largely effective responses to the pandemic. City mayors, local government administrations, village authorities, and even individual neighbourhoods (often supported by politically progressive non-government organisations or NGOs) began to respond from "the bottom up" by initiating their own surprisingly effective pandemic measures. The low level of COVID infections reported throughout April and May 2020 can be explained in terms of the effectiveness of these responses (Lindsey & Wilson, 2020).

Local initiatives against COVID

Locally inspired initiatives included reporting of COVID symptoms (in the absence of laboratory testing), hard neighbourhood lockdowns, self-imposed social distancing, the wearing of locally manufactured cloth masks, as well as the production of antibacterial hand rubs (often utilising locally sourced herbal ingredients) and even communal food kitchens. Most of these initiatives were summarily overruled by the central government, which then required individual authorities to re-apply for permission to submit their strategies for approval to the now military and police-controlled authorities.

Here a critical fault line quickly emerged between President Widodo's election platform of streamlining bureaucracy and a direct challenge to the government's authority through local self-organisation and what was effectively informal de-bureaucratisation. In contrast to the President's policy of reducing 'red tape', the government's response delayed effective action against COVID. The prestigious *Frontiers in Public Health* journal referenced Indonesia's pandemic response from January 2020 to July 2020 as "the 4th worse in the world" and as "messy" and "uncoordinated", with the worst COVID-19 testing performance in the world after Bangladesh (Ayuningtyas et al., 2021).

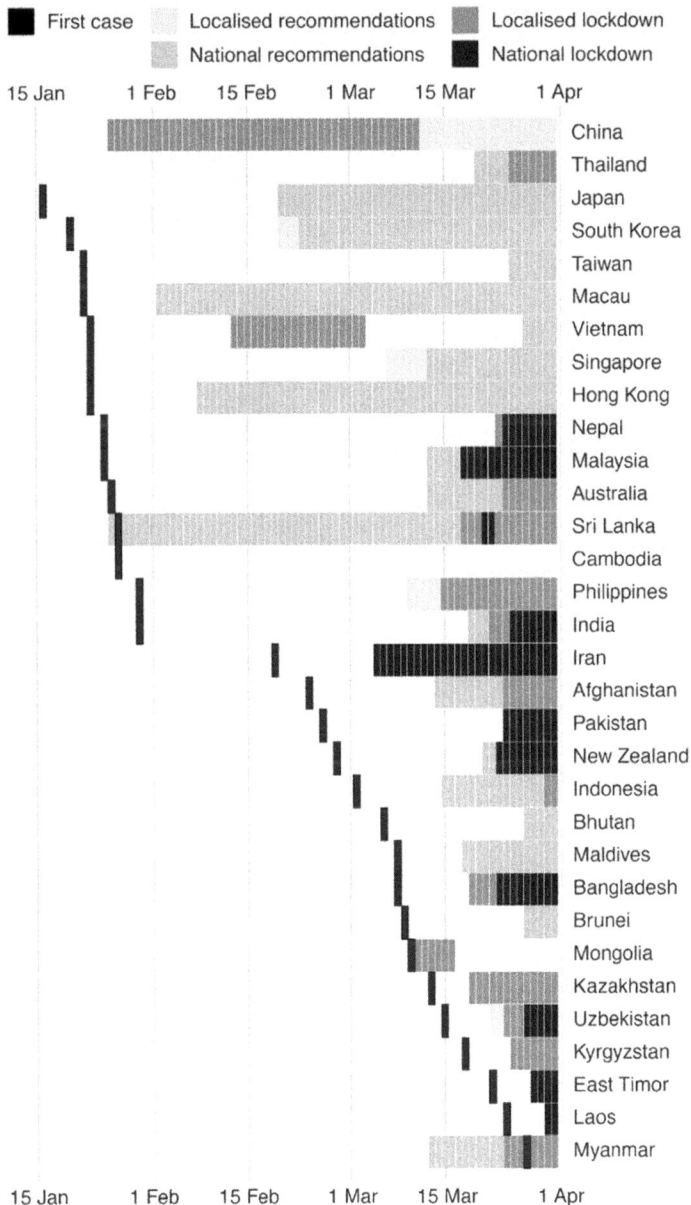

Figure 2.3 Dates and severity of restricted internal movement by country.

Source: Oxford COVID-19 Government Research Tracker, BBC Research (2022).

Note: China and Thailand confirmed their first cases prior to 15 January 2020

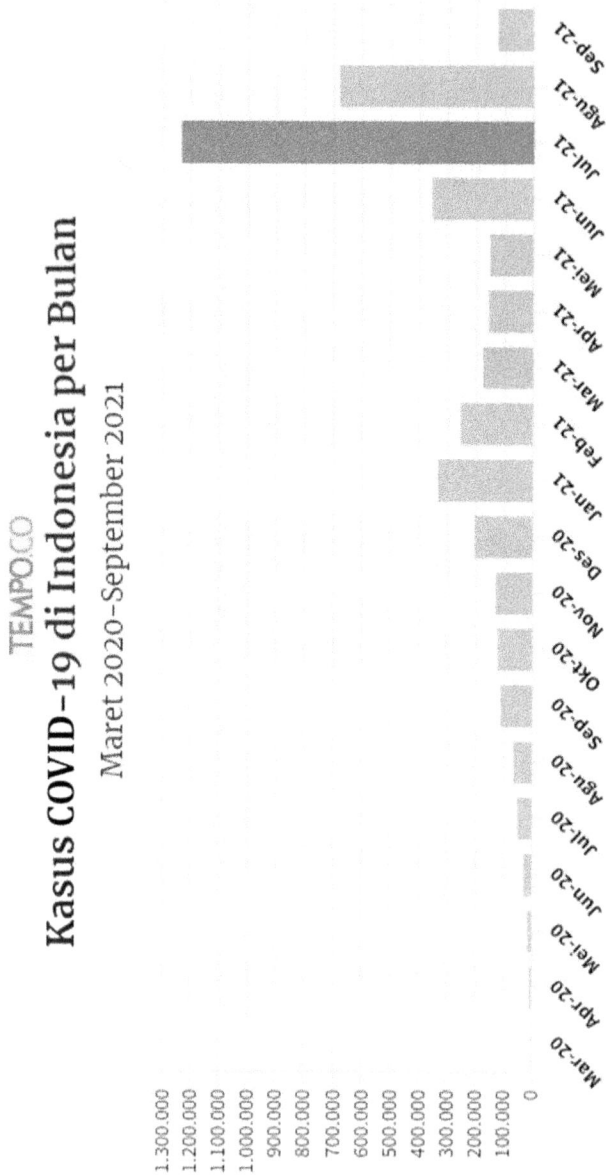

Figure 2.4 Confirmed COVID-19 cases from March 2020 to September 2021.

Source: Javier (2021).

The situation was further complicated by political friction between central and local government authorities as increasing case numbers coincided with the holy month of Ramadan and the distinctively Indonesian festival of *Mudik*, where tens of millions of city-dwellers return to their villages of origin for *Idul Fitri* the public holiday that marks the breaking of the monthlong fast of Ramadan. In response to rising COVID-19 numbers, between 6 and 17 May 2020, the Widodo government ordered an official ban on *Mudik*. The *Mudik* ban was, however, deliberately constructed in such a way as not to provoke a backlash from the President's most important organisational supporter, the 90 million-strong *Nahdlatul Ulama* (NU) [Revival of the Ulama], the largest Islamic organisation in the world (Esposito, 2013: 570). This approach set the ambiguous tone for all future 'lockdowns', to which the President was consistently opposed on the grounds that they would damage the economy. Rather, Indonesia initiated a four-level public decentralised activity restrictions system (PPKM) based on what were, as argued in this chapter, significantly underreported, or deliberately not reported, case numbers (Gaduh et al., 2022).

Despite the deployment of large numbers of police and soldiers to enforce it, the *Mudik* ban was clearly designed to be ineffective. On 12 May 2020, less than a week into the proscribed period, the ban was relaxed, and *Mudik* travel resumed. The seemingly contradictory messaging from the government neutralised the President's political adversaries by denying them the opportunity of claiming that he was "hostile to Islam". The result was that COVID-19 numbers continued to rise. However, paradoxically, this increase was mostly felt by the urban elite, and not by the urban and rural poor. Middle and upper-middle-class Indonesians were, in fact, spreading the virus because of their social mobility, especially through large numbers of domestic tourists who became the chief vectors. In contrast, the poor, who are less mobile geographically because of their economic circumstances, were less at risk, with impoverished urban and rural neighbourhoods reporting very low case numbers (Lindsey & Wilson, 2020).

One year later, in July 2021, Indonesia recorded its biggest one-day increase in new cases, with more than 47,000 infections. Three days later, this record was again broken with 56,000 infections. The islands of Java and Bali both experienced record-breaking numbers of new cases and deaths (Budiman, 2021). In response, the government announced new "micro-level social restrictions" for Java and Bali. However, in a positive move by the government, this utilised an effective neighbourhood-based zoning system to enforce local lockdowns. These restrictions were extended nationwide while the government prepared to roll out a mass vaccination programme in the absence of robust testing and contact tracing, or an effective system of isolating positive cases.

During the July 2021 peak of clinical cases (see Figure 2.5), Indonesian and international epidemiologists warned that the caseload in Indonesia could be as much as eight times higher than what the government was reporting. Seroprevalence studies have since confirmed that, by late 2021, at least ten percent

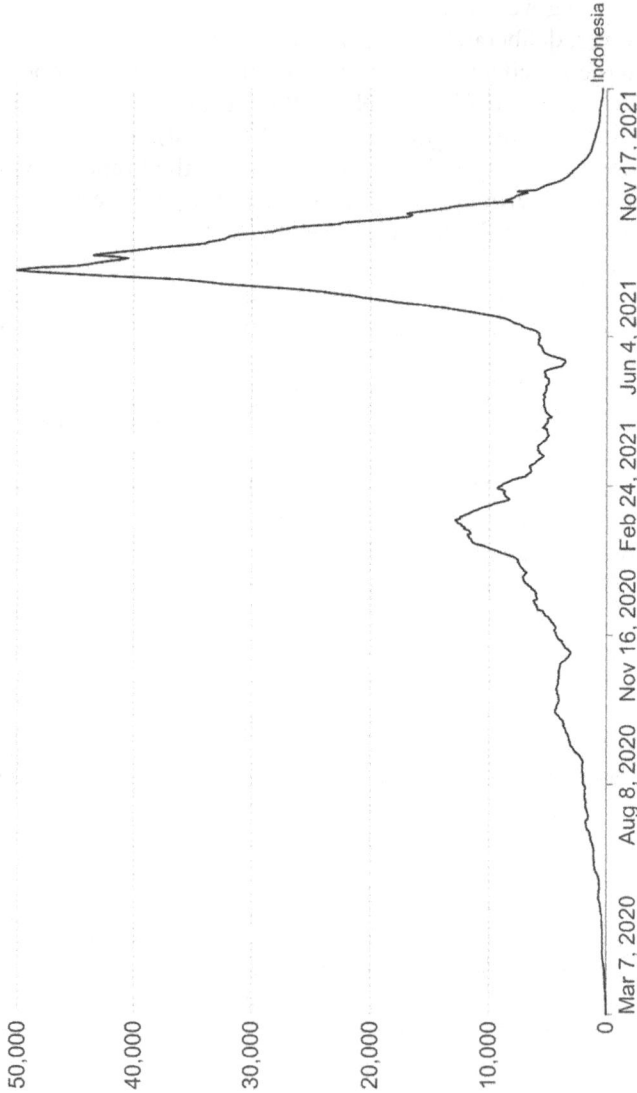

Daily new confirmed COVID-19 cases

Seven-day rolling average. Due to limited testing, the number of confirmed cases is lower than the true number of infections.

Figure 2.5 Daily confirmed COVID-19 cases, Indonesia, March 2020–November 2021.
Source: (Budiman, 2021).

of Indonesia's 270 million residents had been infected with the more contagious second-wave Delta variant (Jaffrey, 2021). In response, in July 2021, the
government imposed broad emergency restrictions on both travel and nones-
sential work. These rules were however relaxed within weeks, and Indonesia
returned to implementing less economically damaging micro-restrictions.

Paradoxically, even as the government sought to minimise economic disruption through largely ineffective restrictions, it was also introducing an aggressive and well-coordinated national vaccination programme. Then, as
restrictions eased, the government (under Minister Luhut Pandjaitan's coordination) rolled out its ambitious vaccination effort, which at its peak adminis-
trated over one million inoculations a day (Jaffrey, 2021). This programme
was divided into two phases: the first ran from January to April 2021 and targeted 40.2 million healthcare workers, public servants, and the elderly. The
second phase ran from April 2021 to March 2022 and targeted the public.
The vaccination campaign mostly utilised the Chinese-produced (and
WHO-endorsed) vaccines Sinovac and Sinopharm. The campaign was however hampered by vaccine supply problems, inadequate cold chain storage
(Nugraha et al., 2021) as well as questions about the safety and overall efficacy
of the chosen vaccines (Pearson, 2021).

Notwithstanding criticisms of the 'securitisation' response, the National
Disaster Mitigation Agency's priority of targeting vulnerable groups for vaccination in the most populated islands of Java and Bali, as well as in geographical
isolated regions such as Papua (where there are also high transmission rates),
has been largely effective. In May 2022, Luhut Pandjaitan reported that because of the national vaccination programme, COVID deaths had decreased
by 98% with COVID positive hospital rates of less than 3% (Wardani & Ferdinan, 2022).

Vaccination has clearly been the mainstay of the Indonesian government's
COVID response, and for the national vaccination programme to achieve sustained coverage, it will require better supply chain management, the elimination of distribution bottlenecks, and a strategy to confront growing vaccine
hesitancy. It will also require the fair distribution of the global vaccine stock-
pile, which has consistently held back the Indonesian programme (Jaffrey,
2021).

Impacts of the COVID-19 epidemic on Indonesian civil society

Having set out the preliminary background to the pandemic in Indonesia, we
now explore some of the impacts of the pandemic on Indonesian civil society.
This section draws heavily on an analysis of UNICEF data (UNICEF, 2021a)
from a landmark Indonesian survey that captured comprehensive data sets
from over 12,000 families across 34 provinces and 274 administrative districts.
That research was undertaken from October 2020 until December 2020 (well
before the peak of cases in July 2021 and as such, the report's conclusions can
be seen as representing a pre-peak mean). The research was undertaken with

special reference to women, families with children, boarding house residents (who often are not reflected in such research), and people with disabilities. There were several key areas that reflect the ongoing social consequences of the pandemic on ordinary Indonesians that are discussed in the following sections.

Family finances and employment

COVID-19 has had a significant effect on family finances across Indonesia. The most telling feature of the UNICEF survey is that three out of four households in Indonesia have experienced a decrease in income during the pandemic. Some 44% of urban households have experienced a decreased income of more than 25%, while in rural areas, the rate of decrease reached 34%. The loss of income caused by job losses, as well as reduced paid working hours, occurred in all sectors from hospitality to mining. This has been particularly felt in the informal sector (Dekker, 2020). Small businesses have suffered the most from reduced customer numbers, with dramatic decreases in income and increased costs. Indeed, many previously secure middle-income households have fallen into poverty (UNICEF, 2021a: 6).

According to UNICEF (2021a: 6) around "three-quarters of households (74.3%) interviewed in October and November 2020 said they were earning less than they were in January 2020". This is a concerning finding as the proportion of low-income households with children in Indonesia is 75.3%, and those living in urban areas is 78.3%.

Households in urban areas also experienced a greater decline in income, and in many cases, this was a larger decline than for households in rural areas. Households across all income groups, from the poorest to the richest, experienced a decrease in revenue by a similar percentage. As the report states,

> This decline in proportion appeared in all expenditure groups, with the largest drop occurring between the full-scale survey and the first monitoring survey, and among the Bottom 40% and the Middle 40% welfare groups.
>
> One in two households reported experiencing income fluctuation while one third of respondents experienced a continuous decrease in income throughout the survey period.
>
> (UNICEF, 2021a, pp. 2–3)

According to the report, many households that previously enjoyed a secure income stream became poor or were at risk of becoming poorer. However, for many, loss of income was not the only challenge. Rather, almost a quarter of respondents (24.4%) said that their expenditure also increased significantly, with material price increases being the major contributor to increases in household spending. There was also a much higher proportion of households with children (65%) that spent more money on internet costs or mobile phone credit (related to homeschooling) compared to homes without children (28.9%) (UNICEF, 2021b: 3).

During the UNICEF survey period, only a small fraction (14%) of family breadwinners changed jobs due to COVID-19. Despite this, almost half (47.3%) of those who changed jobs switched from the formal to the informal sector, and thus from more secure to less secure employment. Half of total households (51.5%) did not have any savings whatsoever, and so had no contingency funds. More than a quarter (27.3%) of households had to pawn property to survive. A quarter (25.3%) of families interviewed were forced by circumstances to borrow money from family or friends (UNICEF, 2021a: 6).

Social assistance

Of the households (85.3%) that received at least one form of social assistance—whether direct grants or the in-house provision of material goods such as food staples—half (50.8%) received direct cash assistance from the government. The poorest households received the most assistance. More than 90% accepted at least one form of assistance, and more than 60% received cash assistance. Most households that were economically safe before the pandemic, but lost income, also received government assistance (70%). Assistance included tax deferral, subsidy credit, and internet quota assistance targeting newly affected households. Two-thirds (67.4%) of recipients of government assistance said that this helped overcome the impact on their home finances. However, more than a third (38%) of households did not receive cash assistance from October to November 2020. Very few households (7.5%) that ran small businesses received business support from the government at the time of the survey, and four out of ten business owners said they did not know about government assistance (UNICEF, 2021a: 6-7).

Schooling

Almost three out of four parents reported that they were worried about lost learning opportunities for their children. In Indonesia, access to reliable internet remains the main obstacle to a child's success in learning from home. This was reported to be a major problem for 57.3% of households with children. Poorer households in rural areas faced even greater problems connecting to the internet than urban and wealthier households. Many parents reported that they did not have enough time (28.7%) and/or did not have the capacity (25.3%) to support their children in learning from home. Even before the pandemic, Indonesia faced serious learning challenges because 70% of 15-year-olds did not achieve minimum proficiency in reading and mathematics (UNICEF, 2021a: 7).

During the pandemic in 2020–2021, most distance learning in Indonesia was conducted via the WhatsApp platform, thus limiting face-to-face interaction between teachers and students. According to UNICEF data, the average time spent per day on distance learning has varied greatly, with 3.5 hours in Jakarta to 2.2 hours outside of the island of Java. On average, students in elementary schools, students in rural areas, and those who are included in the 40% income group at the bottom of society all spent less time every day involved in distance learning. Almost half of all parents expressed concern about the limited access to the internet and electronic devices and the lack of time and capacity needed to help teach their children. Some 38% of adolescents stated that the main challenge they faced in distance learning was a lack of guidance from teachers. Meanwhile, 31% of teenagers said that boredom was the main challenge (UNICEF, 2021b: 3).

Of all households, 3.45% reported having at least one child cease schooling, particularly where there was a child with disabilities involved, although the actual overall dropout rate is estimated to be much higher (Satriana et al., 2021). A number of households stopped the education of their children temporarily, whilst one in five households did not want to continue it under COVID circumstances. As many as 7.15% of households reported that at least one of their children had worked for wages during the pandemic, with 2.5% of children starting work for the first time since the pandemic began. Although the availability of specific official data is limited, an increase in school dropout rates places children at risk of early marriage and involvement in dangerous and exploitative activities (UNICEF, 2021b: 3).

Healthcare

Even though the death rate of children due to COVID-19 is relatively low, the disruption of basic and routine health services (including support for anxiety and depression) poses long-term risks to indirect mortality for children in Indonesia. Preliminary estimates suggest that disturbances in healthcare systems and reduced access to food have resulted in an additional 30,560 deaths of children under five in just six months. Disruption to child health services, immunisation programmes, the monitoring of child development, family planning programmes and antenatal care is a health problem primarily for children and women. Immunisation services, birth control, antenatal care, delivery, and postpartum decreased by 7% with the decline in urban areas reaching almost 10% in 2020 (UNICEF, 2021b: 4).

The data also shows that households with children were reluctant to access healthcare. One of the main reasons given was that they were afraid of contracting COVID-19. More than one in ten households with children under the age of five years of age said that they did not bring their children to an immunisation clinic for that reason. School closures, social isolation, and uncertain economic prospects also exposed children to other risks. The survey found that 45% of homes reported behavioural problems in their children. Of the total sample, 20.5% stated that children had more difficulty concentrating, 12.9% became more irritable, and 6.5% had difficulty sleeping. Interestingly, the data revealed a gender imbalance in assisting children to learn at home due to COVID school closures—women were three times more likely than men to spend time with their home-schooled children: 71.5% to 22% of households. Half of the home schooling women also held down paid work to support their families (UNICEF, 2021b: 4).

Mental health

Like elsewhere in the world, the pandemic has caused significant disruption to basic health services in Indonesia because health personnel and budgets have been diverted to respond to COVID-19, away from what were already struggling primary health care services. As early as July 2020, concerning evidence of a serious rise in pandemic-related mental health conditions associated with fear, loneliness, frustration, and sadness was also emerging (Nasir, 2020) putting a further burden on already overstretched services. Due to the COVID pandemic, there are now millions of 'disturbed adolescents' with diminished access to health services, nutrition, and protection.

Basic levels of inequality are also increasing across Indonesia, especially with respect to gender and disability. The COVID pandemic has had a significant secondary impact on around 80 million Indonesian children and their daily lives. The number of children and adolescents who have fallen into greater poverty due to the COVID-19 pandemic compared to other age groups is significant. About 33% of the Indonesian population are children under the age of 18 years, and this represents "nearly 40% of the population who fell into poverty in 2020" (UNICEF, 2021b: 2).

Conclusions

The Indonesian government responded to the COVID pandemic by attempting to protect the economy to ensure relative social stability. It initially paid less attention to a vaccine rollout, and at the time of writing (mid-2022), has been only mildly interested in boosters or new vaccines to address future COVID variants. Despite government financial support, especially for poorer families, the negative impacts of the pandemic on Indonesian civil society have been more prominent among women and children, as well as the rural and urban poor. Increasing levels of absolute poverty and extreme income disparity have occurred alongside the overburdening of an already under-resourced healthcare system. The proper funding of critical care equipment, such as mechanical ventilators and oxygen concentrators for future outbreaks, is essential. Indeed, if improvements to unwell patient treatment outcomes during spikes in clinical presentations are to be achieved and trust is to be established in the safety and effectiveness of both primary and tertiary healthcare, training and retention of skilled healthcare workers are necessary, and this applies to both critical care trained and primary healthcare nurses.

Recent government initiatives to promote regional cooperation in Southeast Asia are also important to deal with COVID-19 over the long term. This is because managing a longer pandemic characterised by ever-emerging variant stains will require continued supplies of new vaccines, as well as more advanced therapeutics. The government's recent partnership agreements to establish vaccine and antiviral manufacturing plants in Indonesia are important steps in this direction and, despite shortcomings in track, trace, and isolate strategies, it reflects how far the Indonesian government has come since early 2020.

Notes
1 For a detailed discussion of COVID testing issues including track and trace, see Binnicker (2020) and Ritchie et al. (2020).
2 The positive rate is obtained by dividing the number of people who have tested positive for COVID-19 by the number of tests carried out.

References

Asian Development Bank. (2022). Poverty Data: Indonesia. Available at: https://www.adb.org/countries/indonesia/poverty.

A'yun, R.Q. and Mudhoffir, A.M. (2022, March 21). Reproducing Indonesia's Illiberal Legalism amid COVID-19: Public Health Crisis as a Means of Accumulation. *Aust. J. Asian Law*, 22(2), Article 03, 21–44. Available at SSRN: https://ssrn.com/abstract=4063331.

Ayuningtyas, D., Haq, H.U., Utami, R.R.M., and Susilia, S. (2021, May). Requestioning the Indonesia Government's Public Policy Response to the COVID-19 Pandemic: Black Box Analysis for the Period of January–July 2020. *Front. Public Health*, https://doi.org/10.3389/fpubh.2021.612994.

BBC Research. (2022). Oxford COVID-19 Government Research Tracker.

Binnicker, M.J. (2020, October 21). Challenges and Controversies to Testing for COVID-19 American Society for Microbiology. *J. Clin. Microbiol.*, 58(11), https://doi.org/10.1128/JCM.01695-20.

Bland, B. (2020). Indonesia: Covid-19 Crisis Reveals Cracks in Jokowi's Ad Hoc Politics. *The Interpreter*. Available at: https://www.lowyinstitute.org/the-interpreter/indonesia-covid-19-crisis-reveals-cracks-jokowi-s-ad-hoc-politics.

Bone, A. (2016). Indonesian Breaking Down Taboos. *SBS*. Available at: https://www.sbs.com.au/topics/voices/health/article/2016/05/05/hiv-indonesia-breaking-down-taboos.

Boonto, K. and Julliand, V. (2021, June 8). Forty Years On, Far too Many Indonesians Are Still Dying from AIDS, *Jakarta Post*.

Budiman, D. (2021). Indonesia mencatat peningkatan tertinggi dalam kasus COVID — dan jumlahnya mungkin akan naik lagi sebelum turun. *The Convertaion*. Available at: https://theconversation.com/indonesia-mencatat-peningkatan-tertinggi-dalam-kasus-covid-dan-jumlahnya-mungkin-akan-naik-lagi-sebelum-turun-164559.

Cahya, G.H. (2021). 'I've Seen Too Many Bodies': Jakarta Gravediggers Chart Indonesia's Covid Battle. *The Guardian*. Available at: https://www.theguardian.com/world/2021/jun/27/ive-seen-too-many-bodies-jakarta-gravediggers-chart-indonesias-covid-battle.

Dekker, B. (2020). The Impact of Covid-19 Measures on Indonesian Value Chains. Available at: https://www.clingendael.org/publication/impact-covid-19-measures-indonesian-value-chains

Esposito, J. (2013). *Oxford Handbook of Islam and Politics*, OUP, New York.

Gaduh, A., Hanna, R., Kreindler, G., and Olken, B. (2022). Lockdown and Mobility in Indonesia. Available at: https://histecon.fas.harvard.edu/climate-loss/indonesia/index.html

Hermawan, A. (2020). Let's Not Kid Ourselves. Indonesia Is Unlikely to be COVID-19-Free. And That's Not Our Biggest Problem. *The Jakarta Post*. Available at: https://www.thejakartapost.com/academia/2020/02/29/lets-not-kid-ourselves-indonesia-is-unlikely-to-be-covid-19-free-and-thats-not-our-biggest-problem.html.

Hidayana, I. and Larasati, A. (2021). Why Securitization of COVID-19 Response Sets Dangerous Precedent. *The Jakarta Post*. Available at: https://www.thejakartapost.com/academia/2021/11/02/why-securitization-of-covid-19-response-sets-dangerous-precedent.html.

Islamaj, E. et al. (2021). Lives versus Livelihoods during the COVID-19 Pandemic: How Testing Softens the Trade-Off. Policy Research Working Paper No. 9696. World Bank. Available at: https://openknowledge.worldbank.org/handle/10986/35766 License: CC BY 3.0 IGO.

Jaffrey, S. (2021). How the Global Vaccine Divide Is Fuelling Indonesia's Corona Virus Catastrophe. *Carnegie Endowment of International Peace*. Available at: https://carnegieendowment.org/2021/08/05/how-global-vaccine-divide-is-fueling-indonesia-s-coronavirus-catastrophe-pub-85107.

Jakarta, Globe. (2019, May 19). Can Indonesia Leverage a 'Golden Moment' in Its Economy?, https://jakartaglobe.id/context/can-indonesia-leverage-a-golden-moment-in-its-economy.

Javier, F. (2021). Jumlah Kasus Covid-19 September 2021 Menurun 82 Persen Dibanding Bulan Sebelumnya. *Tempo*. Available at: https://data.tempo.co/data/1225/jumlah-kasus-covid-19-september-2021-menurun-82-persen-dibanding-bulan-sebelumnya.

Karunia, A.M. (2020). Luhut Temukan Manajemen Data Covid-19 yang Tak Sesuai antara Pusat dan Daerah. *KOMPAS*. Available at: https://money.kompas.com/read/2020/11/05/051735926/luhut-temukan-manajemen-data-covid-19-yang-tak-sesuai-antara-pusat-dan-daerah.

Kurnia, S. et al. (2021). Three Reasons Why COVID-19 Data in Indonesia Are Unreliable and How to Fix Them. *The Conversation*. Available at: https://theconversation.com/three-reasons-why-covid-19-data-in-indonesia-are-unreliable-and-how-to-fix-them-157056.

Kyle, J. et al. (2018). Populists in Power Around the World. *Tony Blair Institute for Global Change*. Available at: https://institute.global/policy/populists-power-around-world.

Lindsey, T. and Man, T. (2020). Indonesia: The Not So Good News. *The Interpreter*. Available at: https://www.lowyinstitute.org/the-interpreter/indonesia-not-so-good-news.

Lindsey, T. and Wilson, I. (2020). Is Indonesia's Covid-19 Response too Little, too Late?, Ear to Asia Podcast, https://arts.unimelb.edu.au/__data/assets/pdf_file/0011/3386909/ETA-Episode-69-transcript.pdf.

Nasir, S. (2020). Covid and Mental Health in Indonesia. Asia and the Pacific Policy Society. Available at: https://www.policyforum.net/covid-19-and-mental-health-in-indonesia/.

Nugraha, R.R., Miranda, A.V., Ahmadi, A. et al. (2021). Accelerating Indonesian COVID-19 Vaccination Rollout: A Critical Task Amid the Second Wave. *Trop. Med. Health.*, 49, 76, https://doi.org/10.1186/s41182-021-00367-3.

Osuna, J.J.O. (2020). From Chasing Populists to Deconstructing Populism: A New Multidimensional Approach to Understanding and Comparing Populism. *Eur. J. Polit. Res.*, 60(4), https://doi.org/10.1111/1475-6765.12428.

Parker, E. (2019). What Does Jokowi's Win Mean for Indonesia's Economy? *The Diplomat.* Available at: https://thediplomat.com/2019/04/what-does-jokowis-win-mean-for-indonesias-economy/.

Pearson, C. (2021, December). China Promotes Vaccines Around the World, but Critics Point to Lower Efficacy. *Voice of America.* Available at https://www.voanews.com/a/china-promotes-vaccines-around-the-world-but-critics-point-to-lower-efficacy-/6355437.html.

Ratcliffe, R. (2020). First Coronavirus Cases Confirmed in Indonesia Amid Fears Nation Is Ill-Prepared for an Outbreak. *The Guardian.* Available at: https://www.theguardian.com/world/2020/mar/02/first-coronavirus-cases-confirmed-in-indonesia-amid-fears-nation-is-ill-prepared-for-outbreak.

Riono, P. and Jazant, S. (2004). The Current Situation of the HIV/AIDS Epidemic in Indonesia. *AIDS Educ. Prev.*, 16(3 Suppl A), 78–90.

Ritchie, H., Mathieu, E., Rodés-Guirao, L., Appel, C., Giattino, C., Ortiz-Ospina, E., Hasell, J., Macdonald, B., Beltekian, D., and Roser, M. (2020). Coronavirus Pandemic (COVID-19). *Published online at OurWorldInData.org.* Available at: https://ourworldindata.org/coronavirus [Online Resource].

Rochmyaningsih, D. (2021). Lack of Testing May Mask a "Silent Epidemic" in the World's Fourth Most Populous Country. *Science.* Available at: https://www.science.org/content/article/indonesia-finally-reports-two-coronavirus-cases-scientists-worry-it-has-many-more.

Satcher, D. and Higginbotham, E.J. (2008, March). The Public Health Approach to Eliminating Disparities in Health. *Am. J. Public Health*, 98(3), 400–403.

Satriana, S., Huda, K., Saadah, N., Hidayati, D.N., and Zulkarnaen, A. (2021). Covid-19 Impacts on People With Disabilities in Indonesia: An In-Depth Look, https://www.dfat.gov.au/sites/default/files/covid19-impact-pwd-indonesia.pdf.

Tarigan, E. (2021). Rapid Virus Spread through Indonesia Taxes Health Workers. *AP News.* Available at: https://apnews.com/article/asia-pacific-business-health-indonesia-coronavirus-pandemic-0f1f3fe5157a977d1cbfcf9340584843.

UNICEF Report. (2021a). Analisis Dampak Sosial dan Ekonomi COVID-19 pada Rumah Tangga di Indonesia. *The Interpreter.* Available at: https://www.unicef.org/indonesia/id/laporan/analisis-dampak-sosial-dan-ekonomi-covid-19-pada-rumah-tangga-di-indonesia.

UNICEF Report. (2021b). Menuju respons dan pemulihan COVID-19 yang berfokus pada anak. Available at: https://www.unicef.org/indonesia/id/laporan/menuju-respons-dan-pemulihan-covid-19-yang-berfokus-padaanak?gclid=CjwKCAiA1uKMBhAGEiwAxzvX9_rSnvudMnhg6Sjxr9kUmUmVuQur0ZGwglaQ5WKxEJRlJFFON_1M5hoCyyUQAvD_BwE.

Vieten, M.U. (2020). The "New Normal" and "Pandemic Populism": The COVID-19 Crisis and Anti-Hygienic Mobilisation of the Far-Right. *Soc. Sci.*, 9, 165, https://doi.org/10.3390/socsci9090165.

Wardani, D. and Ferdinan. (2022). Luhut Brings Good News, COVID-19 Hospital Occupancy Is Currently Only 2 Percent. *VOI.* Available at: https://voi.id/en/news/165300/luhut-bawa-kabar-baik-keterisian-rs-covid-19-saat-ini-hanya-2-persen.

Witoelar, F. and Utomo, A. (2021). Diagnosing Indonesia's Health Challenges. *The Interpreter.* Available at: https://www.lowyinstitute.org/the-interpreter/diagnosing-indonesia-s-health-challenges.

Wolfe, D. and Dale, D. (2020). It's Going to Disappear: A Timeline of Trump's Claims that Covid-19 Will Vanish. *CNN*. Available at: https://edition.cnn.com/interactive/2020/10/politics/covid-disappearing-trump-comment-tracker/.

World Bank Report. (2021). Indonesian Economic Prospects: A Green Horizon: Toward a High Growth and Low Carbon Economy. Available at: https://openknowledge.worldbank.org/bitstream/handle/10986/36732/166956.pdf.

3 Pandemic, migrant workers, and the economy of Bangladesh

Mamta B. Chowdhury

Introduction

Like any other country, Bangladesh has been impacted considerably by the COVID-19 pandemic and has gone through various health and socio-economic challenges. Although the country was lagging in its control strategy, prevention, and vaccine diplomacy in the early phase of the pandemic, by mid-2021, it could manage the health and economic crisis and overcome a shortage of vaccination doses. As of May 2022, a total of 256.2 million doses had been administered in Bangladesh, which is equivalent to 71% population of the country being fully vaccinated (Our World in Data, 2022). During the last two years of the pandemic, the government of the country implemented various strategies to combat the virus, as well as the socio-economic disruptions, and the country's economy is showing resilience to the unprecedented simultaneous supply and demand shocks.

The economy has displayed a strong recovery from the pandemic and in 2021 achieved a real gross domestic product (GDP) growth of 6.9%, up from 3.4% in 2020. The two major export-earning sectors—ready-made garments (RMG) and migrant human resource services—recovered considerably after a period of severe upheaval due to the global pandemic and earned US$35.6 billion and US$22.1 billion, respectively, in 2021. This chapter highlights the impact of COVID-19 on the Bangladesh economy, with a particular focus on the migrant workers and the flow of remittances to the country, which is the second-largest source of foreign exchange earnings for Bangladesh after RMG export income. The chapter will conclude with a discussion of the strategies and policies that the government of Bangladesh has taken to combat the pandemic and achieve a remarkable recovery from the COVID-19 pandemic.

Economic structure

The People's Republic of Bangladesh, commonly known as Bangladesh, became independent on 26 March 1971 with its capital in Dhaka. Bangladesh is the world's eighth most populous state with 167.7 million people in 2022, equivalent to 2.11% of the world population. Its more limited land area has led

DOI: 10.4324/9781003311522-3

to a high population density— an average of 1,265 people per km². Two major religions dominate Bangladesh: Islam (89.1%) and Hinduism (10%) with the remaining 0.9% identifying as Buddhist or Christian. About 39.4% of the population are urban dwellers, and the median age is 27.6 years. The vast majority (98%) of Bangladesh's population belongs to the Bengali ethnic and linguistic group. Politically, the ruling Awami League and its prime minister, Sheikh Hasina, led Bangladesh throughout the period under consideration.

Since independence, Bangladesh has become one of the fastest-growing economies in the world supported by export-led growth, averaging higher than 6% GDP growth since 1996, despite domestic political and institutional unrest, structural constraints, global economic and financial market uncertainties, and the coronavirus pandemic. The growth rate of the economy was 8.2% in 2019, which slumped to 3.5% in 2020 and then recovered quickly. In 2021 the GDP per capita was equivalent to US$5,139 (World Bank, 2022a).

Over the last three decades, and when compared to its South Asian neighbours, Bangladesh has been performing progressively stronger in terms of its economic and social indicators. Table 3.1 indicates that by 2020, Bangladesh had a high life expectancy (73 years) compared to the average for South Asian countries[1] (70 years).

Bangladesh has also been reducing its poverty headcount ratio—measured at $1.90 a day as a percentage of the population—from 34.2% in 2000 to 14% in 2016, meaning there are fewer people living in poverty. Also, in terms of secondary school enrolment, fixed broadband subscriptions, basic drinking water and sanitation facilities, and hospital beds per 1,000 people, Bangladesh is progressing well on some South Asian indicators.

The economy of Bangladesh is mainly comprised of agricultural, industrial, and services sectors and has remained almost the same over the last decade from 2010 to 2020. The services sector is the largest, and at 53.5% of the economy, it is unchanged since 2010. The agricultural sector's contribution to GDP has shrunk from 17% in 2010 to 13% in 2020, whereas the industry sector has grown from 25% in 2010 to 30% in 2020.

In 2021, the value of Bangladesh's exports grew by 31.6% to USD$44.22 billion from the previous year. Bangladesh is the second-largest exporter of knit and non-knit-RMG in the world, earning USD$31.5 billion in 2021. Other exports from Bangladesh include agricultural products and fish, pharmaceuticals, plastic, rubber, leather and leather products, ceramic tablewares, jute, cotton and cotton products, electronics and electrical products, software and ICT products, and ships and vessels. The major destination countries of exports include Germany ($6.69 billion), the United States of America ($6.25 billion), the United Kingdom ($3.05 billion), Spain ($2.95 billion), and Poland ($2.27 billion), Switzerland ($108 million) and Turkey ($53.9 million) in 2020 (OEC, 2020). The Kingdom of Saudi Arabia (74.08%), Oman (8.91%), United Arab Emirates (4.73%), Singapore (4.52%), and Qatar (1.81%) are the major countries for recruiting migrant workers in 2021 (BMET, 2022). Bangladesh imports rice and wheat, milk and cream, fertiliser,

Table 3.1 Socio-economic indicators of South Asia and Bangladesh (selected years)

	South Asia					Bangladesh				
	1985	2000	2015	2018	2020	1985	2000	2015	2018	2020
Population (person million)	1,010	1,390	1,750	1,927	1981	93	128	161	163	165
GDP (constant 2015 US$, million)	497	1,090	2,700	3,298	3236	2.23	83.5	195	274	324
Gross National Income (GNI) (PPP, current international $)	1,200	2,061	5,104	6,169	6,094	850	1,370	3,790	4,750	5,138
GDP growth	5.4	4.1	7.4	6.4	-5.7	3.3	5.3	6.6	7.9	3.5
Inflation (GDP deflator)	6.6	4.5	2.1	3.6	4.4	18.5	3.4	5.9	5.6	4.1
Exports/GDP	6.3	13.6	18.7	18.5	17.1	5.4	12.3	17.3	15	12
Remittances (current billion US$)	5.8	17	118	132	147	0.50	2	15.4	16.4	21.7
Remittances/GDP	1.98	2.7	4.3	3.8	4.3	2.6	3.7	8.7	5.7	6.7
Life expectancy	56	63	68	69	70	56	65	71	72	73
Net Official Development Assistance (ODA) received (% gross capital formation)	6.1	2.3	1.9	1.1	1.4	27.8	7.7	4.6	3.6	4.7
Gross enrolment ratio, secondary, both sexes (%)	33	43	67	69	70	20	50	64	73	74
Fixed broadband subscriptions (per 100 people)	—	—	1.4	1.7	2.1	—	—	3.13	5	6.1

Basic drinking water (% population with access)	70	81.7	88.6	89.9	90.7	67	95	97	97.4	97.7
People using basic sanitation facilities (% population with access)	18	18.3	56.3	64	69.3	18	23.7	46.7	51.2	54.2
Poverty headcount ratio at $1.90 a day (% of population)	50	40 (2002)	15	15	15	34.5	34	18	14.8	14.3 (2016)
Carbon dioxide (CO_2) emissions (metric tonnes per capita)	0.49	0.77	1.38	1.5	—	0.11	0.17	0.46	0.51	—
Hospital beds (per 1,000 people)	0.71	0.68	0.6	0.58	—	0.29	0.3	0.77	0.79	—
Bribery index	—	—	—	—	24.8	—	—	—	47.7 (2013)	—

Source: Compiled and constructed by the author using World Bank: World Bank Online (2022b) data.

raw cotton, refined petroleum, iron and steel, machinery and electrical appliances, man-made fibre, and woven cotton, mainly from China, India, the United States of America, Australia, Singapore, and Indonesia.

Workers are a key export for Bangladesh, and despite various disruptions in the movement of migrant workers from Bangladesh from early 2020 due to the sudden breakout of the COVID-19 pandemic, the workers' remittances contributed USD$22.1 billion to the economy in 2021 and supported many low-income, remittances-recipient families during the downturn of economic activities.

History of migrant workers and remittance flows to Bangladesh

The movement of people in and out of the Bengal Delta region in search of employment, education, religious missions, travelling, and trade has been taking place over centuries. Under British rule, migration from and through what became Bangladesh and even East Pakistan in the 1960s, a small number of migrant workers were employed by the Kingdom of Saudi Arabia and Qatar, mostly by private initiatives (Chowdhury, 2011). Since independence in 1971 and negotiations between Bangladesh and recruiting countries between 1972 and 1975, the recruitment of Bangladeshi workers to Middle Eastern countries has been facilitated by delegates from recruiting countries (Chowdhury and Chowdhury, 1991). Capitalising on the Gulf States' need for labour and on its own excess supply of human resources, Bangladesh has expanded the labour market beyond its boundaries. Bangladesh emerged as a major human resource exporting country globally in the late 1980s as globalisation created employment opportunities for migrant workers to various other Southeast Asian countries, including Malaysia and Singapore. In response, the Bangladesh government established the Bureau of Human Resources, Employment, and Training (BMET) to export its labour resources in a more coordinated manner, and to devise policies to support what has over time become a vital source of foreign exchange earnings, growing to over one million overseas workers (Figure 3.1).

Currently, about 14 million Bangladeshi workers are employed in overseas countries and contributed more than US$22.1 billion to the country in 2021. The total number of migrant workers rose from only 6,087 in 1976 to 103,814 in 1990, and the remittances income increased from a mere US$24 million in 1976 to US$782 million in 1990 (BMET, 2022). In ten years, the total recruitment increased by 115% to 222,686 people, yielding about US$2 billion in remittances. By the year 2000, remittances had become a stable source of income for many families with members working overseas. Both the recruitment of migrant workers and remittances increased dramatically over the next decade.

In 2010, workers' remittances of over US$11 billion contributed to 12% of the GDP of the country, which reduced the pressure on the domestic labour market, as well as supporting economic growth and social development. These massive remittance flows increased household savings, investment, and consumption (Chowdhury, 2011), and alleviated the poverty level by 6% in

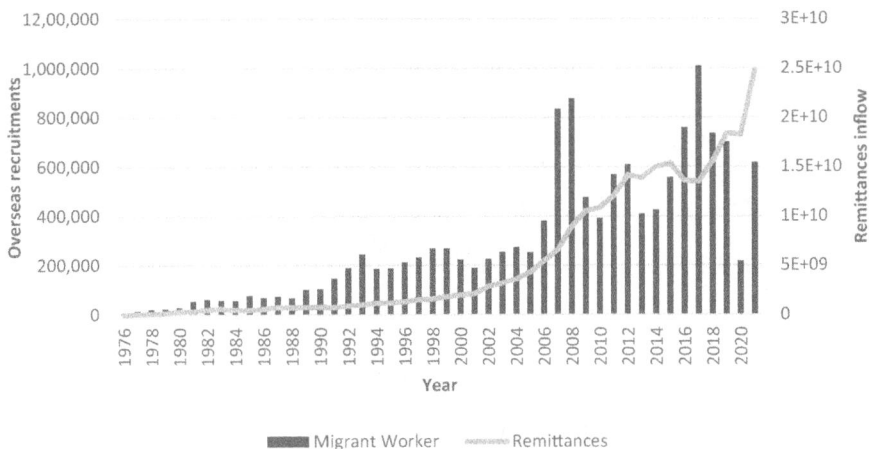

Figure 3.1 Overseas recruitments and remittances flow to Bangladesh 1976–2021.
Source: Constructed by the author using BMET data (2022 Online).

Bangladesh (World Bank, 2006). By 2019, both the number of migrant workers and the flow of remittances showed an upward trend. In 2017, more than a million migrant workers were recruited by overseas employers, who sent US$13.7 billion to the country. In early 2020, the global COVID-19 pandemic suddenly disrupted the flow of human resource services and brought various health and movement restrictions for migrant workers. However, it is interesting to note that even after the recruitment of migrant workers fell by 69% in 2020 from 2019 levels, remittance flow increased by 18.5% to US$21.8 billion, showing resilience (BMET, 2022).

Remittances are also increasingly using formal mechanisms. In 2014, the World Bank (2014) reported that 76.1% of remittances were coming into the country through formal channels, compared to only 46% in 2006; however, 24.9% of remittances are hand-carried by friends and relatives or come through the hundi[2] system, and 4% of remittances are made in-kind. The main reasons for using informal channels to send remittances are that people believe them to be inexpensive, speedy, and require no documentation (Mahmud, 2012).

Destination countries and the skill composition of the migrant workers

Between 1976 and 2020, about 14.1 million Bangladeshi migrant workers were recruited, about 82% by the Gulf countries and the Arab States, and the rest by Malaysia, Singapore, South Korea, the United Kingdom, Italy, Japan, Egypt, Libya, Lebanon, Jordan, Sudan, Brunei, Mauritius, Iraq, the United States of America, Germany, and Australia (Figure 3.2). One in four of the migrant workers originated from just five districts—Cumilla, Bramhmanbaria, Tangail, Dhaka, and Chattogram.

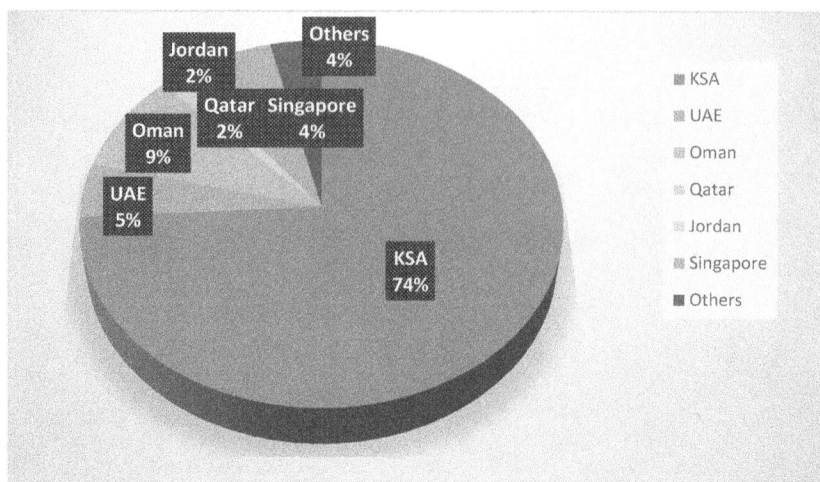

Figure 3.2 Overseas recruitment of migrant workers, 2021 (by country).

Source: Constructed by the author using BMET data (online).

Migrant workers from Bangladesh are usually recruited through short-term contracts and are predominantly male, with only 15% female in 2019. The average age of female workers is 27 years, and 94% of all workers are aged between 18 and 50 years. It is believed that a large number of female workers in the Middle East and Asian countries are undocumented (IOM, 2009). Between 1976 and 2019, on average, 46.5% of migrant workers were less skilled, 15.54% were semi-skilled, 35.54% were skilled,[3] and only about 1.84% were professionals (BMET, 2022).

COVID-19 and Bangladesh economy

Bangladesh identified its first COVID-19 case on 8 March, and the first COVID death was confirmed on 18 March 2020. Despite its inadequate healthcare facilities and emergency policies, lack of ICU beds and ventilators, and poor information and preparedness to deal with the disease, the government gradually started to put in place various measures to contain the spread of the virus and implemented the first nationwide lockdown between 26 and 30 May 2020. The number of cases was relatively low in March 2020 but increased rapidly from early April 2020 as international travellers continued to move in and out of the country. At the same time, around 11 million people, especially people working in the informal sector, left the capital city of Dhaka due to the fear of infection and the shutdown of economic activities.

The total number of infections increased from three on 8 March to 160,000 (with 2,000 deaths) by early July 2020. Then the country experienced its first 'wave' of coronavirus infections in August 2020. In Bangladesh, 55% of people infected were aged between 21 and 40 years, and 17% of infected people were over 50 years. In this older cohort, 71% of those infected were male. The death rate for infections over 50 years was 30% with 77% male and 23% female. It is interesting to note media reports that many high- and middle-income people in large cities in Bangladesh died from COVID-19 (BBC News/Bangla, 2020). The reason for this is not known conclusively; however, this could be because of a low rate of testing among low-income people or because pre-existing health conditions such as higher incidence of diabetes or high blood pressure/heart disease are less prevalent among younger, low-income people. It is also suspected that herd immunity developed relatively quickly among the population living in high-density slums in Bangladesh.

The spread of the COVID-19 pandemic severely disrupted socio-economic conditions in Bangladesh during 2020 and 2021. The country experienced a public health crisis, and economic demand and supply shock at the same time as domestic and international trade and financial activities declined rapidly during the first half of 2020. As the population of the country became more aware of the nature and the management of the virus, many city dwellers started wearing masks and maintaining personal hygiene to participate in social and economic activities.

As household income declined due to massive job losses in the informal sector, the number of people under the poverty line increased. Positive growth continued, but it was lower than it had been—growth in the industry and services sectors declined from 3.8% and 3.5%, respectively, in 2019 to 1.2% and 2.0% in 2020, although the agricultural sector remained constant. As a result, the national growth rate of GDP fell from 8% in 2019 to 3.4% in 2020 (World Bank Online 2022a). A BRAC[4] (2020) report suggested that the agricultural sector lost BDT565.4 million, equivalent to US$6.5 million, during the first lockdown of 45 days in 2020. The price of necessities increased rapidly due to supply chain disruption domestically and internationally. By 24 March, 650 million pieces of RMG orders, valued at US$3.18 billion, had been cancelled by foreign buyers. The RMG sector lost around 84% of its export earnings in April 2020 compared to 2019 as more than 1000 RMG factories closed down, and about 2.2 million workers lost their jobs (BGMEA, 2021).

After infections declined in November 2020, the daily cases of COVID-19 increased rapidly from March 2021, suggesting a second wave of coronavirus. As a consequence, another nationwide lockdown started in mid-April 2021, although this time the majority of public and private offices and businesses remained open. A stricter total lockdown of all public, private, and business was then imposed for a week between 1 and 7 July as new cases increased rapidly. Transportation movements at border areas were controlled to contain virus-carrying travellers moving to and from the neighbouring countries, especially from India, where COVID-19 incidence was high.

Bangladesh began a nationwide COVID-19 vaccination programme on 7 February 2021 with the first recipients being frontline health workers, government workers, police, teachers, and people above the age of 40 years. The vaccination programme is free. By 10 May 2021, about 6 million Bangladeshis had received at least one vaccine, and 3.9 million had received two doses of Oxford-Astra Zeneca Vaccine under the name CovidShield purchased from the Serum Institute of India (World Health Organization, 2021). India also gifted 1.2 million doses of the AstraZeneca vaccine to Bangladesh in March 2021 (Paul, 2021). However, India enacted a temporary freeze on its vaccine exports to Bangladesh as its COVID-19 cases went out of control by the end of May 2021. As a result, Bangladesh had to suspend its vaccination programme from late April 2021. Bangladesh approved three vaccines for emergency use—namely, China's BBIBP-CorV, Russian Sputnik V, and the Pfizer-BioNTech vaccine. By the end of June 2021, Bangladesh also approved the Moderna vaccine for the country (Khatun, 2021). The World Bank provided $500 million to support the vaccination rollout programme in March 2021, which helped the country to procure 15 million doses of Astra Zeneca in administering the vaccines (World Bank, 2022b).

Impact of COVID-19 on migrant workers

Over the last five decades, Bangladesh has benefited enormously from the increasing foreign exchange earnings sent by its migrant workers, and remittances have become a vital source of economic and development support. In recent years, an average of 700,000 workers are employed annually by overseas employers, however, the sudden breakout of COVID-19 brought massive disruption to this human resource exporting sector. As the coronavirus pandemic adversely affected global economic activities, the host countries' economies also slowed down in the first half of 2020. Shrinking economies and falling oil prices compelled the major Middle Eastern recruiting countries to reduce the demand for labour and lay off a large number of Bangladeshi migrant workers. However, the extent of job loss was associated with the sectors in which they were employed and with the overall economic condition of the host country. In the Gulf States, the retail and wholesale trade, hospitality and recreation, and manufacturing sectors were hit hard, and a large number of Bangladeshis lost their jobs. It was reported that about 666,000 registered workers were sent back home, and around two million undocumented workers faced possible deportation (TBS, 2020). Bangladeshi workers employed in the construction sector in various host countries before the pandemic lived in densely populated residences. There were 1.2 million workers alone in Saudi Arabia at risk of losing their employment. It was reported in various local media that the Bangladesh Embassies and High Commissions were informed by authorities of host states about the gloomy economic scenarios their countries were facing, and they asked Bangladesh to take its migrant workers back, especially the undocumented ones (UNDP, 2020). Many of these employing countries deported their less-skilled and semi-skilled unemployed, and undocumented, workers. Those who stayed in the destination countries were then subject to various difficulties, including long hours of forced work without proper payment, termination of allocated houses, lack of access to healthcare services, compromised occupational health and safety, food deprivation, and wage theft, as well as physical and sexual abuse (Sahai, at el., 2021). BRAC estimated that around 275,000 migrant workers returned to Bangladesh between February and September 2020 (Star Online Report, 2020).

The migrant workers, especially those who returned home from Italy, China, and other Middle Eastern countries, were blamed for bringing the virus into the country (Khan and Georgeou, 2021: 83–84). Returnee workers thus faced various economic and social discrimination in their home state—everything from unemployment, financial difficulties, a lack of social acceptance, problems in readjusting without any income, social stigma as carriers of the virus, denial of medical treatment, and a lack of proper and supportive quarantine or medical facilities. Different forms of discrimination have been compounded by the mental stresses of the migrant workers due to their uncertain prospects of future employment, and threats to their livelihoods. Migrant workers' families who had previously depended on remittances faced the highest risk and during the pandemic have been forced to spend less on basic necessities, like food, clothing, education, and healthcare (Khan and Georgeou, 2021). As international travel bans were imposed by many host countries, returned Bangladeshi migrant workers faced the prospect of losing their jobs, especially in the transport sector in the host countries (Chowdhury and Chakraborty, 2021). Most of the female returnee workers fell into a dire situation. Although BRAC tried to set up a catering service for female returnees from Saudi Arabia, it could not make it prosper due to the prolonged lockdown. A 2020 BRAC survey report indicated that about 87% of the respondents revealed that they lost their overseas employment and currently did not have any alternate source of income, 34% indicated that they had no savings; 74% stated that they were suffering from fear and a sense of uncertainty, extreme stress, and mental trauma; and 91% stated that they did not receive any support from the government or non-government organisations (BRAC, 2020; Chowdhury and Chakraborty, 2021).

Debt repayment during COVID-19 was another critical issue for returnee migrants. The majority of migrant workers from low-income families usually take loans to cover the initial migration cost. Returnee migrants, those who lost their jobs, could not service the interest on their debt and thus faced various social harassment. During the first phase of the pandemic, returnee migrants were not welcomed in the rural communities where job prospects were already low. Future job uncertainty and unemployment compelled some migrant households to engage in a distressed asset sale to pay for food, education, and healthcare for their children and repayment of debt (Chowdhury and Chakraborty, 2021).

Bangladeshis who stayed overseas were also affected by COVID. By July 2020, more than 70,000 Bangladeshi migrant workers had been infected in 186 countries, largely because they could not afford to maintain social distancing in congested, unhealthy, and unhygienic residences. By 2020 September, 53,795 migrant workers in Singapore were found to be COVID-positive, among them about 23,000 were Bangladeshi migrant workers. The incidence of COVID infections was however relatively low among female migrant workers. According to the BRAC Migration Program, COVID-19 had claimed the lives of around 2,700 Bangladeshi migrant workers by June 2020. The highest number of deaths (1,200 people) occurred in Saudi Arabia and only two in Singapore. Although the COVID treatment was free for both legal and undocumented workers in the Kingdom of Saudi Arabia and Singapore, a large number of undocumented migrant workers did not go for the treatment due to a lack of access to the information and fearing deportation (TBS, 2020).

International travel restrictions in various host countries affected the mobility of Bangladeshi workers. It was reported that between January and April 2020, some 400,000 workers returned home for different reasons, but they could not then return to their workplaces due to travel restrictions. The monthly overseas recruitment and commencement numbers started falling, from 69,988 people in January 2020 to 52,091 people in March 2020. Between April and June, there were no official employment records. However, from July 2020, workers started returning to their overseas jobs, and the number of returning employees rebounded from just 16 people in July to 28,398 people in December 2020 (BMET, 2022), but still well short of figures from earlier in the year.

Defying the negative forecasts of a massive decline in remittances, inflow to Bangladesh actually grew by 18.5% in 2020 compared to 2019 levels. During the height of the first phase of the pandemic, the inflow of remittances increased sharply from May to July 2020—after falling by 14% in April, remittances increased by 138% to US$2.6 million in July 2020. This surge in remittances at a time when overseas employment had virtually stopped can likely be explained by several factors: an intended increase in family support from those still working overseas; the two largest Muslim religious festivals, Eid-ul-Fitr in May and Eid-ul-Adha in July; and the repatriation of bank savings from host countries due to uncertainties relating to the global pandemic (Chowdhury and Chakraborty, 2021; BMET, 2022).

Government policies, support, and recovery

The macroeconomic picture shows economic activity was restored in the second half of 2021, which contributed to GDP growth of 6.9% in 2021. The economy getting back on track by the middle of 2021 was due to both public- and private-sector initiatives and support during the early phase of COVID-19, as well as effective and timely policy implementation. By the first half of 2021, effective dissemination of information about the management of the pandemic and public awareness and practices of personal hygiene, social distancing, and wearing a mask increased consumer confidence in the market. As a result, in 2021, both exports and imports had positive growth from the previous year, consumption increased by 5.7%, and investment by 2.6% (World Bank Online, 2022b).

Government stimulus packages and policies

The government of Bangladesh implemented various policies to combat the health and economic shocks created by the pandemic. To contain the rapid spread of the virus, the government decided to close all educational institutions from 23 March and imposed a nationwide first lockdown for two months, starting on 26 March 2020. Government organisations and the Ministry of Health started publishing the statistics of infected cases, testing, and deaths from the disease daily to alert and inform people about the severity of the disease. Public alertness and information about the nature and prevention of the disease were regularly posted on all media. Authorities also suspended all domestic air, water, and train travel from 24 March and restricted movement via public transport from 26 March 2020 (Kamruzzaman and Sakib, 2020).

The government announced seven economic stimulus packages in April 2020, costing a combined total of around US$11.5 billion. The Ministry of Finance allocated about US$667 million to fund the Preparedness and Response Plan, delegated to the Ministry of Health for buying, conservation, and distribution of vaccines. The prime minister of Bangladesh announced US$251 million under a housing scheme for the homeless and US$177 million to support vulnerable groups in the informal sectors, like day labourers, rickshaw pullers, and roadside vegetable vendors who lost their livelihood due to the lockdown (IMF, 2022). Under this programme, half a million tonnes of rice and 0.1 million tonnes of flour were distributed among the very low-income group, and to anyone who was in need. Authorities also sold rice in the open market at a fixed low price of BDT10 per kilo to support the poor. The Ministry of Finance pledged US$588 million to the export industries for paying the wages to four million workers over four months and US$11,472 million for the health insurance of the workers in the export-oriented industries (KPMG, 2020). Another US$105.2 million was allocated by the government in the second round of cash support to those who lost their jobs due to the lockdown. A further US$2.2 billion fiscal stimulus was disbursed from the US$4.6 billion which was initially pledged by the government of Bangladesh (IMF, 2022).

Bangladesh Bank, the central bank of Bangladesh, reduced the cash rate from 5% to 4% and relaxed the advances-to-deposit ratio from 83.5% to 87% to increase the amount of credit in the market. As a result, the country's broad money reserve growth also increased. Bangladesh Bank's foreign exchange intervention limits the appreciation of the domestic currency (the Bangladeshi Taka) to keep the exchange rate stable and support its export sectors (IMF, 2022).

Support provided to migrant workers

The government of Bangladesh has taken several measures to support migrant workers in host countries through various programmes. The government allocated a special budget of US$1.2 million to its overseas missions to support stranded migrant workers with food, emergency needs, and other facilities. Each migrant worker was given BDT500 (equivalent to US$67) at the airport upon arrival from the destination countries during the COVID-19 breakout. The government allocated US$27 million to provide medium- to long-run support in the form of a loan of between US$1,333 and US$6,667 at a 4% interest rate to the returnee migrants and their families (OHCHR, 2022). The government also announced a stimulus package of US$229.5 million to support the migrant workers, rural population, and unemployed youth during the crisis (Kumar and Pinky, 2020).

A total of US$85 million for returnee migrant workers was committed for soft loans, cash support, and skills training. To encourage the migrant workers to remit through formal channels, the government also allocated US$386 million to pay a 2% cashback payment to remit foreign earnings through government banks, which cost around US$361 million to the government. Many other financial institutions provided an additional 2% cash benefit while sending remittances through the formal banking system (Borgen Magazine, 2021). Probashi Kallyan Bank provided a loan of US$62.5 million at low rates to the migrant workers who lost their employment due to the pandemic (Chowdhury and Chakraborty, 2021).

Bangladesh Bank provided loans of up to US$6,250 to each deported worker's family. A one-off cash payment of US$3,750 was given to all migrant families, regardless of their visa status (Chowdhury and Chakraborty, 2021). The government instructed its Embassies and High Commissions to provide food support to migrant workers during the pandemic, especially in the Gulf countries and Southeast Asian countries, where most Bangladesh workers are employed. The Bangladesh government also provided financial support to the families of deceased migrant workers, as it usually provides financial support of BDT300,000 (US$4,000) to the family of a deceased migrant worker, and pays BDT35,000 (US$435) for bringing the dead body back to the country (Daily Bangladesh, 2019).

Support provided by local NGOs and international organisations

Besides the Bangladesh government, non-government organisations (NGOs) extended their support to affected communities through cash, loans, food, and health services. NGOs provided around US$1.8 billion in cash support between 5 and 25 May 2020 (Kumar and Pinky, 2020). Bidyanondo Foundation, a volunteer organisation, has been providing food support to a large number of people daily, and it set up a makeshift hospital in the port city of Chittagong and supplied 5,000 pieces of personal protective equipment (PPE) in the public hospital and hand sanitisers in the public transport to contain the spread of the disease. Gonoshashatho Kendra, a well-known Bangladeshi NGO, developed a COVID-19 rapid testing kit, which was claimed to be much cheaper and more effective than market competitors. Several other local

NGO and corporate groups, like Summit Group, Navana Group, Akij Group, Bashundhara Group, Beximco Pharmaceuticals, BRAC, and Green University, have all either donated support to the prime minister's funds, provided cash and in-kind support, medical equipment, or temporary hospital places to tackle the COVID-19 pandemic (BUILD Bangladesh, 2020; Kumar and Pinky, 2020). BRAC, the largest NGO in Bangladesh, delivered various cash grants and counselling support to 35,000 returnee migrant workers (Bergen Magazine, 2021).

Bangladesh economic recovery in Fiscal Year (FY) 2021

The extensive stimulus packages and accommodative macroeconomic and exchange rate policies and measures, along with the support from various international agencies, proved to be effective and successful in bringing back domestic demand and stabilising economic activity after the initial phase of the pandemic. As the global economy rebounded and the national vaccination programme started in January 2021, demand for migrant workers gradually increased. By this time, migrant workers were aware of the nature of the virus and of the need for management of personal hygiene and isolation when affected. So armed, they started to again go abroad for employment. The total number of migrant recruitments increased from 35,732 in January 2021 to 131,316 in December 2021. This figure represented a 184% increase in recruitment from 217,669 people in 2020 to 617,209 people in 2021. As a result, remittances sent by migrant workers in 2021 rebounded to US$24.8 billion. In the first four months of 2022, the recruitment of Bangladeshi workers has increased spectacularly to 426,558 people, 63% of whom are employed by the Kingdom of Saudi Arabia. The total remittance income recorded over the first four months of 2022 was US$7.1 billion (BMET, 2022).

   Various international organisations have been working closely with the local NGOs and supporting the returnee migrant workers to reintegrate during the COVID-pandemic. International Labour Organisation (ILO) provided technical support and shared knowledge of migrant workers' conditions to the government of Bangladesh for policy design and implementation. The Asian Development Bank set up a fund of US$650 million to support stranded Bangladeshi migrant workers financially in different host countries. The United Nations Development Programme (UNDP) provided various support services to migrant workers, including free cash and financial education, and it reduced the cost of sending remittances to source countries. Probash Bondhu, a Saudi telemedical service provided medical consultation to migrant workers. Saudi Arabia, Qatar, and the United Arab Emirates provided COVID-19 treatment irrespective of the visa status of the migrant workers. UNDP also took initiatives to minimise the stigma and discrimination toward migrant workers through a project called Digital Khichuri Challenge[5] (Borgen Magazine, 2021). To promote private investment and develop new software technology, the World Bank granted US$500 million to the Private Investment and Digital

Entrepreneurship (PRIDE) programme, a key objective of which was to combat COVID-19 in Bangladesh, in addition to creating 150,000 jobs. Another US$250 million was contributed by the World Bank to support the economic recovery of Bangladesh (Borgen Magazine, 2021).

Discussion and policy recommendations

The government of Bangladesh provided various methods of economic support to accelerate the country's recovery and to restore the livelihoods of the people, including for the returned migrant workers. Bangladesh's GDP grew 6.9% in 2021, supported by the rebound of major international trade sectors, as well as private-sector investment; the revival of domestic economic consumption and activity; and the implementation of government and international stimulus packages. Exports of RMG increased by 31%, and migrant worker recruitment more than doubled in the first eight months of the 2021–2022 fiscal year compared to the same period of the previous fiscal year.

Despite the concerted efforts by the national government to revive its economy and support its human resource sector to mitigate the effects of the pandemic, there remain various gaps in the implementation of supportive policies for migrant workers, especially in the areas of reintegrating returnee workers and creating opportunities to utilise their skills in the domestic economy (Sahai, et al., 2021). As reported by IMF (2022), by April 2021, 52% of fiscal stimulus had still not been disbursed. During 2022, the sudden and rapid surges in petroleum prices, the impact of the Russia-Ukraine war, and the uncertainty in the global economy have been fuelling price spirals in Bangladesh. The inflation rate increased to 6.2% in March 2022, one of the highest rates since October 2020. Several economists in Bangladesh differ with the published inflation rate of the Bangladesh Bureau of Statistics (BBS), citing rapid price increases for wheat, cooking oil, and food products since late 2021. Also, the value of Bangladesh's currency, the Taka, has depreciated in recent times. As Bangladesh is a food importer, this has led to increased prices for food items and has depleted foreign exchange reserves (The Financial Express, 2022; The Daily New Nation, 2022).

The Centre for Policy Dialogue has estimated that current inflation is around 12%, so rising prices are likely to continue into 2022 (The Daily New Nation). Returned migrant workers' families were already experiencing a drop in their purchasing power, but with inflation, a large number of people in the country are heading back towards the poverty line. The World Bank has projected that fuel prices will increase by 50%, and food prices may increase by 23%, as the wheat price has already increased by 40% in 2022, which is the highest since 2008 (World Bank, 2022b). The United Nations has warned of a food crisis and global famine due to the shortage of grain and fertiliser in the coming years, a result of the Russia-Ukraine war, which can make the Bangladeshi low-income group, including migrant workers' families even more vulnerable (The Guardian, 2022).

The gloomy and uncertain global economic outlook for Bangladesh may impact adversely on employment opportunities for migrant workers and therefore on the volume of remittances income in the coming years. Thus, current national policies should be cohesive and inclusive of the socio-economic and psychological needs of returned migrants, especially given their contribution to the economy both before and during the COVID-19 pandemic. In addition to the current pandemic support to the economy and especially to the migrant workers, the authorities should design and implement additional support measures. The policymakers should proactively prepare guidelines to deal with any socio-economic shocks and allocate a budget for the current and future global health and economic crisis, including the predicted food crisis. Priority healthcare services should be provided to migrant workers and returnees to increase their acceptance by the domestic and international markets as valuable labour assets. Furthermore, to address the current vulnerability of the major macroeconomic variables, the government must devise policies to mitigate prolonged adverse impacts on the wider economy, starting with rapidly increasing inflationary pressure and the projected food crisis. Government spending should be prioritised on health, education, training, and capacity-building areas while reducing foreign borrowing and debt levels with high-interest servicing.

Government should also emphasise supporting skill-building programmes and business development activities of the migrant workers, as their remittance incomes are crucial to supporting 60% of the daily expenses of migrant families.

The COVID-19 pandemic has created a demand for workers in various new areas, including the health services area, which can be availed by Bangladeshi semi-skilled and skilled workers given proper training and education. Authorities should fund demand-based training to prepare their human resources so as to supply the overseas market with workers with the skillsets required for recovery from the pandemic. Thus, Bangladesh should adjust its human resource policies and training to take advantage of job opportunities that have been created by the coronavirus pandemic in the health care, information technology (IT), domestic care, transport, and agricultural sectors. Increased training for lab technicians, other supplementary health service–related work, social care, training for light mechanics and transport, and IT and data-input-related training for an increasingly digital global economy.

With respect to migrant labour, the government has to make an effort to eliminate the bottlenecks in the recruitment process in the country, including administrative irregularities, corruption in the system, and the involvement of middlemen in taking advantage of low-skilled and less-educated potential workers by charging recruitment fees several times higher than the official rates, undocumented migration, female trafficking and abuse (including sexual abuse) in the disguise of overseas employment. Stricter implementation of these measures will reduce the cost of migration for overseas employment and increase the flow of remittances to the country.

Relevant authorities should create a comprehensive database and monitoring system to keep a record of the current and returnee migrant workers and to provide current recruitment information and training to them so that they can be ready to be deployed for any available opportunities. Government should design and implement the reintegration policy framework to utilise the skills of the returnee, especially for female returnee workers in the domestic hospitality sector. The private sector should be given incentives to recruit returnee migrants with advanced skills.

Following the success of the 2% cashback incentive scheme while remitting through official banking channels, the government has raised the cash incentive to 2.5% from January 2022. A safer and fast fund remittance transfer to the remittance recipients' households can be done via further simplified digitalisation of the remittance procedure for both the sender and the receiver. In this regard, funding the programmes to improve the financial literacy of migrant workers will increase the potential remittance flow officially to the country.

The government should design sustainable programmes aimed at the economic, psychological, and social support of migrant workers, based on an assessment of their long-term and short-term vulnerabilities. Bilateral cooperation between the home county and the host country and engaging in dialogues and negotiations to protect workers' rights, health, and safety, and providing them with clear and detailed job specifications, will be supportive in the expansion of the human resources trade between countries. It would be beneficial for both host and home countries to provide support and restore the employment of migrant workers during and after the pandemic, which would minimise the labour market gap in the host countries and provide valuable foreign exchange earnings to the home country.

Conclusion

A number of scholars and commentators have been highly critical of Bangladesh's slow response to the pandemic and the disorganised way that support was rolled out to different sectors (Siddiqui, 2021). Despite the slow responses and lack of preparedness by the government of Bangladesh at the onset of the COVID-19 pandemic in early 2020, various policy responses, along with support from international organisations, brought the economy back on track by mid-2021. Although the Health Ministry of Bangladesh was not fully aware of the extent of the virus like many other countries and could not deploy fully organised plans for the management of the disease, the government imposed a nationwide lockdown from late March 2020 for more than two months to contain the spread of the virus in the early stage. The government pledged a total of US$11.5 billion for the preparedness and fight against the virus, a vaccination programme, and support of vulnerable groups in the informal sector. Various other financial stimulus packages were provided to keep the economy active. The government of Bangladesh, along with NGOs and international organisations, provided considerable financial support, including soft loans, cash support, skill training, and mental health support to the returnee workers who were stranded in Bangladesh and became unemployed. The central bank, Bangladesh Bank, also encouraged the migrant workers to remit through the banking channels via the 2% cash back method, which was a reasonable cash support too.

As the vaccination programme started in early 2021 and the mobility of migrant workers increased, the remittance inflows started contributing positively to the rising economic indicators of the country.

Since COVID-19 has brought unprecedented health and economic shocks worldwide, it is not easy to mitigate the adverse effects in a country of 165 million people and 12 million migrant workers. There remain various administrative, operational, implementation, and budget-related issues and their consequences on the people, especially migrant workers. More support and stimulus packages need to be disbursed given the current Russian-Ukraine war, energy and food crisis, fast-rising inflation, and interest rates (World Bank, 2022c). Authorities need to proactively formulate a holistic policy for migrant human resources, including their mental health and psychological support, in order to secure valuable foreign exchange earnings to sustain the livelihood of a large group of low-income families and the overall economic welfare of the country.

Notes

1 South Asia consists of eight states: Afghanistan, Bangladesh, Bhutan, India, Maldives, Pakistan, Nepal, and Sri Lanka. The figures for South Asia in Table 3.1 are a regional average of all eight states.
2 Hundi or *hawala* (trust) is an old informal way of transferring money or settling accounts, believed to have originated in India. It involves communication between linked businesses so that one will accept money on behalf of a customer in one state, and the money will be passed to the family by a linked business in another. The hawala system bypasses banks, thus avoiding tax.
3 The 'skilled migrant workers' category includes doctors, engineers, and accountants who usually have the ability to work and apply their knowledge independently. The semi-skilled category includes workers who take some specific training before they go overseas for employment. Their skill level is based on their educational attainment of at least up to higher secondary level. The 'less skilled' category includes workers without specific skills, including construction workers, petty traders, cleaners, domestic workers, cooks, and people working in agricultural and light manufacturing sector, who learn skills by doing their jobs.
4 BRAC is the largest NGO in Bangladesh.
5 Digital Khichuri Challenge (DKC) is a competition for young creative Bangladeshi change makers who seek to promote peace and make the digital space more tolerant and safer by actively countering hateful narratives. The DKC started in 2016, organised by UNDP Bangladesh and supported by Facebook and ICT Division.

References

BBC News/Bangla. (2020, July 13). করোনা ভাইরাস: যমুনা গ্রুপের মালিক নুরুল ইসলাম বাবুল কোভিড-১৯ রোগে মারা গেছেন, https://www.bbc.com/bengali/news-53388379 (Viewed 30 March 2022).

BGMEA. (2021). 'The Apparel Story: COVID-19 and the RMG Industry', https://www.bgmea.com.bd/uploads/newsletters/apparel-story-january-february-2021.pdf.

BMET. (2022). 'Online, Overseas Employment and Remittances, 1976 to 2022', http://www.old.bmet.gov.bd/BMET/viewStatReport.action?reportnumber=24.

Borgen Magazine. (2021). 'COVID-19 Impacts on Bangladeshi Diaspora', https://www.borgenmagazine.com/covid-19-impacts-on-the-bangladeshi-diaspora/ (Viewed 4 April 2022).

BRAC. (2020). 'A Rapid Assessment Vulnerabilities of Agricultural Producers during COVID-19 Pandemic', http://www.brac.net/program/wp-content/uploads/2021/03/Report-A-rapid-assessment-Vulnerabilities-of-agricultural-producers-during-COVID-19-pandemic.pdf.

BUILD Bangladesh. (2020). 'COVID-19 Impact and Responses: Bangladesh', https://gsgii.org/wp-content/uploads/2020/05/Bangladesh-NAB_COVID-19-Impact-and-Responses_April-2020.pdf.

Chowdhury, M. B. (2011). 'Remittances Flow and Financial Development in Bangladesh'. *Economic Modelling*, 28, pp. 2600–2608.

Chowdhury, M. B. and Chakraborty, M. (2021). 'The Impact of Covid-19 on the Migrant Workers and Remittances Flow to Bangladesh'. *South Asian Survey*, 28(1), pp. 38–56, https://doi.org/10.1177/0971523121995365.

Chowdhury, M. B. and Chowdhury, K. (1991). 'Trade in Labour Services and Its Macroeconomic Effects on a Small Economy: Evidence from Bangladesh'. *Proceedings of the 14th International Symposium on Asian Studies*, 6, pp. 327–334.

Daily Bangladesh. (2019, September 27). 'Death in Abroad: Govt Donates Tk 3 Lakh to Families', https://www.daily-bangladesh.com/english/Death-in-abroad-Govt-donates-Tk-3-lakh-to-families/29113 (Viewed 30 April 2022).

IMF. (2022). 'Policy Responses to Covid-19', https://www.imf.org/en/Topics/imf-and-covid19/Policy-Responses-to-COVID-19#B.

IOM. (2009). 'IOM Backs Training for Bangladesh's Women Migrant Workers'. IOeM Press Briefing Notes, International Organisation for Migration, posted on Friday 07/08/2009, http://www.iom.nt/jahia/media/press-briefing-notes/pbnAS/.

Kamruzzaman, M. and Sakib, S. N. (2020). 'Bangladesh Imposes Total Lock-down Over COVID-19', https://www.aa.com.tr/en/asia-pacific/bangladesh-imposes-total-lockdown-over-covid-19/1778272 (Viewed 30 March 2022).

Khan, A. A. R. and Georgeou, N. (2021). 'Returned Migrant Workers: The Need for Psychosocial Support', in Eds. Titumir, R, Georgeou, N, and Chowdhury, A., *COVID-19 and Bangladesh: Response, Rights and Resilience*, University Press Ltd. Dhaka, Bangladesh. pp. 82–87.

Khatun, F. (2021). 'The COVID-19 Vaccination Agenda in Bangladesh: Increase Supply, Reduce Hesitancy', https://www.orfonline.org/research/covid-19-vaccination-agenda-in-bangladesh/ (Viewed 31 March 2022).

KPMG, (2020). 'Bangladesh Government Measures in Response to COVID-19', https://home.kpmg/xx/en/home/insights/2020/04/bangladesh-government-and-institution-measures-in-response-tocovid (Viewed 3 April 2022).

Kumar, B. and Pinky, S.D. (2020), 'Addressing Economic and Health Challenges of COVID-19 in Bangladesh: Preparation and Response'. *Journal of Public Affairs*, https://doi.org/10.1002/pa.2556.

Mahmud, S.A.S.M. (2012). *Determinants Behind the Use of Informal Channels for Remitting Money from Overseas by the Wage Earners of Bangladesh*, http://www.bankingandfinance.ait.asia/sites/default/files/report/report_sharifmahmud.pdf.

OEC. (2020). 'Bangladesh, Online', https://oec.world/en/profile/country/bgd#:~:text=The%20most%20common%20destination%20for,and%20Poland%20(%242.27B).

OHCHR. (2022). Contribution of Government of Bangladesh to UN Secretary General's Report under General Assembly Resolution, A/RES/74/148 on the Protection of migrants. Available at: https://www.ohchr.org/sites/default/files/Documents/Issues/Migration/GA76thSession/States/Bangladesh.pdf.

Our World in Data. (2022). 'Coronavirus (COVID-19), Vaccinations', https://ourworldindata.org/covid-vaccinations.

Paul, R. (2021, March 28). 'India's Modi Gifts Bangladesh 1.2 Million Doses of AsraZeneca Vaccine'. *Reuters*, https://www.reuters.com/article/us-health-coronavirus-india-bangladesh-idUSKBN2BJ0KC.

Sahai, R., Bansal, V., Sikder, M. J. U., and Kysia, K. (2021). 'Shattered Dreams: Bangladeshi Migrant Workers during a Global Pandemic'. *Journal of Modern Slavery*, 6(2), 106–132.

Siddiqui, T. (2021). *The Other Face of Globalisation: COVID-19, International Labour Migrants and Left-Behind Families in Bangladesh*, http://www.rmmru.org/newsite/wp-content/uploads/2021/04/The-Other-Face-of-Globalisation.pdf.

Star Online Report. (2020, September 9). 'Covid-19 Fallout: Number of Migrant Workers Returning to Bangladesh not 'Alarming', Says Minister'. *The Daily Star*, https://www.thedailystar.net/country/news/covid-19-fallout-number-migrant-workers-returningbangladesh-not-alarming-says-minister-1958513.

TBS (The Business Standard). (2020). '20 Lakh Bangladeshi Migrants May Face Deportation'. 10 July, www.tbsnews.net (Viewed 15 January 2021).

The Daily New Nation. (2022, May 17). 'Economists Differ with 6.22 Per cent Inflation Rate Rather It Is About 12 Per cent', https://thedailynewnation.com/news/322996/Economists-differ-with-6.22-per-cent-inflation-rate-rather-it-is-about-12-per-cent (Viewed 20 May 2022).

The Financial Express. (2022, May 9). 'Rising Inflation in Bangladesh', https://thefinancialexpress.com.bd/views/rising-inflation-in-bangladesh-1651934433 (Viewed 15 May 2022).

The Guardian. (2022, May 19). 'Ukraine Has Stoked Global Food Crisis That Could Last Years, Says UN'. | Ukraine | *The Guardian* (Viewed 3 June 2022).

UNDP (United Nations Development Programme). (2020). 'Covid-19: An Uncertain Homecoming for Bangladeshi Migrant Workers'. *UNDP Bangladesh*, www.bd.undp.org/content/bangladesh/en/home/stories/covid-19--an-uncertain-homecoming-for-bangladeshi-migrant-worker.html (Viewed 3 November 2020).

World Bank. (2006). *Global Economic Prospects: Economic Implications of Remittances and Migration*. World Bank, Washington.

World Bank. (2014). 'Migration and Remittances – Recent Developments and Outlook', *Migration and Development Brief 25*.

World Bank. (2022a). 'Bangladesh Development Update: Recovery and Resilience amid Global Uncertainty', https://thedocs.worldbank.org/en/doc/2a191d9c8a9de1a31c642cf3dfb00a74-0310062022/original/Bangladesh-Development-Update-Spring-2022.pdf.

World Bank. (2022b). *A Timely Response and Vaccination Program Help Bangladesh Contain the COVID-19 Pandemic*, https://www.worldbank.org/en/news/feature/2022/04/06/a-timely-response-and-vaccination-program-help-bangladesh-contain-the-covid-19-pandemic.

World Bank. (2022c). 'Food and Energy Price Shocks from Ukraine War Could Last for Years', https://www.worldbank.org/en/news/press-release/2022/04/26/food-and-energy-price-shocks-from-ukraine-war.

World Bank Online. (2022a). 'GDP Per Capita, PPP (Current international dollar) – Bangladesh', https://data.worldbank.org/indicator/NY.GDP.PCAP.PP.CD?locations=BD.

World Bank Online. (2022b). 'World Development Indicators', https://databank.worldbank.org/source/world-development-indicators.

World Health Organization. (2021). 'COVID-19 Vaccination: WHO Supports an Effective Campaign in Bangladesh while Strengthening Vaccine Roll-Out Preparedness for Rohingya', https://www.who.int/bangladesh/news/detail/20-05-2021-covid-19-vaccination-who-supports-an-effective-campaign-in-bangladesh-while-strengthening-vaccine-roll-out-preparedness-for-rohingya.

4 Japan
Moralised politics in countering COVID-19

Yukiko Nishikawa

Introduction

Between January 2020–January 2022, the Japanese government declared a coronavirus 'state of emergency' on four occasions, either nationwide or in particular areas of the country. Importantly, since 2020, the Japanese government has relied on ordinary legislation without exercising emergency powers such as applying martial law or suspending civil law. In this 'rule-of-law' context, the number of COVID-19 infections in Japan remained comparatively low, particularly in 2020, before the government amended laws to include tighter measures to prevent the spread of the virus. During 2020, many journalists described Japan's low number of cases and lack of strict measures as a 'puzzling mystery' or as a "mysterious pandemic success" story (Sturmer and Asada 2020; Sposato 2020). The remarkable speed of vaccination and the high percentage of the population that was inoculated by late 2021, despite the slow start of the vaccination campaign, may also be perceived as another 'mysterious success' for Japan.

This chapter explores the first two years of the pandemic in Japan and explains how and why Japan was able to achieve this 'mysterious success' compared to other states. Understanding Japan's "mysterious pandemic success" reveals an interesting combination of law and politics that shapes a pragmatic rule-of-law system, as well as a 'moralised politics' (Tushnet 2008) that has functioned both to enforce the state's policies and to contain state power during the coronavirus emergency situation in Japan.

Japan's response to COVID-19

Japan's experience with the COVID-19 pandemic has been mild in terms of the number of infected people and deaths, despite the country's high population density and 'super-aged society'.[1] During the first two years of the pandemic, between January 2020- January 2022, Japan had, on average, the lowest death rate per million from COVID-19 among the Group of Seven (G7) countries,[2] and, as Figure 4.1 shows, by late December 2021, Japan had fewer cases of COVID-19 per million population than its G7 peers and some other sizeable economies.

DOI: 10.4324/9781003311522-4

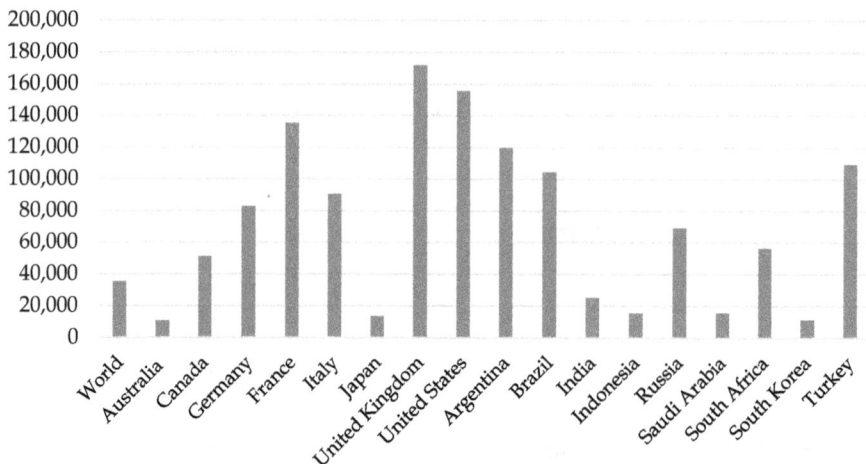

Figure 4.1 Graph showing COVID-19 cases per one million population at 22 December 2021.

Data Source: ECDC, John Hopkins University.

The overall number of infected people in Japan significantly increased in early 2022 owing to the new COVID-19 Omicron variant. Despite this, Japan's total infection rate remained lower than its G7 peers.

Since the first COVID-19 case was discovered in Japan on 16 January 2020, the country has experienced six waves of outbreak measured by the number of infected people in the country between January 2020 and February 2022, although the first two waves were relatively small (see Figure 4.2).

Similarly, deaths from COVID-19 closely followed the waves of infected persons as seen in Figure 4.3.

Throughout 2020 and 2021, the Japanese media regularly reported the daily number of infected people and deaths. Accordingly, people were aware of the pandemic, which often generated overt fear in the population and sometimes resulted in excessive reactions towards those who refused to take preventive measures.

During the period under consideration, a major international sporting event was held in Tokyo—the Games of the XXXII Olympiad (hereinafter 'the Olympics')—which had been due to take place in July/August 2020, however, due to the COVID pandemic, were eventually held in July/August 2021, during which time Tokyo was under a coronavirus 'state of emergency'. Also, between January 2020 and January 2022, the usually politically staid Japan had three prime ministers. Shinzo Abe, who led the Liberal Democratic Party (LDP) in government from September 2012 to September 2020, resigned suddenly and was succeeded by Yoshihide Suga, elected by the LDP to replace Abe as prime minister. Suga served as prime minister for just over a year (September 2020–October 2021) before he too resigned and was then replaced by the LDP's Fumio Kishida, who since October 2021 has served as prime minister of Japan.

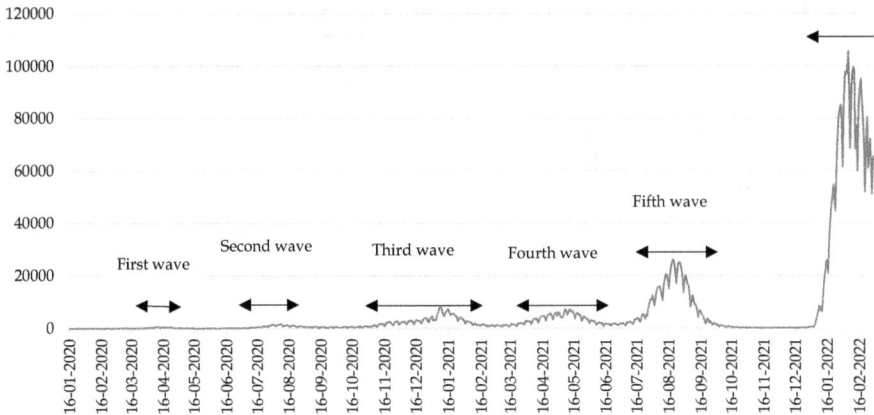

Figure 4.2 Graph showing the number of COVID-19-infected persons (January 2020–February 2022).

Data source: NHK (Japan Broadcasting Corporation) https://nhk3.or.jp/news/special/coronavirus/data-all (accessed on 2 March 2022).

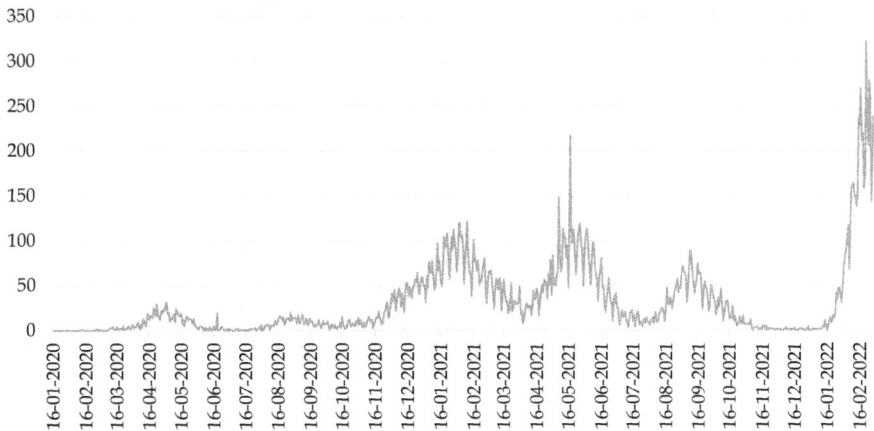

Figure 4.3 Graph showing number of deaths per day (January 2020–February 2022).

Data source: NHK Broadcasting Corporation https://www3.nhk.or.jp/news/special/cpronavirus/data-all (accessed on 2 March 2022).

The government took various economic measures to support economic recovery, jobs, and businesses throughout the years 2020–2021.[3] For example, it announced a package of 'Emergency Economic Measures to Cope with COVID-19' as large as ¥117.1 trillion (equivalent to US$899.73 billion) on 7 April 2020 (see Table 4.1).[4]

Table 4.1 Total expenses of emergency measures (20 April 2020)

	Area of support	Expenses (trillion yen)
I	Measures to prevent the spread of infection, build medical treatment structures, and develop pharmaceuticals	2.5
II	Protecting employment and keeping business viable	88.8
III	Recovery of economic activities as a next phase through public and private cooperation	8.5
IV	Making economic structure resilient	15.7
V	Preparing for the future (establishment of new contingency fund)	1.5
Total		**117.1**

Source: The Cabinet Office (Economic Measures). Available online in Japanese/English. https://www5.cao.go.jp/keizai1/keizaitaisaku/2020/20200420_economic_measures.pdf (2 May 2022).

Table 4.2 Economic stimulus package (8 December 2020)

Pillar	Area of support	Fiscal expense (trillion yen)	Projects (trillion yen)
I	Containment measures for COVID-19	5.9	6
II	Promoting structural change and positive economic cycles for the post-corona era	18.4	51.7
III	Securing safety and relief with respect to disaster management	5.6	5.9
VI	Proper and timely implementation of the reserve fund	10	10
Total		**40**	**73.6**

Source: The Cabinet Office (Economic Measures). Available online in Japanese/English. https://www5.cao.go.jp/keizai1/keizaitaisaku/2020-2/20201208_economic_measures.pdf (2 May 2022).

In December 2020, the cabinet also decided to commit a further ¥113.6 trillion to a series of economic stimulus packages titled the 'Comprehensive Economic Measures to Secure People's Lives and Livelihoods towards Relief and Hope' (see Table 4.2).

These are merely some of the economic measures Japan's government undertook as it confronted the pandemic. Indeed, during the year 2020, the government revised its planned budget spending three times. Much of the revised spending was to take necessary anti-COVID-19 measures, including support for medical institutions and business owners, COVID-19 testing, and loans for small- and medium-sized businesses. It also used the largest amount of money from the national contingency fund (*yobihi*, 予備費) in the year, amounting to about ¥10 trillion, which is a far larger amount than the annual spending from the contingency fund over the last ten years.[5] The spending from the contingency fund was for the cost related to anti-COVID-19 measures. A similar tendency was observed in the budget year 2021.

Legal basis and administrative organisation to counter COVID-19

The government's basic policies for novel coronavirus disease control released in March 2020 identified the following three objectives: (1) slow down the speed of infection by containing clusters and reducing chances of contact; (2) minimise the incidence of severe cases and death through surveillance and appropriate medical care, especially for the elderly; and (3) minimise the impact on society and economy through pandemic prevention and economic and employment measures.[6] Many policies and a legal framework were introduced in March 2020 during the first wave, when the number of people infected started to increase. The then prime minister Shinzo Abe called on schools nationwide to temporarily close from 2 March, while his government enacted the Revised Act on Special Measures for Pandemic Influenza and New Infectious Diseases Preparedness and Response (Law No. 31, 2012)—新型インフルエンザ等特別措置法 (*Shingata Infuruenza tou Tokubetsu Sochihō*) (hereinafter the 'Special Measures Act' as commonly called in Japan)—on 14 March, which provided the principal legal basis for anti-COVID measures in Japan.[7] The Special Measures Act enables the government to declare a state of emergency when an infectious disease is designated as a pandemic. It also allows a prefectural governor to 'request' (*yousei*, 要請) business owners to restrict/suspend the use of their facilities or the holding of events. Such a 'request' has a legislative basis but is not a legal obligation. The Act then stipulates that if the business owner refuses to fulfil such a request without good reason, the governor can 'instruct' (*shiji*, 指示) measures to be taken concerning the request (Article 45-3).[8] As soon as such a request and instruction are made, the governor 'must' announce it publicly (*kōhyō*, 公表) (Article 45-4).[9] Nevertheless, if a governor's instruction is ignored, no penalty is imposed, even though certain detrimental economic effects may be expected by publicising the name of a business. In other words, under the Special Measures Act, prefectural governors can take preventive measures on a 'request' basis, but they cannot issue 'orders' that incur a punishment.

While the first wave 'peaked' on 18 April, the Special Measures Act stayed in effect until January 2021 and was then extended until January 2022.[10] It was amended to enable the government to take necessary countermeasures without having a specific date of expiration and also to include stricter measures, including such things as penalties for non-compliance, which were enacted on 13 February 2021.

Administratively, the government set up the Novel Coronavirus Response Headquarters (NCRH)—新型コロナウイルス感染症対策本部 (*Shingata*

Coronavirus Kansenshou Taisaku Honbu)—headed by the prime minister, which is the highest authority to respond to COVID-19 (see Figure 4.4). The NCRH has its legal basis in Article 15 of the Special Measures Act.

The NCRH is where the basic policies to prevent the spread of COVID-19 and measures to counter it are discussed, and where the government's basic action policy is devised. In so doing, inputs were required from the Expert Meeting on Novel Coronavirus Disease Control (hereinafter the Expert Meeting)—新型コロナウイルス対策専門家会議 (*Shingata Coronavirus Kansenshou Taisaku Senmonka Kaigi*)[11]—a group that provides the prime minister and cabinet with medical opinions and perspective relating to the virus and what it deems necessary countermeasures. The Expert Meeting was comprised of medical experts and academics with expertise on, for example, infectious diseases and public health. Initially, it was established under the NCRH, but in July 2020, it was replaced with the Subcommittee on Novel Coronavirus Disease Control in order to better situate the Expert Meeting within existing laws and also to include experts from wider fields, such as risk communication and representatives from the municipal government.[12] The existing laws are to counter 'pandemic influenza and new infectious diseases' and thus are not always applicable to the newly established bodies to counter 'novel coronavirus'. Local governments and/or prefectural governors are responsible for implementing various countermeasures based on the basic action policy, in cooperation with municipal governments and public health centres.

A slow and cautious start in 2020

The Japanese government's initial reaction to COVID-19 cases was not so swift. There are, at least, three possible reasons why. The first and second reasons are closely intertwined. First, the Abe government maintained its intention to hold the 2020 Tokyo Olympic and Paralympic Games in July and August of 2020, and this remained one of the government's policy priorities until the decision by the International Olympic Committee (IOC) to delay the Olympics by 12 months, or until at least March 2021. Even though some countries decided not to send their national team or athletes to the Games, and two-thirds of Japanese nationals hoped that the Olympics would be postponed, Prime Minister Abe did not want to cancel the event. The most reported reason in the Japanese media for Abe's reluctance to cancel the Olympics was that cancellation would significantly affect Japan's already gloomy economic prospects,[13] while postponing the Olympics left a glimmer of hope for a rebound in tourism. Yet, many analysts speculated Abe's reluctance to cancel had more to do with his personal aspiration (Kingston 2020: 7; Izumi 2020); for if the Olympics were cancelled, Abe's leadership would have been questioned. He was expecting to be Japan's longest-serving prime minister by August 2020, and the LDP's presidential election was due in September 2021.[14] Prime Minister Abe's personal ambition to leave a positive legacy at the end of his premiership, or to hang on for another term by

Ministerial Meeting for Pandemic Influenza and New Infectious Diseases
新型インフルエンザ等対策閣僚会議

Members: All Ministers
Convened by the Prime Minister

Expert Meeting for Pandemic Influenza and New Infectious Diseases
新型インフルエンザ等対策有識者会議

Advisory Committee on the Basic Action Policy

Council for the Promotion of Countermeasures against Novel Influenza and Other Diseases

Subcommittee on Basic Action Policy
基本的対処方針分科会

Subcommittee on Medical and Public Health
医療・公衆衛生に関する分科会

Subcommittee on Social Function
社会機能に関する分科会

Subcommittee on Novel Coronavirus Disease Control (July 2020~)
新型コロナウイルス感染症対策分科会

Cabinet Office

Cabinet Secretariat

Prefectural Response Headquarters
都道府県 対策本部

Municipal Response Headquarters
市町村 対策本部

Set up the headquarters when necessary

Consultation

Opinion

Cabinet

Replaced (July 2020)

Novel Coronavirus Response Headquarters
新型コロナウイルス感染症対策本部

Head: Prime Minister (PM)
Vice Head 1: Chief Cabinet Secretary
Vice Head 2: Minister of Health, Labour and Welfare

Expert Meeting on Novel Coronavirus Disease Control (the Expert Meeting)
新型コロナウイルス感染症等対策専門家会議
PM appoints the members.

Abolished

Advice

Advice

Novel Coronavirus Response Advisory Board (predecessor of the Expert Meeting till Feb 2020.
Restart from July 2020)

Ministry of Health, Labour and Welfare (MHLW)

Prefecture Public Health Centers/Health Bureau
都道府県 保健衛生部・保健所

Municipal Health Centers 市町村 保健センター

Ordinance-Designated Cities
Health Bureau/ Public Health Centers

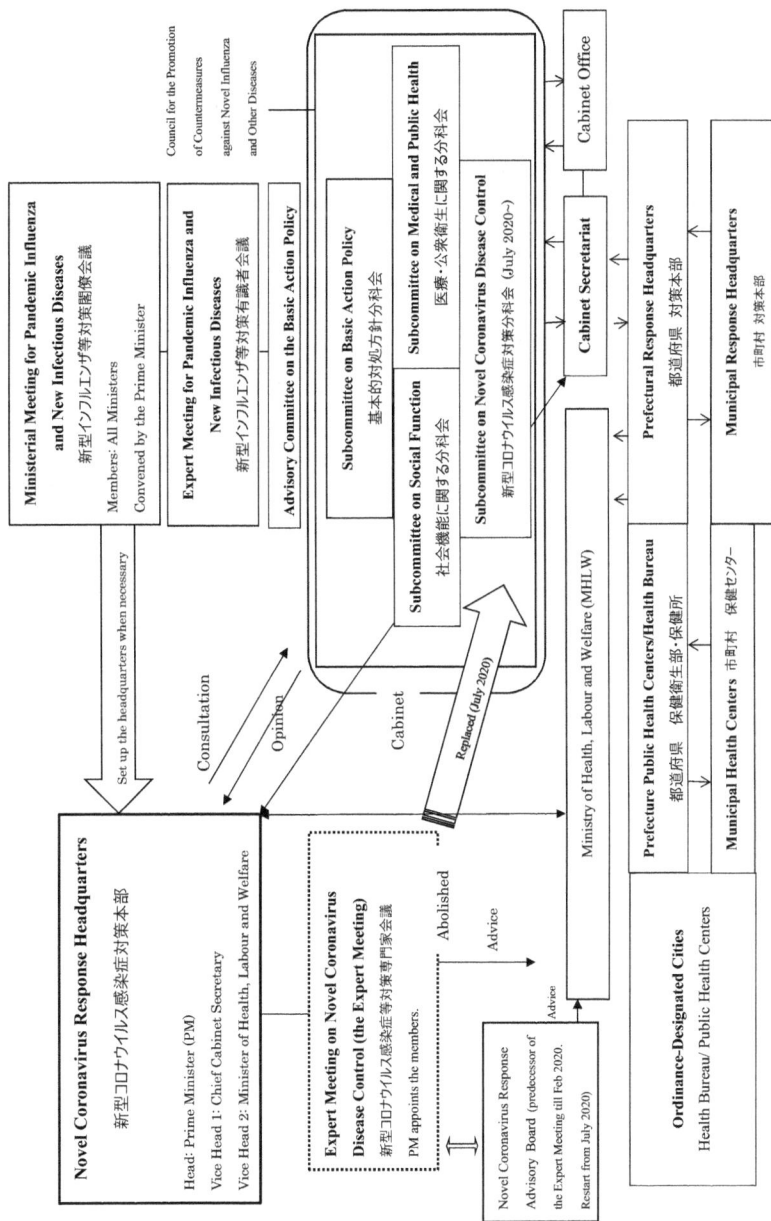

Figure 4.4 Organisational chart for novel coronavirus response in Japan.

Data source: Created by the author based on the information on the following websites: Ministry of Health, Labour and Welfare, (2020), Cabinet Office and Cabinet Secretariat.

changing the party's rules, was a likely factor.[15] Accordingly, until the postponement was officially announced in late March 2020, the government downplayed the risks of coronavirus in an abortive attempt to save the Olympics.

Second, measures to counter COVID-19 have had a significant impact on Japan's economy and its businesses. The Abe government's policy priority had been the revitalisation of the Japanese economy after two decades of deflation. 'Abenomics' is a portmanteau of 'Abe' (the then prime minister's surname) and 'economics', and the main tenets of Abenomics are an aggressive monetary policy, flexible fiscal policy, and a growth strategy. The Abe government was concerned with how the measures designed to prevent the spread of COVID-19, such as restrictions on movement or hours of operation for businesses, would affect the economy. The government, thus, did not declare a state of emergency until early April.

Abe's government indeed pledged an economic stimulus package as large as 20% of economic output to battle the deepening economic fallout from the coronavirus. This decision came in very late March 2020, around the same time that the government decided to postpone the Olympics.[16] The scale of the economic stimulus packages illustrates the extent to which the government prioritised the country's economy in facing COVID-19. Abenomics was closely tied with Abe's political fate, as the LDP has close ties with Japanese companies and the business community (*zaikai*), as evidenced by the receipt of business donations and formal recommendations to relevant ministries and agencies, the dispatching of executive officials to advisory councils and the policy coordination between secretariats of business federations and relevant ministries through informal contacts (Yoshimatsu 1997: 123–126).[17] Holding the Olympics was inseparable from the LDP's goal of economic revitalisation because inbound tourism would provide much-needed economic stimulus for the country beyond 2020. The Abe government's delay of the first emergency declaration was said to be due to his anxiety about the expected impact on the country's economy and business, which was closely linked with the fate of the Abe government.

Third, unlike neighbouring countries South Korea and China, which suffered outbreaks of Severe Acute Respiratory Syndrome (SARS) in 2003 and Middle East Respiratory Syndrome (MERS) in 2012, Japan had little experience in countering epidemics and thus was not well-prepared for the novel coronavirus pandemic (Moon et al., 2021: 661). In fact, the government had to review its laws and made a series of decisions on the legal and administrative structures required to counter COVID-19. It relied on a restrained approach in its early stage of countering COVID-19, such as a 16 January 2020 press release asking people who had some apparent symptoms, for example, fever and coughing, to visit a medical institution (Ministry of Health, Labor and Welfare, 2020). In contrast, South Korea, which had experienced epidemics, already had established independent national agencies that played an autonomous role in handling infectious diseases and took a more proactive approach to testing and treatment (Moon et al., 2021).

During the early stage of the pandemic in 2020, the public was dissatisfied with the Abe government's handling of the virus, largely because of limited testing, poor handling of the coronavirus-stricken cruise ship *Diamond Princess*[18] (which quarantined in the port of Yokohama in February), and its hesitation to impose a state of emergency at either the provincial or national level. The Abe government finally declared a state of emergency in seven prefectures on 7 April 2020 and eventually nationwide on 16 April,[19] which was the first coronavirus state of emergency in the country. Coming three months after the first case of COVID-19 in Japan, and almost a month after the World Health Organization declared the novel coronavirus a global pandemic, many Japanese considered that the government's declaration of a nationwide emergency was "too little too late".[20]

Tighter COVID-19 measures in 2021

Under the Suga administration (September 2020–October 2021), a state of emergency was declared for three consecutive periods in 2021 (January–March, April–June, and July–August) with measures that were stricter than those adopted during the first state of emergency. From early 2021, there were more COVID-19 cases, and Japan experienced the third, fourth, and fifth waves of the outbreak (see Figure 4.2). With the worsening situation, the Special Measures Act was partially amended and came into effect on 13 February 2021 (Act No.5, 2021). The amendment was made for four reasons: (1) to establish new measures entitled 'Area-Focused Intensive Measures for Prevention of the Spread of Infection' for a more targeted and phased approach in specific areas to prevent a nationwide spread, (2) to efficiently support affected business owners, (3) to classify novel coronavirus infectious diseases as 'novel influenza infectious diseases' under the Infectious Disease Act, and (4) to establish legal grounds for making requests for home-based and accommodation-based recovery.[21]

One point that drew the media and public attention concerning the amendment was Article 45. The amended Special Measures Act enables prefectural governors to 'order' (*meirei*, 命令), rather than instruct, and noted they 'may', rather than 'must', publicly announce that cooperation has been requested (Article 45-4 and 5). Also, in cases during a state of emergency where business owners did not comply with a prefectural governor's request and order to suspend the use of their facilities (i.e. administrative order violations), the governor could charge a non-penal fine of up to 300,000 yen (equivalent to US$2,305); however, this would be only 200,000 yen during normal times (see Table 4.3).[22]

Similarly, in case someone refuses to be hospitalised without a justifiable reason or runs away from hospital, a non-penal fine of up to 500,000 yen will be charged (Article 80 of the Infectious Diseases Control Law).[23] Nevertheless, the overall penalties for non-compliance in Japan are modest compared to those implemented in other countries.

Table 4.3 Partial amendments made in the Special Measures Acts (before and after)

	Before amendment	After amendment
No State of Emergency	Article 14-31 Article 24-1: prefectural headquarters can make comprehensive coordination Article 31: prefectural governor can request to provide medical care	Prefectural governor can: • request to change facilities' business hours • order and make a public announcements • charge non-penal fines up to 200,000 yen in cases of violation Article 31 (new): establishes measures entitled 'Area-Focused Intensive Measures for Prevention of the Spread of Infection' to enable the government to take a more targeted and phased approach in specific areas Article 63(2) (new): The government and municipalities shall provide necessary support in financial and other aspects to mitigate the impact on business management and the people's lives
In a State of Emergency	Article 32: Declaration of a State of Emergency Article 45(1): prefectural governor can request for cooperation Article 45(3): prefectural governor can 'instruct' business owners who refuse to meet a request without good reason	Article 32: Declaration of a State of Emergency Article 45(1): prefectural governor can request for cooperation Article 45(3): prefectural governor can 'order' business owners who refused to meet a request without good reason → In case of violation, non-penal fine of up to 300,000 yen

Article 45(4): instruction 'must' be made public

Article 45(4) (new): prefectural governor requires obtaining opinions from experts in advance when making an assessment for request or order
Article 45(5): Whenever the governor requests or orders, such a fact 'may' be publicly announced

Source: The Special Measures Act: Comparison before and after released by the Constitutional Democratic Party of Japan. Originally in Japanese. Note: The author extracted only relevant points of amendments for this chapter.

Other major points of amendment include, among others, stipulating the government's responsibility to provide necessary financial and other support to affected business owners, defining the responsibility of national and prefectural governments to prevent discrimination against patients and medical staff, and providing statutory status for the Council for the Promotion of Countermeasures against Novel Influenza and Other Diseases under the cabinet.[24] This move reflected the prolonged pandemic situation, which in mid-2022 still seriously affected business owners, and the increasing number of COVID-19 cases, which had by then exceeded the capacity of medical institutions and national health centres.

Between July and August 2021 when COVID-19 cases peaked, Japan was in a coronavirus state of emergency. Japan hosted the Olympics even though many Japanese people still had not had their first vaccination. The Suga cabinet was widely criticised by people who were frustrated about being unable to receive vaccination and for its general mishandling of the COVID-19 pandemic. By 9 May 2021, just 2.59% of the Japanese population had received at least their first vaccination, a figure that compared poorly to the 52.25% of people vaccinated at least once in the United Kingdom (Eiraku and Aizawa 2021). Public disapproval of the measures enacted to counter COVID-19 mirrored the gradually decreasing political support for Suga and his government, even though his political party, the LDP, maintained public support (Mizorogi 2021). The decreasing support for Suga's government dated from before the Olympics began in July 2021, mainly from street protests outside the National Stadium in Tokyo, where the opening ceremony was to be held, protests that demanded the Olympics be cancelled.[25] In fact, in a survey conducted by *Asahi Shinbun* or *Asahi Newspaper* released on 17 May 2021, a total of 83% of those polled said that they did not want Tokyo to hold the Olympic Games.[26]

Government's appeals for preventive measures and voluntary restraint (*Jishuku*, 自粛)

The Japanese government relied heavily on citizens' self-restraint or voluntary restraint to prevent the spread of the coronavirus. The government or government officials vigorously promoted three main actions or policies as preventive measures, and advised voluntary restraint to protect oneself and others, particularly for those over the age of 65 with chronic disease. The public extensively shared information and appeals through traditional and social media. One of the important campaigns launched by Japanese officials was to "Avoid the Three Cs" (*san-mitsu* or *mittsu no mitsu*, 三蜜 or 三つの蜜): (1) crowded places with many people nearby, (2) closed spaces with poor ventilation, and (3) close-contact settings, such as close-range conversations.[27] The public health and sanitation campaign was transmitted through government speeches and public service announcement campaigns, as well as flyers and posters made by the Prime Minister's Office and the Ministry of Health, Labour and

Welfare. In fact, the planned national budget allocation for public relations expenses for the budget year 2020 doubled compared with that of previous years, and thus there was a fierce debate between the ruling and opposition parties during the budgetary discussion in the National Diet (The House of Representatives 2020).[28] The actual spending for the budget year 2020 re-leased by the Ministry of Finance shows that the government spent a total of 5 billion yen (equivalent to US$38.4 million) from the contingency fund for strengthening counter-COVID-19 public relations.[29] Notably, the seriousness of the pandemic along with the message "Avoid the Three Cs" was shared nationwide, but only after the decision to postpone the Olympics had been publicly announced.

Second, the government emphasised the importance of wearing a mask to prevent the spread of the virus.[30] A team at the Massachusetts Institute of Technology (United States) revealed that Japan's rate of mask wearing was more than 95% (Lu et al. 2021).[31] This high rate was achieved without any legal measure put in place providing for fines or sanctions for non-compliance. The high rate of mask wearing is in part because of the Japanese custom of wearing masks—a practice that long preceded the COVID-19 pandemic—during illness or allergy season, and Japanese people frequently wear a mask as a common method to protect themselves and others from infection.

Third, the Japanese government also appealed to people to reduce the ex-tent of their physical contact by 80%.[32] The idea was suggested by a theoretical epidemiologist who made a mathematical estimation that a sharp decline in the number of infected people would be seen after two weeks if the 80% reduc-tion had been achieved. A health expert defined close 'contact' as being within "a distance where people can touch each other if they extend their arms; more specifically, having someone within two meters of you".[33] Companies also at-tempted to achieve an 80% decrease in their staff social contacts. Notably, a study conducted by Japanese scholars revealed a more than 70% reduction in social contact in Tokyo following the government's message (Yabe et al. 2020: 5–6).[34] The study shows that voluntary restraint (*jishuku*, 自粛) worked in Tokyo to a certain extent; however, even before late March 2020, many peo-ple had started reducing their physical contact (by around 40%) when the number of cases of COVID-19 from abroad had started to increase (Yabe et al. 2020: 6).

There were other government policies, such as encouraging telework (or remote work),[35] and the various economic stimulus measures, touted as the country's "biggest-ever stimulus package", and employment-related measures. All of these policies may have contributed to low infection rates; however, vac-cination is thought to have been one of the most important factors in the significant reduction in COVID-19 cases and deaths that occurred in the fifth wave of the outbreak after October 2021.[36] Despite the initial slow start, the pace of vaccinations quickened with Prime Minister Suga's goal of "one mil-lion doses administered per day". This goal was indeed realised by June 2021 (Jackman 2021). Eventually, more than 70% of the population was fully vaccinated against COVID-19 by October 2021. Among people over 80 years old, the rate of double vaccination reached 95%, the highest among the G7 countries.[37] Most Japanese voluntarily vaccinated. Unlike some other countries, one's vaccination status did not become a political question in Japan, nor was vaccination viewed as a trade-off against individual rights and freedoms. This is largely because the government did not make vaccination mandatory. The people were vaccinated at their own discretion for fear of being infected or of passing the infection on to others, particularly to aged people. While Japan was similar to other countries in that there were anti-vaccination demonstrations and calls against mask use in many places, particularly in major cities like Tokyo and Osaka (Manabe 2022), people could decide to be vaccinated, use masks, or stay at home at their own discretion.

Political and social practice that filled the legal vacuum

As Japanese responses to COVID-19 were often characterised by self-restraint, the presence of emergency powers was barely perceptible over the first two years of the pandemic. This is largely because in the Constitution of Japan and other laws of the country, there is no legal provision that stipulates emergency powers.[38] Japan's post-war Constitution was drafted during the occupation period, and it does not stipulate any emergency powers, so as to deny excessive power to the state. The Japanese legal system has emerged as a historical amalgam of contradictory indigenous and foreign influences, mixing Anglo-American ideas and French/German legal traditions (Nishikawa 2020). Nevertheless, why Japan's measures were less strict in law and practice than those in many other countries cannot be explained merely by the absence of legal provisions concerning emergency powers.

Among government officials and citizens, since 1945, there has been a tendency to avoid granting excessive power to the executive, mainly because of Japan's wartime experience where centralised government resulted in dictatorship. For Japanese citizens, Japanese socio-political practice tends to collectively enforce certain policies and decisions; in effect, socio-cultural practice provides majority support in an extra-legal manner and strengthens executive power. Both political and social tendencies seem to have worked together to prevent an unnecessary legal or constitutional strengthening of the power of authorities, even while Japan experienced the COVID-19 emergency situation. Paradoxically this socio-political tendency helped constrain executive power among Japan's political leaders at the same time as it enhanced citizen compliance with the government's policies during the coronavirus emergency situation.

Historical legacies and continuing post-War politics

Japanese politicians and political leaders have divided views on the COVID emergency powers, a legal instrument not stipulated in the Constitution of Japan (Nishikawa 2020). The foundational and key principles of the

Constitution of Japan were laid out by the General Headquarters (GHQ) led by the supreme commander for the Allied Powers during the occupation period after World War II and enacted in 1947. The Japanese Constitution is grounded in the rule of law, and it establishes the notion that government power will be bound by the "will of the people" (Urabe 1990: 64). It also entails the perpetuity and inviolability of fundamental human rights (Article 97), the status of the Constitution as the supreme law (Article 98), the establishment of the system of judicial review (Article 81), and due process (Article 31). Nevertheless, at the most fundamental level, the legitimacy of the Constitution is still debated, primarily whether it is a 'Japanese' constitution or a constitution imposed by the occupying powers. For this reason, views and interpretations on different points of the Constitution do not involve a simple dichotomy. Instead, various opinions exist around different issues that divide politicians, political leaders, and legal experts, as well as citizens.

Whether or not a Japanese government can actually exercise emergency powers is one of the issues for which no single interpretation exists (Nishikawa 2020). All parties agree that Japan's pre-war and wartime experience, particularly the government's oppression of democratic movements before and during World War II,[39] should not be repeated. Many are cautious about any tendency that gives excessive power to the executive, and generally, politicians are aware that any political movement that attempts to amend the constitution, in general, and strengthen executive power, in particular, divides the nation and leads to a loss of public support for their party or regime (Nishikawa 2018: 115–131). Reflecting such political considerations among Japanese politicians, a supplementary resolution was attached when the Special Measures Act was amended. This resolution stipulates that citizens' rights and freedoms should not be unfairly infringed even when the amended Special Measures Act is applied, particularly when imposing penalties.[40]

Prime Minister Fumio Kishida may have thus been concerned that giving excessive power to the executive threatened his regime's fate. In October 2021, in response to a question from an opposition party member in the Lower House, Kishida stated that

> hard lockdowns (or mandatory mass quarantines), which rigorously restrict certain conduct, and the violation of which results in punishment, such as those applied in some countries in Europe or the US, do not suit Japan (or Japanese culture and practice).[41]

He emphasised that his government would strengthen Japan's crisis management by reinforcing policy coordination and enhancing stay-at-home requests instead of considering the introduction of further tighter measures.

Japanese political leaders are sensitive to popular will (or *min'i*, 民意) as it directly affects their electoral fate. Indeed, public opinion polling concerning the constitutional revision conducted by the Nippon Hōsō Kyōkai (NHK) [Japan Broadcasting Corporation] on 3 May 2022 indicates that 35% of people support the revision with 19% opposed, while 42% neither agree nor disagree. The rest (4%) is those who did not answer. Public opinion over the last ten years has also been divided between those who support, those who oppose, and those who neither agree nor disagree with the revision (Nishikawa 2018: 91). Many past prime ministers of post–World War II Japan, mostly from the LDP, were well aware of the sensitivity of the issue and they thus focused on improving the economy instead of placing the constitutional amendment at the centre of their policies, even though a constitutional revision has been part of the LDP's policy platform since its establishment in 1946 (Nishikawa 2018: 125).

Peer pressure that enforces government policies

In April 2020, when the first state of emergency was declared, all measures were adopted on a request basis. Important questions thus concern the 'how' and 'why' of Japan's reliance on self-restraint when managing the country's response to the COVID-19 pandemic. Although the Special Measures Act was amended and eventually included tighter measures with a possible administrative penalty (not criminal penalty in administration), emphasis is placed on the application of such measures being the 'minimum necessary' to enable COVID countermeasures (Article 5 of the Special Measures Act). In fact, many government policies and decisions were expected to be *voluntarily* realised, such as mask wearing, avoiding the 'Three Cs', reducing social contacts, and even being vaccinated. These measures were relatively successful at containing the spread of the virus, and the balance between the power of the authorities and people's rights and freedoms was partly maintained because the population voluntarily complied.

There were however some individuals, institutions, or facilities that ignored the requests of prefectural governors, even during the emergency period. Some owners of restaurants and leisure facilities refused to close their businesses, and some COVID-infected people refused to be hospitalised or disappeared from the designated quarantine hotels or accommodations prepared by the local government. For these reasons, the amended Special Measures Act allows the prefectural governor both to 'request' (*yousei*, 要請) cooperation from individuals and facilities (Article 24-9 and 45-2) and to 'order' (*meirei*, 命令) them to obey, if owners of facilities defy the request (Article 45-3) (see Table 4.2). Prefectural governors 'may' publicly announce the fact whenever they 'request' and 'order' facilities to close (Article 45-5). If the infected individuals refuse the request and the order of hospitalisation, or escape from the hospital without appropriate reasons, the governor can fine them (Article 80 of the Infectious Diseases Control Law).

Before the amendment of the Special Measures Act, the prefectural governor had to publicly announce without delay if a request or instruction for cooperation had been issued and not followed, as stipulated in Articles 45-2 and 45-3 (Article 45-4). In Osaka, in April 2020, the governor, therefore, publicly announced the names and addresses of the six facilities that had not complied with the request. Some of the named facilities then received a number of telephone calls from members of the public who criticised or intimidated them, leading them to close.[42] Similar cases occurred in other prefectures, including Hyogo and Tokyo. In these contexts, the public announcement was an administrative means to urge the business owners to fulfil the requests and instructions issued by the governor.

There are, at least, three possible meanings concerning public announcement in general: (1) public announcement as a sanction, (2) public announcement to ensure effectiveness, and (3) public announcement as information provision (Kimura 2021: 3). The government explained the aim of public announcement was 'to inform users widely about the content of the request, the facility's name and address'.[43] It also explained public announcement as follows:[44]

> The public announcement concerning the governor's request and order to limit facility-use in an emergency was stipulated because it is important to announce to the people widely in advance. The purpose is not to sanction but to ensure the users' rational behaviour. It thus requires considering its influence in order not to be counterproductive in preventing infection or not to cause defamation and false accusations. There are possible cases in which public announcement may not ensure users' reasonable actions, such as attracting more users by public announcement. It is, therefore, important to note that Article 45(5) is amended from 'must publicly announce' to 'may publicly announce'. In latter cases, it is possible not to publicly announce.

As illustrated in the statement, and following the three meanings advanced by Kimura (2021), the aim of public announcement in the Special Measures Act is information provision, rather than sanction. Nevertheless, the actual cases in Osaka and other prefectures exhibited that the administrative means of public announcement worked as a *de facto* sanction. It indicates that public announcement had unintended psychological effects on the people that the government might not have initially expected. The Osaka example shows the difficulty of categorically separating public announcement as information provision and public announcement as sanction. In the study of public policy, public announcement as a sanction is considered to belong to the psychological method of administrative means that functions as a 'nudge' and guides people and their behaviour in the appropriate direction without coercive intervention by the government (Kimura 2021: 4).

In practice, as the case in Osaka demonstrated, public announcement helped to generate 'peer pressure' in the form of shaming and assisting local governments to achieve their objectives. Here 'peer pressure' refers to the direct and indirect influence of peers and social groups on an individual who is influenced to follow the opinions and behaviours of the majority. The individual is, thus, expected to change attitudes, ideas, values, and behaviours to conform to those who have influence or who are dominant in society. The example here illustrates how certain policies were administratively enforced in an extra-legal way.

Similarly, a study by Nakayachi et al. (2020) illustrates how and why Japanese people wear masks, despite the government's refusal to take legal action. Their nationwide survey, conducted in March 2020, revealed that Japanese people wear masks even when there was not a prescription to do so to "conform to societal norms" and that they "felt relief from anxiety" when doing so. Notably, the authors concluded that mask use was not affected by risk reduction expectations (which is to say 'the participants' did not account for the severity of the disease or the efficacy of masks in reducing infection risk, either for themselves or for others). Social psychological motivations or "conformity to the mask norm" provides a significant explanation of mask use among the Japanese. An important implication of this finding is that Japanese people experience a certain social expectation, or even pressure, that obligates them to wear masks, largely because not doing so may jeopardise them socially and may cause them to become a target of intimidation. This practice of mask wearing rationalises how a certain government-promoted policy was extra-legally realised in Japan.

Japan has a history of the extra-legal enforcement of policies in economic, social, and political fields of practice. For example, Japanese administrative agencies use 'administrative guidance' (*gyōsei shidō*, 行政指導), which is non-binding 'advice' or a 'recommendation' by an administrative agency to the public concerning how best to comply with a certain law or regulation, or to persuade private entities to voluntarily cooperate with public officials (Fenwick 2010: 318). Although other states and societies have informal ways of enforcing government policies, the degree of pervasiveness and importance of such methods is unique to Japan (Matsushita 1993: 59–73). Indeed, the practice is often considered a trait of Japanese political culture (Fenwick 2010: 317). While administrative guidance may not necessarily equate to public announcement, among the measures adopted to counter COVID-19, public announcement contributed to generating peer pressure, functioned as an extra-legal method of achieving the authority's objectives, and helped to attain low COVID transmission in the country.

A rule-of-law system in the coronavirus emergency in Japan

Self-restraint was largely effective in Japan during the coronavirus emergency. While tighter measures were adopted with legal backing in some cases, those who disobeyed them were in many cases urged through peer pressure to comply with the prefectural governor's requests. Japanese people recognise that shaming and other social punishments are viable methods to enforce certain policies without necessarily resorting to law or other formal measures. Such administrative practices are well recognised and analysed in public policy studies.

Nevertheless, such practices require the majority of the population's support, thus turning them into forms of 'peer pressure'. Political leaders indeed appealed for support of their policies, which were designed to protect citizens, particularly aged people. In general, Japanese people expressed policy preferences that emerged from the atmosphere created by experts' comments and information provided via media reports. Continuous media coverage of the government's appeals, together with images of those in critical condition due to COVID-19, set a tone for self-restraint and formed a synchronisation of a national mood that was the "dominant opinion monopolizing the public scenes" (Thomas 2008: 371).

This situation is similar to what Mark Tushnet has described as 'moralised politics'—the kind of politics "in which political leaders appeal for support on the basis of moral claims in addition to appealing for support on the basis of constituents' non-moral preferences" (Tushnet 2008: 151). The Japanese peer pressure that appeared in the face of COVID-19 was, in that sense, a symptom and a consequence of moralised politics. In Japan, the majority's support for the government's policies to prevent the spread of COVID-19 influenced members of the public who, intentionally or unintentionally, acted against those who disobey the government's policies. Tomohiro Osaki, for example, while noting that "[v]igilantism during a pandemic is not peculiar to Japan" also reported "an army of coronavirus vigilantes" who harassed potential spreaders of CO-VID-19 (Osaki 2020). In other cases, self-righteous individuals act as 'self-restraint police' (*jishuku keisatsu*, 自粛警察) and aggressively monitor and hunt for cars travelling from outside of their prefecture, or shame anyone breaching 'stay-at-home' requests (Osaki 2020). These are the ways in which public pressure helped to enforce government policies that aimed to prevent the spread of the virus, although their actions have sometimes put others at risk.

The moralised politics observed in countering COVID-19 in Japan helped to overcome the limits of laws and formal measures, particularly in emergency situations. With respect to Japan's absence of the emergency powers common to other states, moralised politics, in a sense, compensated for any legal limitations. Tushnet, indeed, has stated, "Politics is the obvious alternative to law as a means of regulating the exercise of emergency powers—not politics as mere preference or the exercise of power for its own sake" (Tushnet 2008: 147).

In reality, state power is, to a certain extent, regulated through politics, which is normatively infused. Considering the complex and divided nature of interpretations and views on the absence of emergency powers in the Constitution of Japan, moralised politics emerged. In effect, it has provided an alternative to help realise the state's policies while at the same time containing centralised state power. In this sense, at least in Japan, the combination of law and a moralised politics has operated effectively to manage the coronavirus emergency, which may be regarded as evidence of the existence of a rule-of-law system and society. Understanding this rule-of-law system, to a great extent, explains how and why Japan's 'mysterious success' was possible without exercising emergency power.

Some potential drawbacks of moralised politics

While the combination of law and moralised politics succeeded to a large degree in combating COVID-19 in Japan, moralised politics may have certain drawbacks that could increase the unintended threat to the protection of rights and freedoms of certain people, and to democracy in the long run, if such a practice is regularised in non-emergency situations. If moralised politics is practiced frequently, the freedom to express one's opinions and the freedom of choice, for example, would be threatened by intimidation and harassment by certain groups of peers whose opinions are supported by the majority. When public opinion is evenly divided in a society, such risks may be low, whereas when a particular policy choice is clearly supported by a great majority, such risks may be high because moral rhetoric is more likely to be exploited and effective when majority support is granted.

If moral rhetoric is used and a vast majority of people support a certain policy, those with other opinions may be excluded or even be victimised by intimidation. The policy choice emphasised in moralised politics serves to reinforce conformity and denies diverse views; however, the majority view is not always either 'right' or 'good'. In a moralised politics context, those who intimidate others tend to view the national or prefectural government's appeals or requests to the public as an endorsement, and they thus consider their acts and actions of intimidation as legitimate. They often feel a sense of self-righteousness, harassing or intimidating those who do not comply with the 'right' things to do to "contribute to the society" (Ota 2021: 174–176). In fact, Yuichi Inukai explains that the self-restraint police who appeared in Japan during the COVID-19 pandemic viewed their own acts of intimidation in this way, and Inukai considered such acts as "attacks disguised as justice" (Inukai 2021: 127). There was also a report on 'self-restraint police' in Chiba Prefecture, which featured a traditional Japanese sweets shop receiving a note in May 2020 demanding it suspend operations.[45] Again, Inuaki pointed out that such an act was done based on a "sense of justice". Similar cases were reported in Yokohama Prefecture in May 2020.[46] In such cases, the society is intolerant to diverse or minority opinions and, as Toru Takahashi highlights, public opinion cannot fulfil its function of bringing varied themes and views into the political discussion (Takahashi 2016: 13). Accordingly, moralised politics would likely be a platform open to manipulation.

When moral rhetoric is used in a particular policy area in an ordinary political environment, it can obstruct one's freedom to express an opinion against the majority, however, a government advancing a specific policy to the public should not result in the restraint of diverse opinions. Rather, contemporary liberal democracy relies on pluralism and encourages diversity. In a manipulative political environment created by moralised politics, those holding contrary views to the majority are silenced, and they may even become targets of peer intimidation. Therefore, although moralised politics has helped fill the legal vacuum during the COVID-19 emergency in Japan, it potentially increases the risk of generating intolerance towards diverse or minority viewpoints and opinions. As with the peer pressure that permeates Japanese society, moralised politics is a double-edged sword.[47]

Over the two years of 2020–2021, COVID-19 in Japan brought about a range of changes to keep individuals and communities safe. While the 'new normal' requires adapting to constant preventive and protective measures against COVID-19, it is vital to recognise the possible and obscured risks and effects on our society, politics, and ourselves generated by the emergence of moralised politics in a time of prolonged emergency.

Conclusion

Japan's relative success in keeping the number of infected persons and deaths per million lower than in many other industrialised countries is an achievement, especially considering the slow start and the super-aged nature of Japanese society. This success is largely explained by Japanese 'voluntary' compliance with the government's policies and the 'self-restraint' of the population. In reality, both legal measures and citizens' self-restraint worked together to prevent the spread of the virus. This was possible partly because political leaders strenuously emphasised preventive measures, such as mask use and avoiding the Three Cs—avoiding closed spaces, crowded places, and close-contact settings—and appealed to citizens for their support on the basis of moral claims. Such political and moral appeals were widely shared on traditional and social media, and were supported by most Japanese citizens, therefore generating peers who diligently monitored potential spreaders of COVID-19. In this sense, Japan's handling of COVID-19 in 2020 and 2021 may be considered as a situation of what Mark Tushnet calls 'moralised politics'. The government also introduced several tight restrictions with legal backing so that prefectural governments could enforce compliance and impose penalties in cases of violation. While the combination of moralised politics and law constitutes a rule-of-law system, moralised politics may have long-term negative effects if it is integrated into ordinary political practice. It may foster a manipulative political environment that significantly threatens freedom to limit the discussion of different points of view or opinions in political debate. In the long run, self-imposed social restrictions may threaten the quality of Japanese democracy. As the pandemic continues, we may discover that the effects of this 'new normal' on Japanese social relations and society may be far deeper than might have been expected.

Notes

1 A super-aged society means a society in which over 21% of the population is aged 65 or older. The concept is commonly used by the World Health Organization (WHO). If the society's aging rate, which measures the proportion of persons aged 65 or older, surpasses 14%, it is an 'aged society', while if it exceeds 7%, it is an 'aging society'. Japan became a super-aged society in 2007, and now the country's aging rate is expected to reach 30% by 2025 and 40% by 2060.

2 The death rate is based on the actual, expected, and excess deaths of G7 countries in the 12 months up to February 2021 as provided by the Human Mortality Database and World Mortality Dataset. https://health.org.uk/publications/long-reads/comparing-g7-countries-are-excess-deaths-an-objective-measure-of-pandemic-performance (accessed 18 December 2021).

3 Information concerning the government's economic measures is available online at the website of the Cabinet Office of Japan. https://www.cao.go.jp/index-e.html (3 May 2022). Also, for a concise and overall picture of Japan's early economic spending, see Walton (2020).

4 The Emergency Economic Measures were later amended on 20 April 2020. The amount in US dollar was calculated by the author at the exchange rate of 130.15 yen per dollar.

5 The government's spending from the contingency funds per year had been less than 2 trillion yen. The information was obtained from the website of the Ministry of Finance.

6 See the website of the Cabinet Secretariat. https://corona.go.jp/en/news/news_20200510_76.html (2 May 2022).

7 The Act's original version, the Act on Special Measures concerning Pandemic Influenza and New Infectious Diseases Preparedness and Response, was enacted in 2012 to respond to future outbreaks of new strains of influenza. It resulted from lessons learnt from the novel influenza (A/H1N1) outbreak in 2009. The 2012 Act had to be revised to adapt it to the COVID-19 context because COVID-19 was not originally believed to qualify as one of the new infectious diseases defined in the original Act.

8 The term 'instruct' here is meant to show a policy, procedure, and standard among others for a specific action to take. Those who receive the 'instruction' are legally obligated to fulfil the instruction, although the instruction does not incur penalties.

9 Article 45 of the Act does not provide information concerning 'public announcement'. However, a guidance document sent from the chair of the Office for the Promotion of Countermeasures against Novel Coronavirus of the Cabinet Secretariat to governors dated on 23 April 2020 states that 'public announcement' shall include the names and addresses of the facilities of concern, the content of the request and the reason for the request, and shall be publicized on the website of each prefecture.

10 The original Special Measures Act stipulates that it can be applied for a maximum of two years with possible extension for no more than one year.

11 The members of the Expert Meeting were appointed by the prime minister and no more than 40 persons. The list of members is available on the website of the Cabinet Secretariat. The Expert Meeting was held 17 meeting between February and July 2020. It was then removed in July 2020.

12 This reason concerning the replacement was explained by Nishimura Yasutoshi, the then minister in charge of Economic Revitalization. See *The Sankei News*, 24 June 2020 (in Japanese).

13 The estimated economic loss in the case of cancelation was around 190 billion yen (equivalent to 1.46 billion US dollars). The estimation was made by the Nomura Research Institute in March 2021. The amount in US dollars was calculated by the author at the exchange rate of 130.15 yen per dollar.

14 Abe Shinzō became the longest-serving prime minister on 23 August 2020. He served as prime minister for 2,822 consecutive days since 2012, which surpasses his granduncle's record of 2,798 days as prime minister. See, "What Will Be Abe's Legacy as the Longest-Serving Prime Minister?" *The Japan Times*, 27 August, 2020.

15 The president of LDP can serve maximum for three consecutive terms (total nine years). Prime Minister Abe became LDP's president in September 2018 of his third term.

16 David Walton concisely explains the economic packages of the Japanese government. See, Walton (2020). See also "Abe Unveils 'Massive' Coronavirus Stimulus Worth 20% of GDP", *Japan Times*, 6 April 2020. Available online: https://www.japantimes.co.jp/news/2020/04/06/business/shinzo-abe-japan-massive-coronavirus-stimulus (2 May 2022).

17 See also the following news article: "Japan's Ruling Party Gets Lion's Share of Business Donations: Automakers Association Was the Single Largest Donor to Shinzo Abe's LDP in 2016', *Nikkei Asia*, 1 December 2017.

18 The Carnival Corp cruise ship *Diamond Princess* carried 3,711 passengers of whom 712 persons became infected with COVID-19. The Japanese government was harshly criticised for its quarantine measures on the virus-stricken ship.

19 See the website of the Cabinet Secretariat (in Japanese). https://corona.go.jp/news/pdf/kinkyujitai_sengen_0407.pdf (2 May 2022).

20 See the nationwide public opinion poll conducted in August 2020 by the Shakai Chōsa centre. The result shows that among the 1,042 persons who responded, about 90% of them did not support the Abe government's response to COVID-19.

21 A summary of the amendment is available on the website of the Ministry of Health, Labour and Welfare in Japanese online: https://www.mhlw.go.jp/content/10900000/000737689.pdf (2 May 2022).

22 The amount in US dollars was calculated by the author at the exchange rate of 130.15 yen per dollar. Information concerning the penalties related to novel coronavirus in Japan, see the Special Measures Act and the Act on the Prevention of Infectious Diseases and Medical Care for Patients with Infectious Diseases (the Infectious Diseases Control Law).

23 The Infectious Diseases Control Law, together with other laws, was also amended in accordance with the amendment made in the Special Measures Act.

24 See the summary of the amendment. Available in Japanese online: https://www.mhlw.go.jp/content/10900000/000737689.pdf (2 May 2022).

25 The scenes of hundreds of protesters were released in the media report around the world. See, for example, "Stop the Olympics: Hundreds Protest Outside Tokyo 2020 Opening Ceremony" video, *The Guardian*, 23 July 2021. Available online: https://www.theguardian.com/sport/video/2021/jul/23/stop-the-olympics-hundreds-protest-outside-tokyo-2020-opening-ceremony-video (2 May 2022).

26 "Survey: 83% Against Holding Tokyo Olympics This Summer", *The Asahi Shinbun*, 17 May 2021.

27 The poster in English is available online on the website of the Ministry of Health, Labour and Welfare of Japan. https://www.mhlw.go.jp/content/3CS.pdf (27 December 2021). The poster is available in 18 different languages downloadable from the government website. The WHO also promoted the similar idea to avoid"'the Three Cs" (Crowd places, Close-contact setting, and Confined and enclosed spaces) through its Facebook on 18 July 2020. See also Allgayer and Kanemoto (2021).

28 Until 2019, the overall public relations expense in the government had been between 8.2 and 10.3 billion yen. For the budged year 2020, the government planned to add 10 billion yen more.

29 The information is obtained from the Ministry of Finance of Japan. https://www.mof.go.jp (3 May 2022).

30 There was a shortage of face masks in Japan in February and March 2020. To respond to the situation, the Abe government decided to give each household two reusable surgical masks and, indeed, distributed these nationwide by June 2020. The policy was later named 'Abenomask' (meaning 'Abe's mask'). It was harshly criticised and ridiculed as the costs to produce and deliver the masks reached nearly 50 billion yen (440 million US dollars). Even after a year, further criticism of the

policy emerged as 81.3 million Abenomasks remained in storage as of the end of October 2021, costing 600 million yen (5 million US dollars) by the end of March 2021. See Nishimura (2021).

31 The study used two datasets collected by Facebook and other research findings, covering more than 900,000 people.

32 See, for example, the following news article: "How to Reduce Physical Contact with Others by 80%: Japan Medical Experts", *The Mainich*, 10 April 2020.

33 A definition provided by Dr Koji Wada of the International University of Health and Welfare.

34 The study was conducted by using large-scale mobility data collected from mobile phones. The authors used the data to quantify the changes in human mobility behaviour and social contacts during the COVID-19 spread in Tokyo in 2020.

35 Telework, which means 'working from home', was strongly promoted in both private and public companies. Nevertheless, the actual percentage of companies that could accommodate telework remained only 13% in March 2020. See Shaw et al. (2020, p. 6).

36 It is not understood why such a sudden decline in the number of COVID-infected people has occurred since October 2021 in Japan. Scientists considered a mixture of factors to be at work, instead of a single factor.

37 The vaccination rate is based on the rate in November 2021. See also the following reports: Jiji (2021) and Kyodo (2021).

38 The following laws include certain emergency provisions: The Police Act (Article 71 and 74), the Self-Defence Forces Act (Article 76, 78 and 81), and the Basic Act on Disaster Management (Article 105 and 105). Nevertheless, these should not be considered synonymous with emergency powers because there is no agreed interpretation of the significance of these articles to the question of whether the administrative authorities can suspend the constitution and other ordinary laws of the country. See Nishikawa (2020). Experts, therefore, differ on whether the current constitution allows the state to exercise emergency powers. For more details on this point, see Nishikawa (2020).

39 For example, between 1894 and 1925, the government enacted the Public Security Preservation Laws (commonly known as the 'Peace Preservation Laws') and oppressed democratic movements.

40 The ninth point of a supplementary resolution approved at the 204th Diet meeting in the Lower House.

41 Kishida's response was delivered at the question-and-answer session in the Lower House on 11 October 2021 (translation by the author).

42 Several newspaper agencies reported the named facilities. Some of the facilities, after all, decided to close as they received telephone calls to criticize them. See, for example, *Yomiuri Shinbun* on 27 April 2020 (in Japanese). Also, see "Japan's Osaka to Name and Shame Pachinko Parlors Defying Coronavirus Lockdown", *Reuters*, 27 April 2020.

43 An official guidance document to prefectural governors from the chair of the Office for the Promotion of Countermeasures against Novel Coronavirus of the Cabinet Secretariat dated on 23 April 2020 was to provide instructions concerning public announcement based on Article 45. It is in Japanese (translation by the author).

44 This is an explanation in an official document from the Office for the Promotion of Countermeasures against Novel Coronavirus of the Cabinet Secretariat to prefectural governors and designated public institutions dated on 12 February 2021. It is in Japanese (translation by the author). The amendment of the Special Measures Act together with other relevant laws was approved at the Diet on 3 February 2021.

45 "Harassment over Coronavirus Restraints on Rise in Japan", *News from Japan*, 9 May 2020. Available online: https://www.nippon.com/en/news/yjj202005090 0144 (2 May 2022).

46　See, "Self-Restraint Police in Japan Harassing Business Operating Amid Virus Outbreak", *The Mainichi*, 23 May 2020. Available online: https://mainichi.jp/
english/articles/20200522/p2a/00m/0na/023000c (2 May 2022).
47　Many Japanese analysts point out peer pressure as a key explanatory factor of both
positive and negative affairs observed in the Japanese society. While it is considered
contributing to the low crime rate and good public health in Japan, it is also considered an important factor that explains the high suicide rate, bulling in schools,
and workplace moral harassment.

References

Allgayer, S. and Kanemoto, E. (2021). "The <Three Cs> of Japan's Pandemic Response
as an Ideograph", *Frontiers in Communication*, 6: 1–11. Available online: https://
www.frontiersin.org/articles/10.3389/fcomm.2021.595429/full (3 May 2022).

Eiraku, M. and Aizawa, Y. (2021, May 12). "Japan's Vaccine Rollout Slow to Get Off
Ground", *NHK World-Japan*, News. Available online: https://www3.nhk.or.jp/
nhkworld/en/news/backstories/1636 (20 December 2021).

Fenwick, M. (2010). "Emergency Powers and the Limits of Constitutionalism in
Japan". In Ramraj, V. Victor, and Arun K. Thiruvengadam (eds.) *Emergency Powers
in Asia: Exploring the Limits of Legality*, Cambridge: Cambridge University Press.
pp. 314–341.

Inukai, Y. (2021). *Sekentei Kokka, Nihon (Japan, The State That Worries about How
People See Them)*, Tokyo: Koubunsha (originally in Japanese).

Izumi, H. (2020, March 13). "Prime Minister Abe Who Is Brought to Bay Due to
Emerging Opinions to Cancel the Olympics and Paralympics Games". [*Tokyo Gorin
Chūshiron de oitsumerareru Abe Shushou*] (originally in Japanese), *Toyo Keizai
Online*. Available online: https://toyokeizai.net/articles/-/336514 (2 May 2022).

Jackman, S. J. (2021, June 23). "Japan Reaches Suga's Target of 1 Million Vaccine
Doses Per Day", Bloomberg/*The Japan Times*. Available online: https://www.
bloomberg.com/news/articles/2021-06-23/japan-reaches-suga-s-target-of-a-
million-vaccine-doses-per-day#xj4y7vzkg (2 May 2022).

Jiji, K. (2021, October 26). "With over 70% Fully Vaccinated, Japan Ranks in Top
Three among G7", *Japan Times*.

Kimura, S. (2021). "Special Measures Act concerning the New Coronavirus Measures
– A Signpost to the Act on Special Measures for Pandemic Influenza and New Infectious Diseases Preparedness and Reponses and the Administrative Law", *Meiji University Academic Repository*. Available online: https://m-repo.lib.meiji.ac.jp/
dspace/bitstream/10291/21843/1/special_kimura.pdf (3 May 2022).

Kingston, J. (2020). "Abe Prioritized Olympics, Slowing Japan's Pandemic Response",
The Asia-Pacific Journal, 18(7), number 5: 1–8.

Kyodo. (2021, November 19). "Japan leads G7 with COVID-19 Vaccination Rate of
Nearly 76%", *Japan Today*.

Lu, J. G., Jin, P., and English, A.S. (2021). "Collectivism Predicts Mask Use During
COVID-19", *Psychological and Cognitive Sciences*, 118(23): 1–8. Available online:
https://doi.org/10.1073/pnas.2021793118 (27 December 2021).

Manabe, A. (2022, January 29). "The Reason Why 'Anti-Vaccine Movement' Appears
Heterogeneous in Japan". [*Nihon no 'han-wakuchin undō ga doumo ishitsu ni mieru
wake*] (originally in Japanese), *Toyo Keizai Online*. Available online: https://
toyokeizai.net/articles/-/507354 (3 May 2022).

Matsushita, M. (1993). *International Trade and Competition Law in Japan*, Oxford: Oxford University Press.

Minister of Health, Labour and Welfare. (2020, January 16). (in Japanese) "Concerning the outbreak of pneumonia in a patient in conjunction with the new coronavirus (the first case)". Available online: https://www.mhlw.go.jp/stf/newpage_08906.html (2 May 2022).

Mizorogi, T. (2021, August 30). "Japanese Disapproval of Suga's COVID Response Hits Near-Record High", *Nikkei Asia*. Available online: https://asia.nikkei.com/Politics/Japanese-disapproval-of-Suga-s-COVID-response-hits-near-record-high (19 December 2021).

Moon, M.J., Suzuki, K., Park, T.I., and Sakuwa, K. (2021). "A Comparative Study of COVID-19 Responses in South Korea and Japan: Political Nexus Triad and Policy Responses", *International Review of Administrative Sciences*, 87(3): 651–671.

Nakayachi, K., Ozaki, T., Shibata, Y., and Yokoi, R. (2020). "Why Do Japanese People Use Masks against COVID-19, Even though Masks Are Unlikely to Offer Protection from Infection?", *Frontiers in Psychology*, 11:1918.

Nishikawa, Y. (2018). *Political Sociology of Japanese Pacifism*, London: Routledge.

Nishikawa, Y. (2020). "Japanese Response to COVID-19: Politics of Emergency Power, Human Rights and the Rule of Law". In Biddulph, Sarah, Kathryn Taylor, Yukiko Nishikawa, and Sebastien Lafrane (eds.) *Law on the State of Emergency*, Hanoi: Vietnam National University and Melbourne Law School, pp. 234–253.

Nishimura, K. (2021, December 16). "Government: Anyone Want a Free Abenomask? Anyone?", *The Asahi Shinbun*.

Osaki, T. (2020, May 13). "Japan's Vigilantes' Take on Rule-Breakers and Invaders", *The Japan Times*. Available online at: https://www.japantimes.co.jp/news/2020/05/13/national/coronavirus-vigilantes-japan

Ota, H. (2021). *Douchou-Atsuryoku no Shoutai (The True Nature of Peer Pressure)*, Tokyo: PHP Interface (originally in Japanese).

Shaw, R., Kim, Y.-K., and Hua, J. (2020). "Governance, Technology and Citizen Behavior in Pandemic: Lessons from COVID-19 in East Asia", *Progress in Disaster Science*, 6: 1–11.

Sposato, W. (2020, May 14). "Japan's Halfhearted Coronavirus Measures Are Working Anyway: Despite Indifferent Lockdowns and Poor Testing, Japan Seems to Be Skipping the Worst of the Pandemic", *FP*, Argument. Available online: https://foreignpolicy.com/2020/05/14/japan-coronavirus-pandemic-lockdown-testing/ (19 December 2021).

Sturmer, J. and Asada, Y. (2020, May 23). "Japan Was Feared to Be the Next US or Italy. Instead their Coronavirus Success Is a Puzzling 'Mystery'", *The ABC News*. Available online: https://www.abc.net.au/news/2020https://www.abc.net.au/news/2020--0505--23/japan23/japan--waswas--meantmeant-to--bebe--thethe--nextnext--italyitaly--onon--coronavirus/12266912coronavirus/12266912 (19 December 2021).

Takahashi, T. (2016). "Populism and Moralization of Politics in the Age of Systemic Crisis: A Sociocybernetic Case Study of Japanese Politics", *The Chuo Law Review*, 122 (11/12): 1–24.

The House of Representatives. (2020). The Information Concerning the Questions Raised in the Budgetary Discussion on 12 June 2020, available in Japanese, https://www.shugiin.go.jp/internet/itdb_shitsumon.nsf/html/shitsumon/a201266.htm (3 May 2022).

Thomas, J. (2008). "From People Power to Mass Hysteria: Media and Popular Reactions to the Death of Princess Diana", *International Journal of Cultural Studies*, 11(3): 362–376.

Tushnet, M. (2008). "The Political Constitution of Emergency Powers". In Ramraj, V. Victor (ed.) *Emergencies and the Limits of Legality*, Cambridge: Cambridge University Press. pp. 145–155.

Urabe, N. (1990). "Rule of Law and Due Process: A Comparative View of the United States and Japan", *Law and Contemporary Problems*, 53(1): 61–72.

Walton, D. (2020). "Japan". In Georgeou, Nichole and Hawksley, Charles (eds.) *State Reponses to COVID-19: A Global Snapshot at 1 June 2020*, HADRI: Western Sydney University, pp. 52–53. Available online: https://doi.org/10.2183/5ed5a2079cabd (2 May 2022).

Yabe, T., K. Tsubouchi, Fujiwara, N., Wada, T., Sekimoto, Y., and Ukksuri, S. V. (2020). "Non-Compulsory Measures Sufficiently Reduced Human Mobility in Tokyo during the COVID-19 Epidemic", *Scientific Report*, 10 (18053): 1–9. Available online: https://doi.org/10.1038/s41598-020-75033-5 (30 December 2021).

Yoshimatsu, H. (1997). "Business-Government Relations in Japan: The Influence of Business on Policy-Making through Two Routes", *Asian Perspective*, 21(2): 119–146.

5 Making sense of behavioural restrictions and institutional controls

The Philippine COVID-19 experience

*Leslie A. Lopez, Jessica Sandra R. Claudio,
Dennis B. Batangan, Joselito T. Sescon and
Haraya Marikit C. Mendoza*

Introduction

For populist states such as the Philippines, which during the 2020–2021 period was led by President Rodrigo R. Duterte, the pandemic could have been an excellent opportunity to showcase its management and governance prowess. However, the state's segmented responses and shifting policies indicate otherwise. Instead of exploring a more geographically and culturally nuanced COVID-19 management approach, the country followed the bandwagon of using a more technocratic-authoritarian governance approach. Given its recent history of authoritarian leadership, this expansion of state powers in the Philippines, including the securitisation of COVID-19 measures, did not come as a surprise.

This chapter argues that the fluidity of the COVID-19 situation on the ground provides a space for the Philippine state to recalibrate its role vis-a-vis other societal institutions. To trace this, we explore the Philippine state's responses to the COVID-19 pandemic, through its political, economic, and health actions, specifically focusing on the emergence of the uniformed sector as a dominant state functionary over the past two and a half years. We conclude by arguing the political leaders of the Philippines looked to history to militarise what was a complex public health emergency, with predictable results.

Political response

The Philippines dealt with COVID as a security issue, and the state expanded the role of the Philippine National Police (PNP), and the Armed Forces of the Philippines (AFP) from ensuring health protocols and quarantine guidelines to providing technical, administrative, and logistical assistance (Caliwan, 2020) in Social Amelioration Program (SAP) distribution. The PNP and AFP assisted the Department of Social Welfare and Development (DSWD) in distributing aid more efficiently (Gita-Carlos, 2020) and arresting corrupt and dishonest local officials (DILG, 2020), a move that signifies the ubiquity of state security forces in the Philippines' pandemic response. As Migdal

DOI: 10.4324/9781003311522-5

(2001: 15–16) has observed, the state is "a field of power marked by the use and threat of violence and shaped by the image of a coherent, controlling organization in a territory, which represents the people bounded by that territory". Hence, the reshaping of the Philippine state through "the actual practices of its multiple parts" (Migdal, 2001: 16) during the pandemic was to be expected.

The Interagency Task Force on Emerging Infectious Diseases (IATF-EID) was activated on 28 January 2020 through Executive Order No. 168, s. 2014. As an intersectoral body, it is part of the IATF-EID's mandate to provide guidelines on managing COVID-19, including the guidelines on health quarantine referred to as lockdowns. The Department of Health (DOH) chairs this body.[1]

The Philippine government then introduced selective quarantine for returning overseas Filipino workers (OFWs) starting on 2 February 2020, a response measure indicative of globalism and nationalism tension. With increasing COVID-19 cases, President Duterte signed Proclamation 922 (8 March 2020) placing the Philippines under a State of Public Health Emergency. The law was an attempt "to capacitate government agencies and local government units (LGUs) to utilize appropriate resources to implement urgent and critical measures to contain or prevent the spread of COVID-19" (Proclamation 922). However, barely a week had passed when it was superseded by Proclamation 929 (16 March 2020), declaring the whole country under a State of National Calamity. This declaration was initially anticipated to last for only six months (until September 2020), however, it was extended to 12 September 2021 (Proclamation 1021), and eventually to 12 December 2022 (Proclamation 1218).

On 13 March 2020, the government put Metro Manila under Enhanced Community Quarantine (ECQ), considered to be the most stringent type of lockdown. By 17 March, the ECQ had been extended to the entire Luzon region and later to several areas in Visayas and Mindanao. Less stringent forms of community quarantine were also identified, such as the Modified Enhanced Community Quarantine (MECQ), General Community Quarantine (GCQ), and Modified General Community Quarantine (MGCQ). In June 2020, most places eased quarantine restrictions to GCQ. However, the National Capital Region (NCR) and surrounding provinces of Bulacan, Cavite, Laguna, and Rizal were again reclassified to ECQ on 4–18 August 2020 due to an increase in the number of COVID-19 cases.

Throughout the pandemic, provinces across the country vacillated between the different forms of community quarantines. During 2020, the Philippines is even said to have had the "longest and strictest" COVID-19 lockdown in the world (Olanday and Rigby, 2020). The COVID-19 narrative was also muddled by changing lockdown restrictions imposed in small chunks of time by the IATF. From March 2020 to early September 2021, the community quarantine classification system was as follows (Figure 5.1):

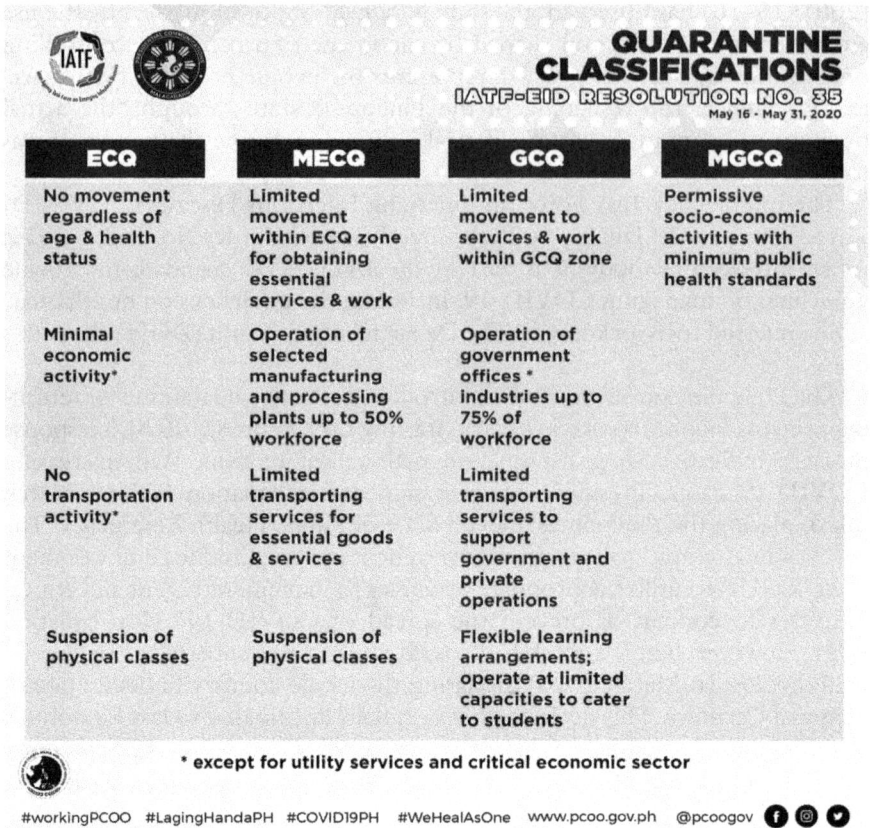

QUARANTINE CLASSIFICATIONS
IATF-EID RESOLUTION NO. 35
May 16 - May 31, 2020

ECQ	MECQ	GCQ	MGCQ
No movement regardless of age & health status	Limited movement within ECQ zone for obtaining essential services & work	Limited movement to services & work within GCQ zone	Permissive socio-economic activities with minimum public health standards
Minimal economic activity*	Operation of selected manufacturing and processing plants up to 50% workforce	Operation of government offices * industries up to 75% of workforce	
No transportation activity*	Limited transporting services for essential goods & services	Limited transporting services to support government and private operations	
Suspension of physical classes	Suspension of physical classes	Flexible learning arrangements; operate at limited capacities to cater to students	

* except for utility services and critical economic sector

#workingPCOO #LagingHandaPH #COVID19PH #WeHealAsOne www.pcoo.gov.ph @pcoogov

Figure 5.1 Quarantine classification system (March 2020–September 2021).
Source: Presidential Communications Operations Office.

In September 2021, however, the national government approved the new alert level and granular lockdown system (see Figure 5.2) to replace the old community quarantine system. The new system became fully implemented (nationwide) in November 2021.

These community lockdowns exacted a stiff toll on many disadvantaged communities, including many informal settlements within the NCR where the lockdowns were most severe.

Beyond these policies, government responses to the pandemic have often been criticised for their framing and methodology. These responses have generally been described as 'militarised' (Imbong, 2022; Gibson-Fall, 2021) and "war-like" (Hapal, 2021; Agojo, 2021), incorporating extensive use of police and military forces in a war with an unforeseen enemy, the coronavirus. The war narrative, however, started prior to the onset of the pandemic, and the country's response to the COVID pandemic is simply a continuation (Hapal,

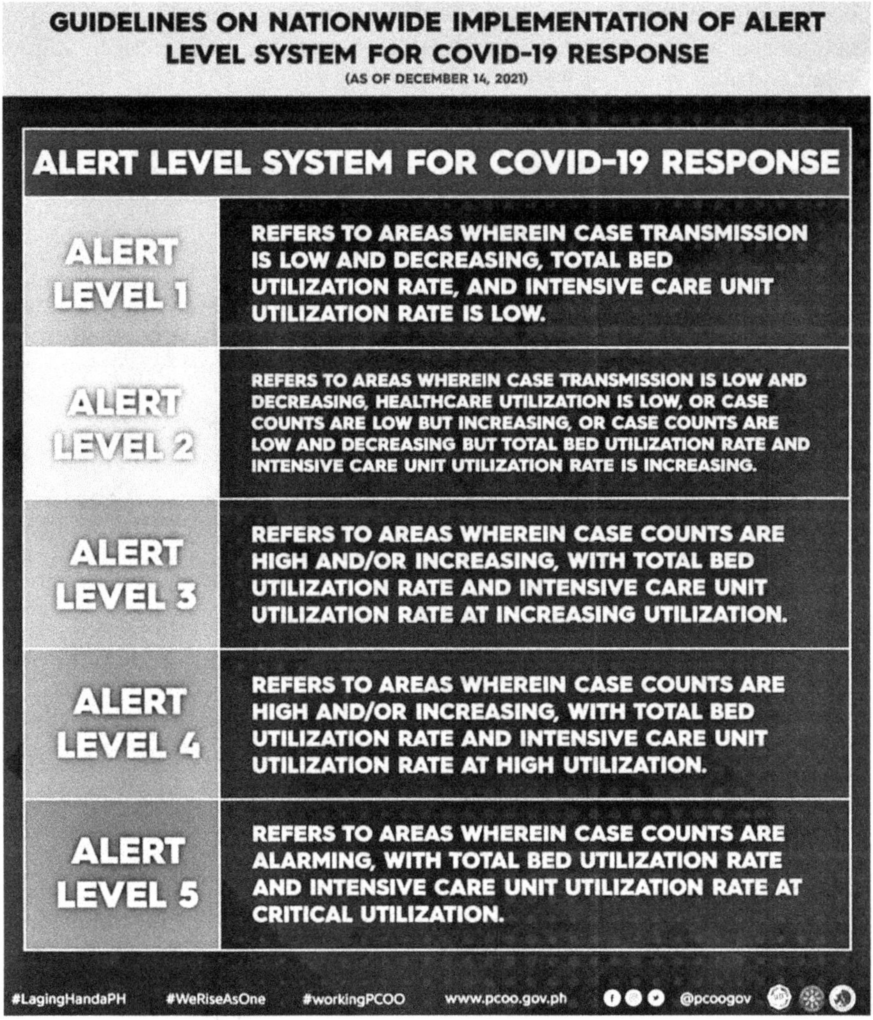

GUIDELINES ON NATIONWIDE IMPLEMENTATION OF ALERT LEVEL SYSTEM FOR COVID-19 RESPONSE
(AS OF DECEMBER 14, 2021)

ALERT LEVEL SYSTEM FOR COVID-19 RESPONSE

ALERT LEVEL 1	REFERS TO AREAS WHEREIN CASE TRANSMISSION IS LOW AND DECREASING, TOTAL BED UTILIZATION RATE, AND INTENSIVE CARE UNIT UTILIZATION RATE IS LOW.
ALERT LEVEL 2	REFERS TO AREAS WHEREIN CASE TRANSMISSION IS LOW AND DECREASING, HEALTHCARE UTILIZATION IS LOW, OR CASE COUNTS ARE LOW BUT INCREASING, OR CASE COUNTS ARE LOW AND DECREASING BUT TOTAL BED UTILIZATION RATE AND INTENSIVE CARE UNIT UTILIZATION RATE IS INCREASING.
ALERT LEVEL 3	REFERS TO AREAS WHEREIN CASE COUNTS ARE HIGH AND/OR INCREASING, WITH TOTAL BED UTILIZATION RATE AND INTENSIVE CARE UNIT UTILIZATION RATE AT INCREASING UTILIZATION.
ALERT LEVEL 4	REFERS TO AREAS WHEREIN CASE COUNTS ARE HIGH AND/OR INCREASING, WITH TOTAL BED UTILIZATION RATE AND INTENSIVE CARE UNIT UTILIZATION RATE AT HIGH UTILIZATION.
ALERT LEVEL 5	REFERS TO AREAS WHEREIN CASE COUNTS ARE ALARMING, WITH TOTAL BED UTILIZATION RATE AND INTENSIVE CARE UNIT UTILIZATION RATE AT CRITICAL UTILIZATION.

#LagingHandaPH   #WeRiseAsOne   #workingPCOO   www.pcoo.gov.ph   @pcoogov

Figure 5.2 COVID-19 alert level and granular lockdown system.
Source: Presidential Communications Operations Office.

2021). Duterte's "War on Drugs" utilised a broad public concern against the drug menace and securitised the issue. Further, he appointed 40 former police and military personnel to various cabinet positions (Maru, 2020) where their influence was initially balanced with that of civilian government leaders. This balance, however, tipped in the favour of former military generals when they were appointed as members of the IATF-EID, initially headed by a civilian, the DOH secretary (Imbong, 2022; Agojo, 2021). Eventually, the IATF-IED was later relegated to a mere policymaking body under the National Task Force (NTF) on COVID-19, which is headed by retired military officers.[2] These arrangements effectively expanded the military's power to areas beyond their traditional expertise, providing them with global powers and effectively subordinating various civilian government agencies (Imbong, 2022).

Analysts view the militarisation of the pandemic as the deployment of Bargu's (2019) biopolitical state apparatus (BSA), which recognises the unique role that police power occupies within Althusser's (1971) twofold classification of state apparatuses—the ideological state apparatus (ISA) and the repressive state apparatus (RSA). Bargu's analysis of police power provides a 'disjunctive synthesis' of Althusser's work, using Foucault's insights. Thus, the BSA 'discriminates' subjects through surveillance (Bargu, 2019) and produces oppositional archetypes (Hapal, 2021), such as the virtuous (personified by frontline workers and law-abiding citizens) and the '*pasaway*' (stubborn, law-breaking citizens). In this narrative, the errant 'pasaway' are justifiably punished by police and military forces. This succinctly describes BSA's work of "regulating subjects as bodies . . . sorted according to the main differential for identifying "good" subjects from "bad" ones" (Bargu, 2019: 314). The IATF-EID, composed primarily of senior military staff, is seen as exacting policing practices that brand citizens as good or bad, in the process marking them for treatment by the ISA or the RSA.

Jensen and Hapal (2018) suggest that this depiction of a 'bifurcated society' is aligned with Duterte's populistic brand of leadership, and it is thus no wonder that the government's pandemic response has closely resembled the "War on Drugs" approach. At the height of the pandemic, Duterte claimed that the military was the backbone of his administration (Dizon, 2020). In early April 2020, in a late-night telecast of his speech, Duterte said,

> I will not hesitate. My orders are to the police and military, as well as village officials, if there is any trouble, or occasions where there's violence, and your lives are in danger, shoot them dead. [. . .] Do not intimidate the government. Do not challenge the government. You will lose.
>
> (Inquirer.net, 2020)

Duterte's speech came after reports that residents in a poor area in Manila were arrested for protesting insufficient government aid. His words, in essence, ensure that bad subjects (the 'pasaway') would be met with punitive measures, creating unnecessary fear and panic among the public. In a two-week period between 6 and 20 August 2021, the PNP reported 149,963 quarantine violators, with omissions ranging from not following minimum health standards such as wearing face shields and masks, to curfew violations, and going out of one's home unnecessarily.

While the military has the organisational structure to respond well to the immediate demands of the pandemic situation, military leadership in national COVID-19 management can have negative consequences on hard-earned civil liberties (Engels 2020). The huge military influence is expected to effectively reduce civil society's participation in major decision-making pertaining to COVID-19. Aside from Duterte's instructions to the police and the military to shoot lockdown violators, there were also documented cases of human rights abuses such as putting violators in dog cages, coffins, or making them sit for hours in the midday sun. The expanded police and military power became normalised during prolonged lockdowns (Chen, 2020). Yet, war and military metaphors are dangerous because they effectively exclude "alternative ways of understanding the disease and what fuels it" (Gibson-Fall, 2021: 168).

Health response and impacts

The COVID pandemic exacerbated the challenges for an already fragmented health system in the Philippines. The first COVID-19 case was reported on 30 January 2020 (a 38-year-old Chinese national). Four imported COVID-19 cases followed before the first cases of local transmission were reported on 5 March 2020—a 62-year-old husband and 59-year-old wife without any recent travel history. On 2 May 2022, the COVID-19 Tracker of the DOH indicates that the Philippines has had about 3.6 million COVID-19 cases since February 2020 (Figure 5.3), and while 98% of those infected recovered, 60,397 people have died from the virus.

Until late February 2022, the Philippines consistently had the second-highest number of COVID-19 cases after Indonesia among the ten member states of the Association of Southeast Asian Nations (ASEAN).[3] In late April 2022, the Philippines ranked fifth among ASEAN in terms of the total number

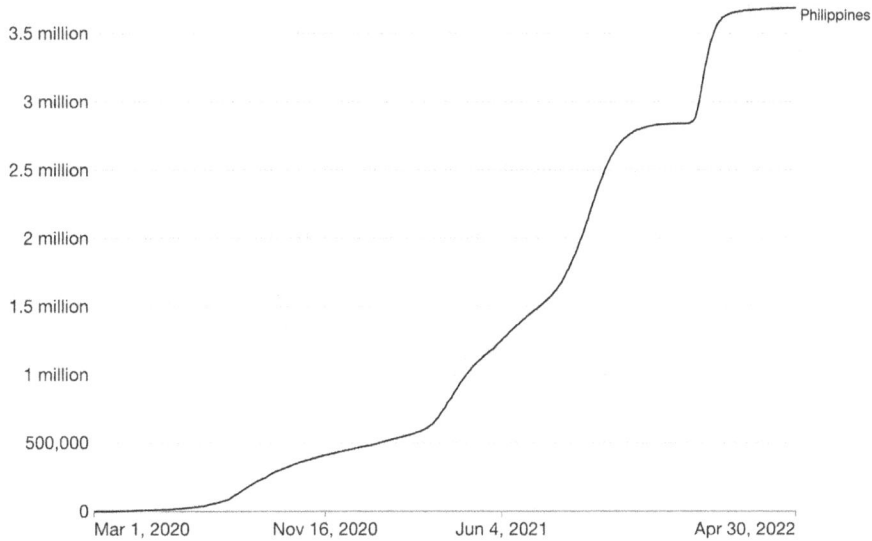

Figure 5.3 Cumulative confirmed COVID-19 cases (Philippines).

Source: Ritchie et al., 2020a (via Our World in Data).

of cases, largely because Vietnam, Malaysia, and Thailand have experienced recent case surges (Figure 5.4) and second in terms of confirmed COVID-19 deaths (Figure 5.5). While Singapore, and to a certain extent Thailand, have robust healthcare systems that enabled them to provide more immediate responses to the pandemic, countries like Indonesia and the Philippines lacked the adequate human resources and equipment to do so. The detection of new COVID-19 variants also hampered government initiatives to restore public health systems to normal. Specifically, two variants (Delta and Omicron) caused significant surges in the number of cases in late 2021 (Delta) and early 2022 (Omicron). The Omicron surge after the new year in 2022 prompted local authorities to enforce stricter protocols.

The emergence of these variants also coincided with the vaccination rollout in the country, an effort that commenced in March 2021. As of 11 May 2022, a total of 148 million doses had been administered—134.48 million initial protocol doses and 13.52 million booster doses (see Figure 5.6) (Ritchie et al. 2020b).

Vaccination efforts were not exempt from implementation challenges. Priority groups of eligible populations (DOH, 2021a) were initially identified for vaccination due to the inadequacy of vaccine supply. This grouping was based on the World Health Organization (WHO) Strategic Advisory Group of Experts on Immunization Values Framework for the Allocation and Prioritization of COVID-19 Vaccination, as well as on the national context, the epidemiologic settings, and the COVID-19 vaccine characteristics and supply (DOH, 2021b).

Historically, the Philippines has consistently had high vaccine confidence. However, the recent (2016–2017) Dengvaxia debacle—over Dengue fever vaccines that induced Dengue—eroded public trust and heightened vaccine hesitancy (Larson, Hartigan-Go, & de Figueiredo, 2018). A survey conducted by the Social Weather Stations (SWS) from 28 April to 2 May 2021 (about two months into the COVID vaccination rollout) indicated that while 51% of Filipinos trusted the government's assessment of the vaccines, only 32% were willing to be vaccinated (SWS, 2021), and the main reasons mentioned were fear of side effects and uncertainty about vaccine safety and efficacy.

Further, and perhaps associated with vaccine hesitancy, there was a notable brand preference for certain COVID-19 vaccines. SWS survey findings suggest that 63% of Filipinos prefer US-manufactured COVID-19 vaccines, while 19% prefer China-manufactured COVID-19 vaccines (Mendoza, 2021). The same survey, however, notes that slightly more (39%) specifically prefer China's Sinovac Biotech, while 33% prefer Pfizer BioNTech.

In response to vaccine brand preference, the DOH directed LGUs to only disclose the brand of COVID-19 vaccine to recipients who are already in the vaccination sites during their vaccination schedule (Abad, 2021b). This "brand agnostic" policy was seen as aligned with the DOH's message of "the best vaccine is the one that is available". Critics, however, pointed out that this policy might cause further vaccine hesitancy (Amit et al., 2022). In addition, the

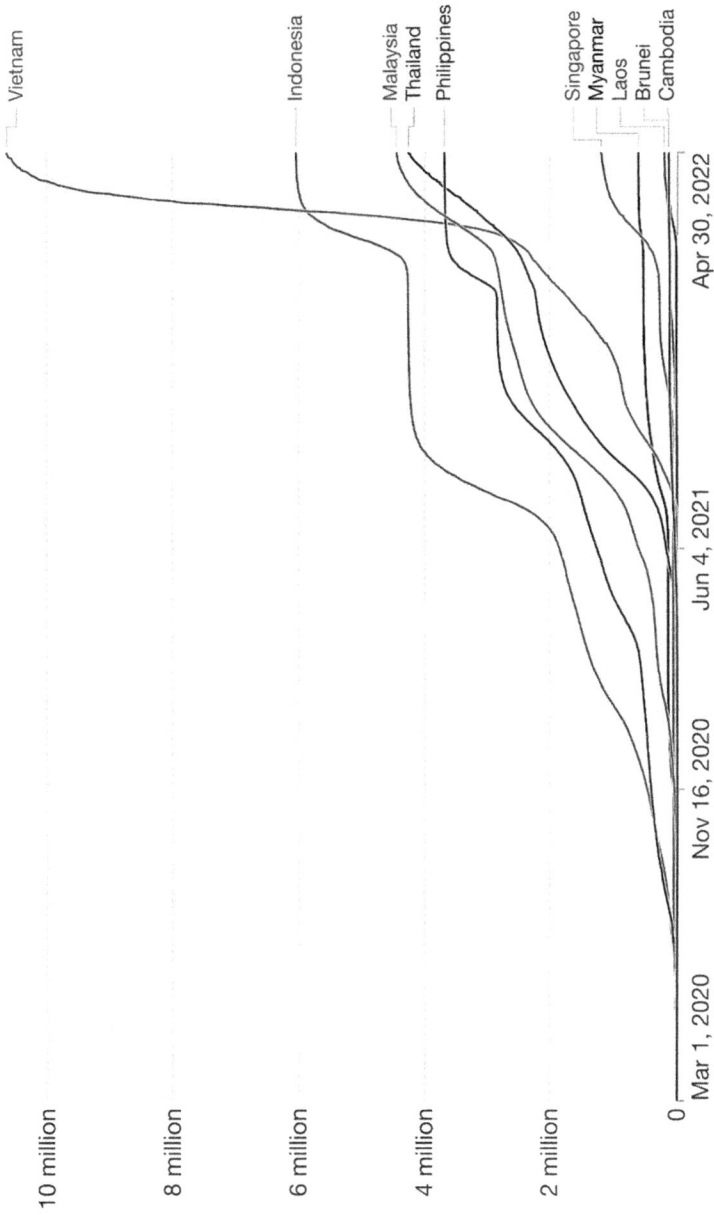

Figure 5.4 Cumulative confirmed COVID-19 cases (Southeast Asia) March 2020–April 2022.

Source: Ritchie et al., 2020a (via Our World in Data).

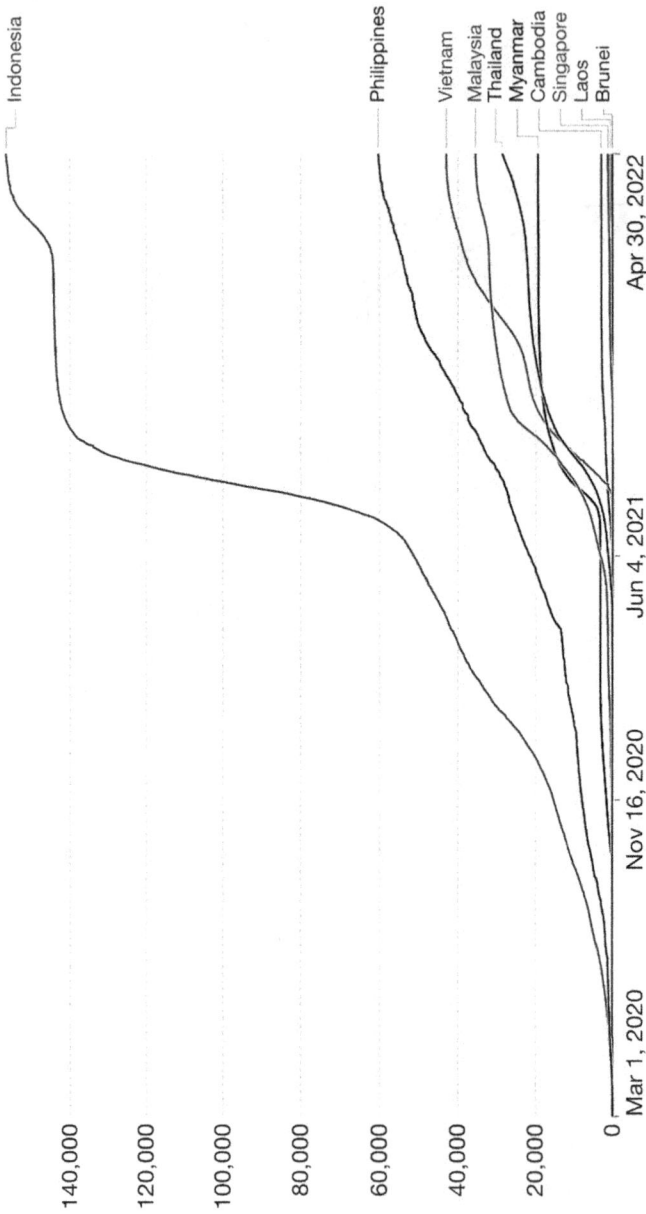

Figure 5.5 Cumulative confirmed COVID-19 deaths (Southeast Asia).

Source: Ritchie et al., 2020a (via Our World in Data).

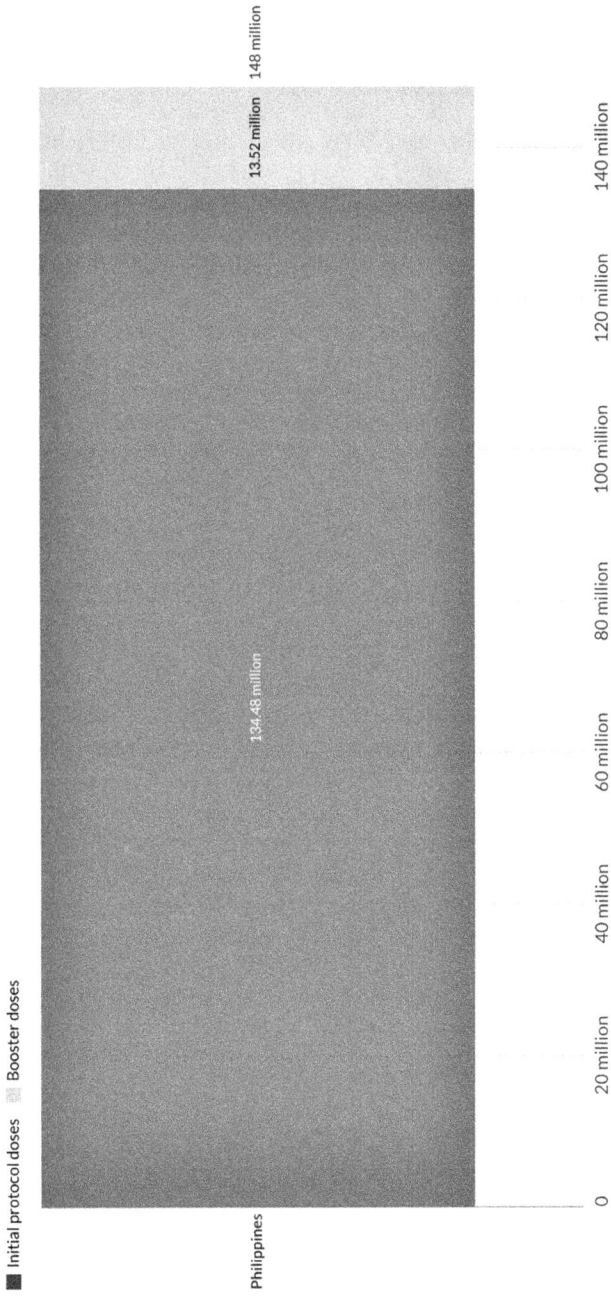

Figure 5.6 COVID-19 vaccination status (initial and booster doses).

Source: Ritchie et al., 2020b (via Our World in Data).

move was also seen as a potential violation of the principles of informed consent and patient autonomy (Aning, Cinco, and Chiu, 2021), and perceived as a curtailment of the patients' civil liberties.

Service delivery and access to medical commodities

Mobility restrictions posed considerable challenges in global health supply chain management, which "plays an important role in equitable access to essential medicines and services in low- and middle-income countries" (Ghaffar et al., 2021). Locally extended community quarantines resulted in widespread disruptions in healthcare delivery and accessibility of medical commodities, especially to geographically isolated and disadvantaged areas and communities. Mobility restrictions prevented clients from accessing health services and prevented health facilities from continuing to provide services.

The pandemic has also brought into focus the scarcity of health resources in the country. The national public health system struggled to cope with the continuous increase in cases due to a shortage of health professionals and underfinanced health infrastructure. The situation further exacerbated the government's limited capacity to conduct mass testing and systematic tracking, preventing quick identification and neutralising emerging disease hot spots. Several hospitals declared full bed capacity in their respective COVID-19 wards, while the lack of ventilators was also highlighted during the pandemic, prompting donations from various countries, including China and the United States. Furthermore, the increased demand for personal protective equipment (PPE) resulted in a general shortage, which further increased the vulnerability of health workers.

Several challenges in human resources for health also emerged due to the pandemic. According to the UP COVID-19 Pandemic Response Team (2020a: 5), "[T]here should ideally be one attending physician for every two patients, and one-on-one nursing, to handle critical cases". Additionally, "there should be one intensivist, pulmonologist, and infectious disease specialist for every five patients". However, data shows that there are only 3.7 doctors and 8.2 nurses per 10,000 population in the Philippines, far below the ratio of 1 doctor and nurse per 1,000 population prescribed by the WHO. The national ratio also varies widely by region (UP COVID-19 Pandemic Response Team (2020a)).

Most health workers were also diverted for the emergency response to the pandemic. As health workers were also at risk of contracting COVID-19, they often had to be apart from their families. The risk of COVID-19 exposure took a toll, not just in terms of health workers' physical health but also on their mental well-being.

Health information system

Inadequate health information and reporting delays worsened the situation. Data that is relevant, accurate, and, more importantly, timely, remains significant in pandemic management. However, data gaps and inconsistencies in DOH and LGU reporting often led to the public's confusion and anxiety (UP

COVID-19 Pandemic Response Team, 2020b). Furthermore, the proliferation of 'fake news' and misinformation also posed a challenge in changing the public's health behaviours in the context of the pandemic.

Health financing

The government likewise redirected financial resources to support the mitigation and control of COVID (DSWD, 2020). Apart from the 'Bayanihan to Heal as One Act'[4] (or *Bayanihan 1*), the Department of Finance (DOF) reported a total of US$25.8 billion in budgetary support, grants, and loan assistance from various international organisations (such as the Asian Development Bank, the World Bank, the US government, the Asian Infrastructure Investment Bank, among others) for COVID-19 response (DOF, 2022). Yet questions remain as to whether this budget is being spent appropriately, noting that the country has not seen improvements in testing, tracing, and treatment, despite the large amount allocated for the COVID-19 response.

Health governance

More importantly, the pandemic threatened the delay of implementation of Republic Act 11223 (or the 'Universal Health Care (UHC) Act'), an initiative much needed within the current context of the pandemic. The Philippine Health Insurance Corporation (PhilHealth) also noted the resulting deficit in funds because of the reduced payment capacities of its contributors. This deficit will not be felt until 2024 (Lozada, 2020; Aguilar, 2020). It is also estimated that in consideration of the pandemic, the UHC Act will now need at least three years for full implementation (Aguilar, 2020). In the Philippine Congress, many lawmakers opposed PhilHealth's statement and emphasised the benefits of a fully implemented UHC Act in times of public health crisis.

Socio-economic impacts

The COVID pandemic caused the Philippines' economic growth to contract. The −0.65% contraction in the first quarter of 2020 was followed by the more serious −16.98% in the second quarter. The economy continued to post negative growth in the following quarters, resulting in a −9.6% annual growth rate for 2020. The steep gross domestic product (GDP) decline in 2020 served to reverse the country's recent gains in poverty reduction. On average, around 26.14 million Filipinos now live below the poverty threshold, estimated at Philippines Pesos (PhP) ₱12,082 for a family of five per month in 2021 (Philippine Statistics Authority, 2021).

The economy started to recover in the second quarter of 2021, with positive growth rates in the succeeding quarters and up until the recently reported 8.3% growth in the first quarter of 2022 (Figure 5.7). Full recovery to 2019 GDP levels was expected to be achieved during 2022 (Philippine Statistics Authority, 2022).

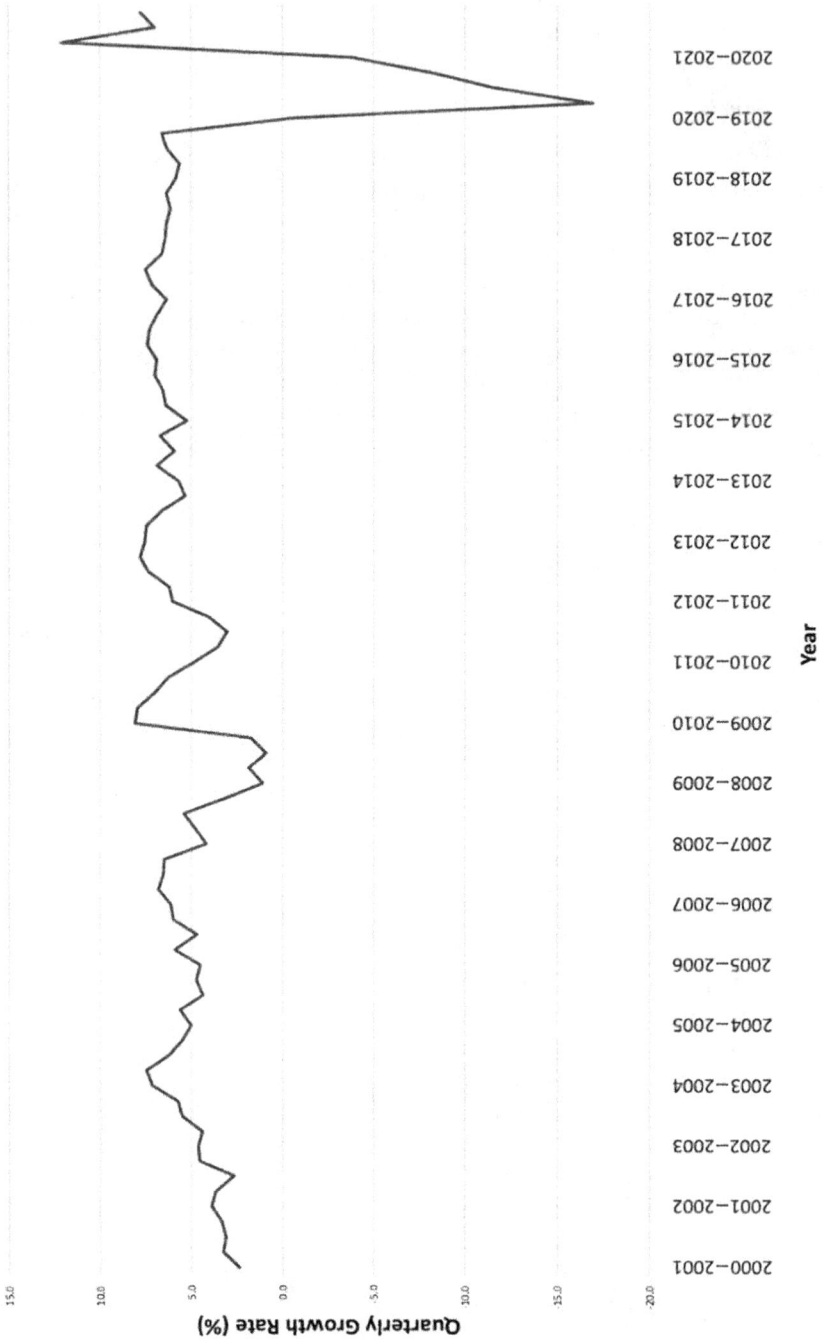

Figure 5.7 Quarterly GDP growth rate (2020–2021, in percentages).

Source: Philippine Statistics Authority, 2022.

The steepest drop in GDP growth happened in the second quarter of 2020, which coincided with the strictest lockdown. In this period, investment expenditures fell by 51.8%, imports by 37.2%, exports by 33.2%, and household consumption by 15.3%. Government expenditures however increased throughout the year, reflecting efforts to pump prime the economy to lessen the impact of the pandemic. In the second quarter of 2020, the services sector, which accounts for 60% of GDP, contracted by 17%, and the industrial sector, which comprises about 30% of GDP, declined by 21.7%. Only agriculture recorded an occasional low positive quarterly growth during the pandemic; however, this sector has had a record of dismal growth for the past two decades (Philippine Statistics Authority, 2022).

The economic figures are partly explained by the strict lockdowns. ECQs were designed to slow down the spread of COVID-19, but they also resulted in great hardship for those who lost their jobs and livelihoods due to mobility restrictions. The impact was felt strongly by individuals and households from highly affected sectors and even more so by those reliant on informal jobs and other non-regular forms of employment (Ducanes et al., 2021).

Due to lockdowns and social distancing measures, a significant share of the population became jobless or underemployed. The World Bank's Philippine Economic Update (Qian et al., 2020: 31–33), reported that the official unemployment rate went to a high of 17.6% in April 2020. Between October 2019 and October 2020, a staggering 2.7 million people lost their jobs. The services sector shed 1.9 million workers and the industry sector around 827,000 as community quarantine and operational capacity requirements were imposed by the government. A quarter of household heads who had a job in February 2020 were no longer working by August 2020. A large share of these remained jobless even after the government started easing restrictions (Qian et al., 2020: 31–33).

Government support programmes

In March 2020, right after the ECQ commenced, the Department of Trade and Industry (DTI) set up the Small Business Corporation with its ₱1 billion Enterprise Rehabilitation Financing facility under the *Pondo sa Pagbabago at Pagasenso*[5] (named COVID-19 P3-ERF) to support micro and small businesses affected, and to cushion the economic impact of the spread of COVID-19 virus in the country. The loan facility is open to micro and small enterprises with at least one-year continuous operation prior to March 2020 and whose businesses suffered "drastic reductions in sales"[6] during the ensuing epidemic. Depending on the asset size of enterprises, micro-enterprises may borrow from ₱10,000 to ₱200,000, while small enterprises may borrow a higher amount not exceeding ₱500,000 (DTI, 2020a). The DTI also issued a memorandum circular granting concession to commercial rents of Micro, Small, and Medium Enterprises ('MSMEs') (DTI, 2020b), a sector with a 99% share of all business enterprises in the country, and one which employs more than 5.4 million people or 63% of total employment in all business enterprises (DTI, 2020c) in the country.

The Philippines' central bank, *Bangko Sentral ng Pilipinas* (BSP), made policy issuances to ease the credit access of MSMEs. These are a combination of adjusting regulation in capital requirements in MSME exposure of financial institutions and reporting of non-performing loans. Overall, these measures are expected to channel liquidity directly to the MSME sector (Caliwan, 2020). Andal et al., however, assessed that MSMEs will be able to provide little help in alleviating the vulnerability of households to income loss during the pandemic (Andal et al., 2021: 244).

Using Philippine Statistics Authority (PSA) national accounts, the authors of this chapter have calculated the national government increased total expenditure by 10%, from 2.34 to ₱2.65 trillion between 2019 and 2020, with the largest increase in the second quarter. This further increased to ₱2.84 trillion in 2021. Like other states, the Philippine government has increased its total debt to ₱12.679 trillion, to bankroll the massive cost of the COVID-19 response, which is an increase in percentage terms from 39.6% of GDP to 63.5% of GDP by 2021. The secretary of the DOF said that the challenge of the new incoming administration of Ferdinand Marcos Jr. (beginning July 2022) is to reduce this debt with at least 6% annual GDP growth over the next five to six years. On monetary policy, the BSP has cut the cash lending rate several quarters in succession to stimulate growth, ultimately down to 2% by 2021. Overall, in 2020 the BSP injected ₱1.9 trillion (about US$39.2 billion) in liquidity into the financial system, equivalent to 9.6% of the country's GDP (Diokno, 2020). However, these monetary policies to ease liquidity in the financial system are seen as unsustainable in 2022–2023 with the increase of inflation brought about by world supply chain problems, the increase in oil and food prices due to the war in Ukraine, and the upward adjustment of policy rates in the United States.

By far the largest government spending to combat COVID was the SAP through the Bayanihan 1 and 2 Acts that were introduced to provide immediate relief to households affected by harsh community quarantine measures. Bayanihan 1 was implemented in April 2020 and grants the President sweeping powers to carry out necessary and proper measures to combat the transmission of the virus further. It mandated the realignment of ₱275 billion (US$5.37 billion) from the 2019 and 2020 national budgets, an act normally disallowed by law, to fund the SAP for vulnerable families. Additionally, Bayanihan 1 enforces provisions against price manipulation and profiteering. Other provisions include support programmes for workers affected by the pandemic, small businesses, and the agriculture sector, as well as augmented LGU resources through the *Bayanihan Grant* (Asian Development Bank, 2021). As Bayanihan 1 expired in June 2020, the government grappled with the potential repercussions of its expiry in implementing COVID-19 responses that the law is supposed to fund. Instead of extending the law's validity, the Philippine Congress worked on and passed new legislation to carry over the economic stimulus measures.

In September 2020, President Duterte signed Republic Act No. 11494 or the "Bayanihan to Recover as One Act" (*Bayanihan 2*) into law, augmenting the country's COVID-19 response fund with an additional ₱165.5 billion (US$3.4 billion) (Cervantes, 2020a). Bayanihan 2 allowed for the continuation of SAP distribution to vulnerable families, cash for work and employment programmes, and support for the agriculture sector and small businesses. It also allocated funds for the health, education, transport, and tourism sectors (Asian Development Bank, 2021). The just-in-time passage of these laws indicates the lack of planning in the state's management of COVID-19, a recurring pattern that was initially noted in the declaration of a health pandemic (Proclamation 922) only to be replaced by another declaration on the State of National Calamity, a week after (Proclamation 929).

As of December 2021, the Department of Budget and Management (DBM) has released a total of ₱602.15 billion (US$11.5 billion) pursuant to the provisions of the two Bayanihan laws (DBM, 2021). This amount is further augmented by appropriations worth ₱114.79 billion (US$2.2 billion) from the 2020 and 2021 national budgets (DBM, 2021). Of the ₱716.95 billion (US$13.69 billion) total funds, about ₱100.93 billion (US$1.9 billion) remains unspent, though ₱42.25 billion (US$806.9 million) of this total are unpaid obligations.

The DSWD led the implementation of the SAP in coordination with the Department of Interior and Local Government (DILG) and LGUs in the country. The SAP is in fact comprised of various schemes (See Table 5.2).

Aside from these payments, the DSWD also regularly provided food and non-food items (e.g., essential personal hygiene and household items).

The SAP's Emergency Subsidy Program (SAP-ESP) implementation attracted mixed responses, with the adequacy of the cash aid most questioned. For a large family living in Manila, where the average cost of living is relatively more expensive compared to its ASEAN counterparts (Simeon, 2021), a sum of ₱8,000.00 a month might not be enough. The SAP-ESP was however only ever supposed to cover two months, even though the ECQ restrictions held until mid-August 2020.

The scale of the SAP, which some commentators lauded (Cho, 2021), also became its weakness in the absence of a pandemic-responsive beneficiary

Table 5.1 Allotment and utilisation of funding sources for the Philippine COVID-19 response (in billions, as of 31 December 2021)

Funding source	Allotment (₱)	Utilised* (₱)	Unspent (₱)
Bayanihan 1	387.93	363.15	24.78
Bayanihan 2	214.22	195.64	18.58
FY 2020 and 2021 General Appropriations Act (GAA)	114.79	57.22	57.57
Total	716.95	616.02	100.93

Source: Department of Budget and Management (2021).

* Based on disbursements. Obligations not included.

Table 5.2 Selected schemes under the SAP implementation of the DSWD

Scheme	Description
Emergency Subsidy Program (ESP)	emergency subsidy to low-income households, amounting to ₱5,000.00–₱8,000.00 a month for two months (April and May 2020) to cover for basic food, medicine, toiletries, and other basic necessities of affected household beneficiaries
Assistance to Individuals in Crisis Situation (AICS)[7]	₱3,000.00 is provided to families with at least one member, or ₱5,000 to families with two or more members of vulnerable or disadvantaged sectors (This includes senior citizens, persons with disability (PWDs), pregnant and lactating women, solo parents, OFWs in distress, indigent IPs, underprivileged sector and homeless citizens, and informal economy workers.) to assist them in providing the basic needs of their families
	families with deceased indigent COVID-19 confirmed cases and PUIs were also granted a cash aid of PHP 25,000 per deceased person to cover burial expenses
Livelihood Assistance Grants (LAG)	provided to assist in the economic recovery and rehabilitation of the beneficiaries of DWSD's Sustainable Livelihood Program (SLP) whose livelihoods were affected by the pandemic
	maximum of ₱15,000, in the form of cash orindividual check, may be given provided that at least one member is a displaced informal economy worker (A family is only qualified to avail of the assistance under the LAG only once.)
Social Pension for Indigent Senior Citizens Program (SocPen)	a monthly stipend in the amount of ₱500.00 provided to eligible senior citizens to assist in providing their basic needs such as food and medicines, among others
Expanded and Enhanced Pantawid Pamilyang PilipinoProgram (4Ps)	provision of assistance in cash or non-cash, to families who have no incomes or savings to draw from, including families working in the informal economy and those who are not currently recipients of the current 4Ps, which amount should be adequate to restore their capacity to purchase basic food and other essential items during the duration of the quarantine

Source: DSWD Memorandum Circular No. 04, Series of 2020; Reyes et al., 2020.

targeting system (Gudmalin et al., 2021; Aceron, 2020). The DSWD used the National Household Targeting System for Poverty Reduction (NHTS-PR) or *Listahanan 2015*[8] to identify its target beneficiaries for the SAP-ESP (Reyes et al., 2020). The same list was used to identify the beneficiaries of the 4Ps programme. However, it was not used for non-4Ps beneficiaries who are eligible to receive SAP-ESP,[9] who comprised 75% of target beneficiaries for the first tranche (Dadap-Cantal et al, 2020). During the SAP distribution, it was discovered that the list contained 675,933 duplicate names (already part of other government cash-aid programmes) and 239,859 ineligible beneficiaries (Cudis, 2020). Because of this, the DSWD had to undergo a validation and deduplication process before releasing the second tranche of the SAP-ESP (Lalu, 2020; Mateo, 2020; Cervantes, 2020b).

Mobility restrictions and health protocols, while necessary in the time of a pandemic, also resulted in delays in SAP distribution (Pedrosa, 2020; Cervantes, 2020b; Cortez, 2020). The allure of cash distributions at a precarious time in people's lives resulted in packed and overcrowded distribution venues and a neglect of physical distancing rules (Malasig, 2020; Pedrajas, 2020a), some of which led to suspension of the payout (Kabagani, 2021) and even to death (Masculino, 2020; Pedrajas, 2020b). Scarce supplies of PPE meant health and security considerations for SAP distributors and implementers were considered paramount. Thus, while the SAP-ESP was initially scheduled to be distributed in April and May 2020, neither the first nor the second tranches of the cash aid had been completed by November 2020 (Reyes et al., 2020). Implementers who contracted COVID-19 were required to undergo a 14-day quarantine, which affected the SAP distribution. These delays also had repercussions in terms of reach, especially for those living in rural and remote areas.

Administrative concerns related to coordination between national and local governments (Reyes et al., 2020) also posed challenges in SAP implementation. Dissonant messages between the two in terms of the delivery mechanisms of the SAP led to public confusion, exasperation, and misinformation (Aceron, 2020). The pandemic also constrained effective communication between the national government (whose policy decisions impacted subnational agencies) and LGUs that managed local SAP distribution. The monitoring, reporting, and auditing of fund disbursements (Gudmalin et al., 2021) also necessitated close coordination between the two but proved to be arduous as field offices at the local level found it difficult to give real-time feedback to the national government.

Issues of politicking and corruption also plagued the SAP implementation as local governments were tasked to disburse the first tranche (under the supervision of the DSWD). In fact, in September 2020, anomalies in the SAP-ESP distribution caused the Office of the Ombudsman to suspend 89 *barangay* (village, district, or ward)[10] chiefs (Rappler.com, 2020). For the SAP-ESP implementation, as mentioned earlier, beneficiary targeting relied on (1) the NHTS-PR for those who were already 4Ps beneficiaries (25% of the target beneficiaries of the SAP-ESP) and (2) local government listings based on Social Amelioration Cards (SACs) distributed to non-4Ps families. Thus, to some extent, the SAP-ESP allowed for the discretionary allocation of funding, a move that appears to have encouraged political clientelism, patronage, and '*palakasan*'—"assertion of personal interest via *lakas* (power or strength) while subtly bypassing prescribed rules and procedures" (Eadie 2022; Abad, 2021a).

Conclusion

This chapter has examined the different political, health, and socio-economic aspects of the COVID-19 pandemic. The over-reliance on the uniformed sector by the Duterte Administration is a confluence of many factors. The securitisation of a broad public concern such as COVID-19 is a natural extension of the administration's attempts to securitise populist issues, such as the War on Drugs. This strategy makes perfect sense given the inadequacy of the government to respond holistically to the problems brought about by the pandemic. Thus, the use of uniformed men, specifically the PNP, was the strategy adopted by the administration of President Duterte to portray an image of invincibility amidst the crisis brought on by the COVID-19 pandemic (Agojo, 2021).

The pandemic highlighted the pitfalls and shortcomings of an already fragmented health system, as seen in the inadequate capacities to weather disruptions in ensuring continuous service and medical commodity delivery, the insufficiency of human resources for health, and the insufficient reliable and accurate health data. The surge of COVID-19 incidents during the initial phase of the pandemic overwhelmed COVID-19 testing centres, hospitals, and health personnel.

Instead of exploring a more geographically and culturally nuanced COVID-19 management approach, the country followed the bandwagon of those states using a more technocratic-authoritarian governance approach. This approach is problematic, as the expansion of state powers is somehow normalised as part of the everyday lives of Filipinos. As the county's history has proven, pushing back against the military sector or an authoritarian regime passing itself off as a populist regime may be difficult to reverse once it has taken a foothold in the consciousness of Filipinos.

Notes

1 Members include representatives from Department of the Interior and Local Government (DILG), Department of Foreign Affairs (DFA), Department of Justice (DOJ), Department of Labor and Employment (DOLE), Department of Transportation (DOTr), Department of Information and Communications Technology (DICT), and Department of Tourism (DOT).
2 The NTF is headed by Secretary Delfin Lorenzana of the Department of National Defense (DND), assisted by the Department of Interior and Local Government (DILG) Secretary Eduardo Ano, and Peace Process Adviser Carlito Galvez as the chief implementer (Agojo, 2021).
3 The ASEAN was founded in 1967 by Indonesia, Malaysia, Singapore, the Philippines, and Thailand. It has since expanded its membership to include Brunei (1984), Vietnam (1995), Myanmar and Lao People's Democratic Republic (1997), and Cambodia (1999).
4 Bayanihan is a Filipino value roughly translating to the "spirit of cooperation" or "solidarity".
5 The Filipino phrase literally translates to "Funds for Change and Progress".
6 There were no specific definitions in terms of figures to further qualify this in the DTI sources encountered by the authors.

7 Recipients of DOLE programs (e.g. Tulong Panghanapbuhay sa Ating Displaced Disadvantaged Workers or TUPAD and COVID-19 Adjustment Measures Program or CAMP) and other social assistance programs by the national government are not eligible for AICS.
8 'The Filipino word "listahan" literally translates to "list".
9 Families eligible for the 4Ps are included in the SAP-ESP implementation via a top-up to the amount that they regularly receive.
10 A barangay is the smallest administrative unit in the Philippines. There are over 42,000 barangays in the Philippines.

References

Abad, M. (2021a, April 8). 'What Went Wrong in 2020 COVID-19 'Ayuda,' Lessons Learned for 2021', *Rappler.com*. Available: https://www.rappler.com/newsbreak/explainers/coronavirus-ayuda-government-aid-what-went-wrong-2020-lessons-learned-2021/ [Viewed: 6 May 2022].

Abad, M. (2021b, May 22). 'DOH: Brand Preferences Have Affected COVID-19 Vaccine Hesitancy', *Rappler.com*. Available: https://www.rappler.com/nation/doh-says-brand-preferences-have-affected-covid-19-vaccine-hesitancy/ [Viewed: 6 May 2022]

Aceron, J. (2020, April 2). '[ANALYSIS] Challenges Facing Social Amelioration for the Coronavirus', *Rappler.com*. Available: https://www.rappler.com/voices/thought-leaders/256782-analysis-challenges-government-social-amelioration-coronavirus/ [Viewed: 5 May 2022].

Agojo, K. (2021). 'Policing a Pandemic: Understanding the State and Political Instrumentalization of the Coercive Apparatus in Duterte's Philippines', *Journal of Developing Societies*, 37(3), pp. 363–386, Available: https://doi.org/10.1177/0169796X21996832 [Viewed: 3 May 2022].

Aguilar, K. (2020, June 19). 'PhilHealth: UHC Law Seen to Be Implemented by mid-2021', *Inquirer.net*. Available: https://newsinfo.inquirer.net/1294172/fwd-philhealth-uhc-law-seen-to-be-implemented-by-mid-2021#ixzz6nX1jN3fd [Viewed: 4 March 2022].

Althusser, L. (1971). 'Ideology and Ideological State Apparatuses (Notes towards an Investigation)'. In *Lenin and Philosophy and Other Essays*, Monthly Review Press, New York, pp. 127–186.

Amit, A.M.L., Pepito, V. C. F., Sumpaico-Tanchanco, L.., and Dayrit, M. M. (2022). 'COVID-19 Vaccine Brand Hesitancy and Other Challenges to Vaccination in the Philippines,' *PLOS Glob Public Health* 2(1), Available: https://doi.org/10.1371/journal.pgph.0000165 [Viewed: 6 May 2022].

Andal, E.G., Bello, A., and Catelo, M.A. (2021). 'Coping Strategies of Selected MSMEs in Laguna One Year after COVID-19,' *The Philippine Economic Review* 58 (1&2), pp. 241–263, Available: https://doi.org/10.37907/10ERP1202JD [Viewed: 3 May 2022].

Aning, J., Cinco, M., and Chiu, P.D.M. (2021, May 20). "Brand Agnostic' Vaccination Eyed after Big Pfizer Crowd,' *Inquirer.net*. Available: https://newsinfo.inquirer.net/1434045/brand-agnostic-vaccination-eyed-after-big-pfizer-crowd [Viewed: 14 May 2022].

Asian Development Bank. (2021, February). Project Number: 54138-001, Republic of the Philippines: COVID-19 Active Response and Expenditure Support Program, *Monitoring Report* (July–December 2020), https://www.adb.org/sites/default/files/project-documents/54138/54138-001-dpta-en.pdf.

Bargu, B. (2019). 'Police Power: The Biopolitical State Apparatus and Differential Interpellations', *Rethinking Marxism: A Journal of Economics, Culture & Society*, 31(3), pp. 291–317, Available: https://doi.org/10.1080/08935696.2019.162919 6 [Viewed: 3 May 2022].

Caliwan, C. (2020, June 18). 'PNP All Set to Secure Distribution of SAP 2nd Tranche', *Philippine News Agency*. Available: https://www.pna.gov.ph/articles/1106252 [Viewed: 6 May 2022].

Cervantes, F. (2020a, September 11). 'Duterte Signs P165.5-B Bayanihan 2 Law', *Philippine News Agency*. Available: https://www.pna.gov.ph/articles/1115210 [Viewed: 5 May 2022].

Cervantes, F. (2020b, June 22). 'Stringent Validation Causes Delay in SAP Distribution: DSWD', *Philippine News Agency*. Available: https://www.pna.gov.ph/articles/1106665 [Viewed: 5 May 2022].

Chen, L.-L. (2020, May 13). 'Human Rights and Democracy Amidst Militarized COVID-19 Responses in Southeast Asia', International Relations, URL: https://www.e-ir.info/2020/05/13/human-rights-and-democracy-amidst-militarized-covid-19-responses-in-southeast-asia/.

Cho, Y. (2021). 'Realizing the "Transformational Trilogy" of Social Protection Delivery in the Philippines', *World Bank Blogs*. Available: https://blogs.worldbank.org/eastasiapacific/realizing-transformational-trilogy-social-protection-delivery-philippines [Viewed: 5 May 2022].

Cortez, K. (2020, August 26). 'Councilor Calls Out Lapses in Distancing during SAP Distribution', *Davao Today*. Available: http://davaotoday.com/main/politics/councilor-calls-out-lapses-in-distancing-during-sap-distribution/ [Viewed: 6 May 2022].

Cudis, C. (2020, December 7). '14.2-M Beneficiaries Get SAP 2 Aid: DSWD', *Philippine News Agency*. Available: https://www.pna.gov.ph/articles/1123981 [Viewed: 5 May 2022].

Dadap-Cantal, E., Fisher, A., and Ramos, C. (2020). 'Ephemeral Universalism in the Social Protection Response to the COVID-19 Lockdown in the Philippines', *ISS Blog on Global Development and Social Justice*. Available: https://issblog.nl/2020/06/26/covid-19-ephemeral-universalism-in-the-social-protection-response-to-the-covid-19-lockdown-in-the-philippines/ [Viewed: 5 May 2022].

Department of Budget and Management (DBM). (2021). 'COVID-19 Budget Utilization Reports as of December 31, 2021 (Summary Report)', Available: https://www.dbm.gov.ph/index.php/programs-projects/status-of-covid-19-releases#summary-report [Viewed: 5 May 2022].

Department of Finance (DOF). (2022). 'Financing Secured for COVID-19 Response (as of January 14, 2022)', Available: https://www.dof.gov.ph/data/fin-agreements/ [Viewed: 20 June 2022].

Department of Health (DOH). (2021a). 'Who Will Be Vaccinated First?' Available: https://doh.gov.ph/node/28118 [Viewed: 28 April 2022].

Department of Health (DOH). (2021b). 'The Philippine National Deployment and Vaccination Plan for COVID-19 Vaccines'. Available: https://doh.gov.ph/sites/default/files/basic-page/The%20Philippine%20National%20COVID-19%20Vaccination%20Deployment%20Plan.pdf [Viewed: 28 April 2022].

Department of Interior and Local Government (DILG). (2020). 'DILG to PNP: Probe and Arrest Corrupt Local Officials in SAP Distribution'. Available: https://dilg.gov.ph/news/DILG-to-PNP-Probe-and-arrest-corrupt-local-officials-in-SAP-distribution/NC-2020-1134?fbclid=IwAR1bnkZ52NHK5_5zJR0wjvPY53_1XEN BUpW-y6ReAdZBTTTc0mt2iblr15U [Viewed: 3].

Department of Social Welfare and Development (DSWD). (2020). 'DSDW Memorandum Circular No. 04, Series of 2020: Special Guidelines on the Provision Amelioration Measures by the Department of Social Welfare and Development to the Most Affected Residents of the Areas Under Community Quarantine and Continuation of the Implementation of the Social Pension for Indigent Senior Citizens and the Supplementary Feeding Programs'. Available: https://www.dswd.gov.ph/issuances/MCs/MC_2020-004.pdf [Viewed: 5 May 2022].

Department of Trade and Industry (DTI). (2020a). 'SB Corporation Opens P1B Loan Facility for MSMEs Affected by COVID-19 Lockdown'. Available: https://www.dti.gov.ph/archives/news-archives/sbcorp-loan-facility-covid-affected-msmes/ [Viewed: 4 May 2022].

Department of Trade and Industry (DTI). (2020b). 'DTI Memorandum Circular 20-12: Guidelines on the Concessions on Residential Rents; Commercial Rents of MSMEs'. Available: https://www.dti.gov.ph/archives/advisories-archives/mc2012 [Viewed: 4 May 2022].

Department of Trade and Industry (DTI). (2020c). '2020 MSME STATISTIC'. Available: https://www.dti.gov.ph/resources/msme-statistics [Viewed: 4 May 2022].

Diokno, B. (2020, October 14). Moody's Credit Rating Call [Speech Transcript]. Bangko Sentral ng Pilipinas, https://www.bsp.gov.ph/SitePages/MediaAndResearch/SpeechesDisp.aspx?ItemId=756.

Dizon, N. (2020, July 31). 'Duterte and His Generals: A Shock and Awe Response to the Pandemic', *Rappler.com*. Available: https://www.rappler.com/newsbreak/in-depth/duterte-shock-and-awe-coronavirus-pandemic-response-generals [Viewed: 2 May 2022].

Ducanes, G., Daway-Ducanes, S.L., and Tan, E. (2021). Targeting the Highly Vulnerable Households during Strict Lockdowns. *Philippine Review of Economics*, 58(1&2), pp. 38–62.

Eadie, P. (2022, January 21). 'COVID-19, Palakasan and the Culture of Clientelism in the Philippines', *New Mandala*. Available: https://www.newmandala.org/covid19-palakasan-and-the-culture-of-clientelism-in-the-philippines [Viewed: 6 May 2022].

Engels, M. (2020). 'Ten Theses on the Coronavirus for the State and Society', *Global Solutions Initiative*. Available: https://www.global-solutions-initiative.org/press-news/ten-theses-coronavirus-state-society [Viewed: 14 May 2022].

Ghaffar, A., Rashidian, A., Khan, W. et al. (2021). 'Verbalising Importance of Supply Chain Management in Access to Health Services', *Journal of Pharmaceutical Policy and Practice* 14(91). Available: https://doi.org/10.1186/s40545-021-00352-5 [Viewed: 3 May 2022].

Gibson-Fall, F. (2021). 'Military Responses to COVID-19, Emerging Trends in Global Civil-Military Engagements', *Review of International Studies*, 47(2), pp. 155–170. Available: https://doi.org/10.1017/S0260210521000048 [Viewed: 6 May 2022].

Gita-Carlos, R. (2020, May 21). 'Palace Says AFP, PNP to Speed Up SAP Aid Distribution,' *Philippine News Agency*. Available: https://www.pna.gov.ph/articles/1103572 [Viewed: 6 May 2022].

Gudmalin, C., Perante-Calina, L., Balbosa, J., Mangahas, J., and Samoza, M. (2021). 'ADBI Development Case Study No. 2021-3: Protecting the Poor and Vulnerable against the Pandemic', *Asian Development Bank Institute*. Available: https://www.adb.org/sites/default/files/publication/736446/adbi-cs2021-03.pdf [Viewed: 5 May 2022].

Hapal, K. (2021). "'The Philippines' COVID-19 Response: Securitising the Pandemic and Disciplining the Pasaway", *Journal of Current Southeast Asian Affairs*, 40(2), pp. 224–244. Available: https://doi.org/10.1177/1868103421994261 [Viewed: 3 May 2022].

Imbong, R. (2022). 'Police Power in the Philippines in the Time of the Pandemic', *Rethinking Marxism: A Journal of Economics, Culture & Society*. Available: https://doi.org/10.1080/08935696.2022.2043721 [Viewed: 6 May 2022].

Inquirer.net. (2020, April 1). *(FULL VIDEO) Duterte Addresses the Nation* [online video]. Available: https://www.youtube.com/watch?v=RDT0PkERGlM&ab_channel=INQUIRER.net [Viewed: 20 June 2022].

Jensen, S. and Hapal, K. (2018). 'Police Violence and Corruption in the Philippines: Violent Exchange and the War on Drugs', *Journal of Current Southeast Asian Affairs*, 37(2), pp. 39–62. Available: https://doi.org/10.1177/186810341803700202 [Viewed: 2 May 2022].

Kabagani, L. (2021, April 13). 'Overcrowding Suspends 'Ayuda' Payout in Taguig Village', *Philippine News Agency*. Available: https://www.pna.gov.ph/articles/1136662 [Viewed: 6 May 2022].

Lalu, G. (2020, June 9). 'Over 3,700 Beneficiaries Have Returned Cash Aid Due to Duplication – DSWD', *Inquirer.net*. Available: https://newsinfo.inquirer.net/1288350/over-3700-beneficiaries-have-returned-cash-aid-due-to-duplication-dswd#ixzz7TL9pduoE [Viewed: 5 May 2022].

Larson, H., Hartigan-Go, K., and de Figueiredo, A. (2018). 'Vaccine Confidence Plummets in the Philippines Following Dengue Vaccine Scare: Why It Matters to Pandemic Preparedness', *Human Vaccines & Immunotherapeutics* 15(3), pp. 625–627, Available: https://doi.org/10.1080/21645515.2018.1522468 [Viewed: 14 May 2022]

Lozada, B. (2020, June 17). 'Delay in UHC Implementation a Step in the Wrong Direction, Says Drilon', *Inquirer.net*. Available: https://newsinfo.inquirer.net/1293106/delay-in-uhc-implementation-a-step-in-the-wrong-direction-says-drilon#ixzz6nX1wNFmF [Viewed: 4 March 2022].

Malasig, J. (2020, May 11). 'Captured: These Photos Show How Social Distancing Rules Were Broken in Queues for Gov't Cash Aid, Orders for Mother's Day', *Interaksyon*. Available: https://interaksyon.philstar.com/politics-issues/2020/05/11/168179/captured-these-photos-show-how-social-distancing-rules-were-broken-in-queues-for-govt-cash-aid-orders-for-mothers-day [Viewed: 5 May 2022].

Maru, D. (2020, July 22). "'F as in Falfak": PH Gov't Gets Failing Marks in COVID-19 Response from These Experts', *ABS-CBN News*. Available: https://news.abs-cbn.com/news/07/22/20/f-as-in-falfak-ph-govt-gets-failing-marks-in-covid-19-response-from-these-experts [Viewed: 15 May 2022].

Masculino, G. (2020, July 25). 'Senior Citizen, 87, Dies while Waiting for SAP Allowance', *Daily Guardian*. Available: https://dailyguardian.com.ph/senior-citizen-87-dies-while-waiting-for-sap-allowance [Viewed: 6 May 2022].

Mateo, J. (2020, August 5). '3 Million Delisted from Cash Aid List', *PhilStar Global*. Available: https://www.philstar.com/headlines/2020/08/05/2033025/3-million-delisted-cash-aid-list [Viewed: 5 May 2022].

Mendoza, J.E. (2021, May 24). 'Most Filipinos Prefer US as Source of Anti-COVID vaccine,' *Inquirer.net*. Available: https://newsinfo.inquirer.net/1436038/most-filipinos-prefer-us-as-source-of-anti-covid-vaccine [Viewed: 14 May 2022]

Migdal, J. (2001). *State in Society: Studying How States and Societies Transform and Constitute One Another*, Cambridge University Press, Cambridge.

Olanday, D. and Rigby, J. (2020, July 11). 'Inside the World's Longest and Strictest Coronavirus Lockdown in the Philippines', *The Telegraph*. Available: https://www.telegraph.co.uk/global-health/science-and-disease/inside-worlds-longest-strictest-coronavirus-lockdown-philippines [Viewed: 2 May 2022].

Pedrajas, J. (2020a, May 7). 'Residents of Bagong Silang in Caloocan Are Still Stuck in Lines Waiting for DSWD SAP Payouts from Barangay Officials', *Manila Bulletin*. Available: https://mb.com.ph/2020/05/07/residents-of-bagong-silang-in-caloocan-are-still-stuck-in-lines-waiting-for-dswd-sap-payouts-from-barangay-officials [Viewed: 6 May 2022].

Pedrajas, J. (2020b, July 3). 'Woman Dies while Waiting in Line for Cash Aid', *Manila Bulletin*. Available: https://mb.com.ph/2020/07/03/woman-dies-while-waiting-in-line-for-cash-aid [Viewed: 6 May 2022].

Pedrosa, M. (2020, July 24). 'Bacolod Barangays Told to Stop SAP distribution if Health Protocols Are Not Met', *SunStar Bacolod*. Available: https://www.sunstar.com.ph/article/1864719/bacolod/local-news/bacolod-barangays-told-to-stop-sap-distribution-if-health-protocols-are-not-met [Viewed: 6 May 2022].

Philippine Statistics Authority (PSA). (2021). 'Proportion of Poor Filipinos Registered at 23.7 Percent in the First Semester of 2021'. Available: https://psa.gov.ph/content/proportion-poor-filipinos-registered-237-percent-first-semester-2021 [Viewed: 2 May 2022].

Philippine Statistics Authority. (2022). 'Quarterly National Accounts Linked Series (Q1 2000 to Q1 2022)'. Available: https://psa.gov.ph/national-accounts/base-2018/data-series [Viewed: 2 May 2022].

Proclamation No. 922. (2020, March 8). Declaring a State of Public Health Emergency Throughout the Philippines. https://www.officialgazette.gov.ph/downloads/2020/02feb/20200308-PROC-922-RRD-1.pdf

Proclamation No. 929. (2020, March 16). Declaring a State of Calamity throughout the Philippines due to Corona Virus Disease 2019. https://www.officialgazette.gov.ph/downloads/2020/03mar/20200316-PROC-929-RRD.pdf.

Proclamation No. 1021. (2020, September 16). Extending the Period of the State of Calamity throughout the Philippines due to Corona Virus Disease 2019 Declared under Proclamation No. 929, S. 2020. https://lawphil.net/executive/proc/proc2020/proc_1021_2020.html

Proclamation No. 1028. (12 September 2022). https://www.officialgazette.gov.ph/downloads/2022/09sep/20220912-PROC-57-FRM.pdf

Qian, R., Chua, K.C., Cruz, K.T.G., Enriquez, K.A.L., Marohombsar, Z., Santos, E.R., Endo, I. L., Belghith, N.B.H., Piza, S.F.A., Cho, Y., Rodriguez, R.R., Kawasoe, Y., Zapanta, A.M.F.S., Signer, B.L., Cordero, L.J.Y., Skalon, T., and Borja, F.B.B. (2020). 'Philippines Economic Update: Building a Resilient Recovery (English),' *World Bank Group*. Available: http://documents.worldbank.org/curated/en/983051607354214738/Philippines-Economic-Update-Building-a-Resilient-Recovery [Viewed: 7 May 2022].

Rappler.com. (2020, September 12). 'Ombudsman Suspends 89 Barangay Chiefs over Alleged Emergency Subsidy Anomalies', *Rappler.com*. Available: https://www.rappler.com/nation/ombudsman-suspends-89-barangay-chiefs-over-alleged-emergency-subsidy-anomalies [Viewed: 6 May 2022].

Republic Act 11469: Bayanihan to Heal as One Act (2020).

Republic Act 11494: Bayanihan to Recover as One Act (2020).

Republic Act No. 11223: Universal Health Care Act (2019).

Reyes, C., Asis, R. A., Arboneda, A., and Vargas, A. (2020). 'Discussion Paper Series No. 2020-55: Mitigating the Impact of COVID-19 Pandemic on Poverty', *Philippine Institute for Development Studies*. Available: https://pidswebs.pids.gov.ph/CDN/PUBLICATIONS/pidsdps2055.pdf [Viewed: 5 May 2022].

Ritchie, H., Mathieu, E., Rodés-Guirao, L., Appel, C., Giattino, C., Ortiz-Ospina, E., Hasell, J., Macdonald, B., Beltekian, D., and Roser, M.. (2020a). 'Coronavirus Pandemic (COVID-19)'. Available: https://ourworldindata.org/coronavirus [Viewed: 2 May 2022].

Ritchie, H., Mathieu, E., Rodés-Guirao, L., Appel, C., Giattino, C., Ortiz-Ospina, E., Hasell, J., Macdonald, B., Beltekian, D., and Roser, M. (2020b). 'A Global Database of COVID-19 Vaccinations', Available: https://ourworldindata.org/covid-vaccinations [Viewed: 2 May 2022].

Simeon, L. (2021, April 23). 'Manila 3rd Most Expensive City to Live in ASEAN', *PhilStar Global*. Available: https://www.philstar.com/business/2021/04/23/2093042/manila-3rd-most-expensive-city-live-asean [Viewed: 6 May 2022].

Social Weather Stations (SWS). (2021, May 20). 'First Quarter 2021 Social Weather Survey: 51% of Adult Filipinos Are Confident, 17% Are Not Confident about the Government's Evaluation of Covid-19 Vaccines,' *Social Weather Stations*. Available: https://www.sws.org.ph/swsmain/artcldisppage/?artcsyscode=ART-20210520103851 [Viewed: 7 May 2022]

UP COVID-19 Pandemic Response Team. (2020a). 'Estimating Local Healthcare Capacity to Deal with COVID-19 Case Surge: Analysis and Recommendations', *University of the Philippines*. Available: https://up.edu.ph/estimating-local-healthcare-capacity-to-deal-with-covid-19-case-surge-analysis-and-recommendations [Viewed: 6 May 2022].

UP COVID-19 Pandemic Response Team. (2020b). 'Prevailing Data Issues in the Time of COVID-19 and the Need for Open Data', *University of the Philippines*. Available: https://up.edu.ph/prevailing-data-issues-in-the-time-of-covid-19-and-the-need-for-open-data [Viewed: 7 March 2022].

6 Vietnam

COVID-19 in Vietnam

Toan Dang

Introduction

When the COVID-19 pandemic first broke out in China in late December 2019, Vietnamese government leaders and ordinary citizens considered that Vietnam would be the most vulnerable country due to its proximity and trade links with China (Duong et al. 2020). Managing the pandemic has indeed tested the capacity of Vietnam's healthcare system and leadership, and since the pandemic began, Vietnam has undergone four waves of COVID-19 infections, with each affecting the country's social to economic spheres (Minh et al. 2021; Nguyen T.C.Y. et al. 2021: 1304).

This chapter will outline Vietnam's experience with COVID, focussing on the non-pharmaceutical response that initially produced excellent containment, in particular a high level of coordination. It then moves to explore the rollout of vaccines and other medicines before discussing the delicate balance between individual rights and community safety. The chapter argues that while certain features of Vietnam's COVID response hark back to its recent war history, its attitude towards Chinese-produced vaccines is related to a longer and more complex relationship with China.

The four waves of COVID in Vietnam

The first wave of COVID broke out in Vietnam on 23 January 2020 (Bouchnita et al. 2021) and a week later the Vietnamese government declared it viewed COVID-19 as a national emergency (Nguyen L.H. et al. 2021), which was one month before the World Health Organization (WHO) declared COIVD a global pandemic (Le et al. 2020). The government imposed the first nationwide lockdown between 1–15 April 2020 (Duong et al. 2020) and announced the end of the first wave on 16 April 2020. By then, Vietnam had recorded a total of 100 positive cases for COVID-19, and no deaths (Minh et al. 2021). The country then enjoyed 99 days without any locally transmitted cases before the second wave broke out in Vietnam's biggest tourist destination, Da Nang, on 25 July 2020 (Vuong et al. 2021). By the declared end of the second wave on 1 December 2020, Vietnam had a total of 554 cases of community

DOI: 10.4324/9781003311522-6

transmission, and 35 deaths (Minh et al. 2021). A month later, the country was hit hard by a third wave, which commenced on 28 January 2021. This time, the pandemic occurred in the northern province of Hai Duong. When it was declared over on 25 March 2021, the country's total stood at 910 positive cases and no deaths (Minh et al. 2021; Tran et al. 2021). The fourth wave of the pandemic, the deadliest one to date, began on 27 April 2021 and has lasted until the time of writing (March 2022). During 2021, this wave of the outbreak was related to the Delta variant, but by late December 2021, the Omicron variant was overtaking Delta in most provinces (WHO 2021). The fourth wave of COVID has dramatically changed the situation across Vietnam and has disrupted the country's weak public healthcare system and economy (Minh et al. 2021). On 1 January 2022, the Vietnamese Ministry of Health (MoH) confirmed the fourth wave as the most complicated and dangerous wave. Overall, from the first outbreak of the pandemic in January 2020 to the end of 2021, Vietnam had confirmed more than 1,731,257 positive COVID cases and close to 28,000 deaths. The worst period of infection was in the first half of 2022. By July 2022, Vietnam had recorded over 10 million infections and over 43,000 deaths due to COVID.

Non-pharmaceutical as a major response to COVID-19

Although the COVID-19 pandemic is a global pandemic with some shared challenges, individual countries have taken different paths in responding to it, depending on their geographic, economic, political, social and cultural contexts. A strategy that is effective in the context of a well-developed country might not necessarily be as effective in the context of a low-middle-income country such as Vietnam. In fact, Vietnam's response to the pandemic has been quite different from that of many countries, even its neighbours in Southeast Asia. In general, Vietnam's response to the outbreaks of the pandemic, especially the first three waves, involved non-pharmaceutical measures that the country developed. These measures include continuous communication about the pandemic, preventing movement of people from areas with an elevated risk of infection, social distancing, school closures, isolating affected individuals and border shutdowns (Nguyen T.V. et al. 2021).

Vietnam's approach can be generally described as a four-level healthcare strategy: central, provincial, district, and commune. At the village or hamlet level, health workers have a good understanding of the villages and villagers, and they participate as part of a grassroots task force (Nguyen T.C.Y. et al. 2021). This task force acts to implement the government's motto, "fighting against the pandemic is like fighting against an enemy" by arming villagers with knowledge and information, in the hope that villagers will unite through common anti-infection measures. To achieve village-based campaigns requires extensive coordination.

On 30 January 2020, during the first wave and a week after the first cases were reported, Vietnam established the National Steering Committee (NSC) which was mandated to function as a multi-ministerial and multisector body.

Led by the deputy prime minister, the NSC aimed to ensure the top-down coordination and implementation of responses to contain the pandemic nationwide. The establishment of such a top-down structure also reflects the country's political culture as a one-party state.

Upon establishment of the NSC at the central level, 63 provincial and 707 district steering committees were also established at the local level (Tran et al. 2021). Vietnam quickly closed its 1,297 km long border with China for fear that a large number of Vietnamese migrant workers would seek to return home from China to shelter from the pandemic, which may have led to massive transmission of the virus in local communities (Nguyen T.C.Y. et al. 2021). Vietnamese Army forces on the border were ordered to increase checks at all entry points with China. In addition, to help enhance its protective measures against the virus, the country required compliance with a 14-day epidemiological check-up and health monitoring procedure for all persons entering the country from China (Tran et al. 2021). Those who were suspected of being infected and/or who had a travel history to/from Wuhan before 1 January 2020, as well as their direct contacts, were traced and required to stay in government-established quarantine facilities (Do et al. 2020).

As the pandemic threat from outside the country increased, Vietnam tightened its border controls even further (Do et al. 2020). Considering international visitors as potential risk carriers, the country revoked aviation licences and restricted visas for international visitors. By pursuing such non-pharmaceutical strategies such as closing borders, promoting tracing of risk carriers and quarantining those identified as risk carriers, Vietnam not only hoped to protect its local populations better from the attack of the virus, but it also believed that the non-pharmaceutical strategies were more contextually appropriate as a low-middle income economy with a weak public healthcare system (Tran et al. 2021). The non-pharmaceutical measures were able to limit and break the transmission of the pandemic effectively in the first three waves (Nguyen L. H. et al. 2021; Tran et al. 2021). However, when the likelihood of the virus mutating increased in a community, local authorities announced a strict compulsory lockdown as the first step. When a lockdown was applied, local residents had to stay indoors until they were informed of the removal of the measure. Public places like schools, business premises, markets and the tourism industry were also required to shut down completely to break the transmission of the virus. It is believed that the more opportunities the virus has to replicate, the more it spreads throughout the community (WHO 2021). Compulsory lockdowns therefore effectively denied the virus the chance to replicate in a community (Tran B.X. et al. 2020).

To ensure better implementation of the government-led response, Vietnam quickly formulated its non-pharmaceutical strategy, which was underpinned by three key interrelated and interdependent principles: (1) isolation, (2) contact tracing, and (3) hospital quarantine. Isolation strategies aimed to prevent local people in the isolated community from going out to other communities, causing risks, and those from other communities entering the suspected community. Contact tracing aimed to identify potential risk carriers in the isolated community and prevent them from contacting others, causing cross-transmission (Do et al. 2020). On completing contact tracing, those clinically identified as positive for COVID-19 are transported to hospitals for treatment, and those identified as close contacts were isolated (Do et al. 2020).

To help classify levels of risks systematically, Vietnam defined risk carriers using the letter "F", a letter commonly used in genetics, with a numeral:

- F0 is understood as the clinically confirmed source of infections for COVID-19
- F1 is used to refer to those who have had direct contact with a confirmed case (F0)
- F2 refers to those who have had close contact with F1
- F3 is used to describe those who have had contact with F2

and so on (Tran et al. 2021). Those classified as F0 are treated in hospitals, while those confirmed as F1 are required to undertake a 14-day mandatory quarantine in a state-subsidised treatment facility for treatment (Do et al. 2020). If they are clinically confirmed positive for COVID-19, they are treated. Those identified as F2 and F3 and even F4 are required to self-quarantine in their homes for 14 days (Tran B.X. et al. 2020).

At a later stage of the pandemic, Vietnam further developed its state-led response strategy into a kind of a formula known as the '5 K' principle (K being the first letter of each command) to make five state directives.

- Không tụ tập/no assembly in public places
- Khẩu trang/wear a gauze masks
- Khoảng cách/keep your distance
- Khử khuẩn/disinfection
- Khai báo/health declaration

(Lam and Nam 2021)

The use of the 5 Ks aimed to make it easier for local populations to practice and memorise these phrases as Vietnam continued to rely on these non-pharmaceutical measures as the best defence to contain the disease, and to achieve its desired goal of "zero COVID-19".

Realising the vital role of technology as a key factor in winning the fight against the pandemic, Vietnam added an additional measure—an internet-based health declaration system for local citizens. Using their mobile phones, citizens can voluntarily report their own perceived health symptoms and/or potential risk carriers (Do et al. 2020). This technology-based measure has also encouraged local participation as another major factor in the government-led strategy against the pandemic.

To reflect the changing context of the pandemic, Vietnam kept reinforcing its non-pharmaceutical strategy, for example, by mandating wearing facemasks in public places for all citizens at all times. Failure to comply resulted in a fine from 100,000 VND to 300,000 VND. In addition, the country established the disease surveillance system, mandatory health regulations and movement restrictions. Thermal screening and health checkpoints were set up at all immigration ports (air, sea and land borders) to identify potential risk carriers (Quach and Hoang 2020). Anyone from abroad was required to stay in government-established quarantine facilities for 14 days (Tran et al. 2021).

Vietnam was considered as a success story in containing the virus in the first three waves of the pandemic but the country was then hit by a fourth wave. As with other states, the more infectious Delta variant not only spread quickly through Vietnam but was also far deadlier than in the previous three COVID outbreaks. The government realised that achieving "zero COVID-19" was neither a realistic goal nor practically possible. Continued pursuance of the goal would only further disrupt the nation's economy, making it a bigger challenge for it to overcome in the post-pandemic period. In addition, the government realised that the strategy that was once successful in its previous fights against the pandemic would not necessarily be successful again. So, continued reliance upon non-pharmaceutical measures alone, such as facemasks, social distancing, isolation and lockdowns, was not seen as a sustainable way out. The measures could only help slow down or break transmission of the virus in communities, but they could not remove the COVID virus from the communities. Vietnam would have to learn to live with COVID.

A combination of the non-pharmaceutical and pharmaceutical measures

Realising that continued reliance on the non-pharmaceutical preventive strategies or on the 5 K principles was not enough to contain the Delta variant, Vietnam moved to combine non-pharmaceutical and pharmaceutical measures with a focus on vaccines. As a result, the 5 K principle has now been upgraded into '5 K plus', with the 'plus' being vaccines. The government believes that, with the radical change in its strategy, it will better pave the way for its economy, which has been dramatically disrupted by the pandemic, to be re-opened sustainably (Nguyen T.C.Y. et al. 2021).

Vietnam officially commenced its vaccination campaign on 8 March 2021, and it is free to all Vietnamese citizens. The government made full use of its diplomatic relations to promote and purchase vaccines from many countries around the world, including from the United States and the United Kingdom, to provide for its population. At the same time, it also promoted its "made in Vietnam" vaccines, hoping that it would reduce its dependency upon external sources of supply (Nguyen T.C.Y. et al. 2021). Locally produced vaccines were a way to better assist Vietnam combat the virus. However, prior to being able to purchase enough vaccines to provide for the population, the government identified 11 priority groups to be vaccinated first, which included frontline health workers, the elderly, and those at high risk of exposure to COVID-19 (Nguyen T.C.Y. et al. 2021).

By September 2021, Vietnam had licenced eight types of COVID-19 vaccines for the national vaccination programme: AstraZenneca, Sputnik V, Vero Cell, Comirnaty (Pfizer), Moderna, Janssen, Hayat-Vax and Abdala (Doan et al. 2023). Like in many other countries worldwide, people in Vietnam were concerned with vaccine safety, especially because the vaccines were developed and delivered rapidly and there was little understanding of the potential long-term effects of Messenger Ribonucleic acid (mRNA) vaccines. Also undermining public trust was the fact that the information and recommendations about vaccine use for particular age groups often changed. For example, AstraZeneca was at first recommended for all age groups, but this recommendation was then revised, and it was recommended only to people aged over 60 years. This led to confusion, and people were understandably 'vaccine hesitant'.

At the outset of the vaccination programme, the provenance of the vaccine also led to concerns over safety. While generally there was less hesitancy towards Western-made vaccines like AstraZenneca, Comirnaty and Moderna, many people showed strong hesitancy towards the China-made Vero Cell. Vaccine hesitancy in Vietnam was built on a long history of conflict and violence between China and Vietnam. This history has resulted in a deep mistrust of the Chinese government, but it also extends to any products made in China. There is a common conception that goods produced in China are of poor quality and may in fact result in negative health outcomes. As a consequence of this historical legacy, vaccine hesitancy in Vietnam was directed squarely at the Chinese Vero Cell vaccine, with many Vietnamese refusing to be vaccinated with this particular vaccine (Zaini and Hoang 2021).

With its booster programme underway, Vietnam announced it aimed to achieve its full vaccination target for all its citizens aged over 18 years in the first quarter of 2022 (MoH). As of January 2022, more than 160 million doses have been given, bringing the country's coverage rate for those 18 years and older to 99.7% for one shot, while 91.1% have been fully vaccinated (two shots). With a high percentage of the adult population double vaccinated, the theory is the country will return to a 'new normal' where there was no "zero COVID-19" but a policy of "flexibly and effectively adapting to the pandemic".

Impacts of the non-pharmaceutical preventive measures

The physical and mental well-being of local populations was negatively impacted by the COVID-19 preventive measures, and there is a relationship between how local populations responded to the pandemic and what they have suffered (Hoang et al. 2021). Long-term adherence to preventive measures, as well as negative information about the epidemic, such as increasing numbers of deaths, affects physical and mental well-being. This was especially the case for those classified as socially and economically vulnerable—the poor, women, the unemployed and low-income people like unskilled labourers (Hoang et al. 2021). Studies evaluating mental health during the lockdown periods in Austria and the United States showed that people in these social groups seemed to be more stressed than those in other groups (Hoang et al. 2021). The epidemic itself and the mandatory measures to limit its transmission in the community need to be understood against a backdrop of increasing mental health issues for vulnerable groups in Vietnam (Le et al. 2020).

In Vietnam, the government-imposed non-pharmaceutical measures to contain the COVID-19 pandemic, however social distancing, compulsory prolonged quarantine and lockdown have been a double-edged sword. While these deliberate pre-emptive measures have resulted in significantly limited transmission of the virus in communities, it is evident that they have also resulted in negative impacts on local populations, including cramped confinement, boredom, tiredness, stress, depression, anxiety, post-traumatic distress (Le et al. 2020; Pham 2021).

The prolonged lockdown, for example, is believed to have produced the most adverse impacts on local populations, especially the most socially vulnerable groups, such as the urban poor, workers and women in cities (Le et al. 2020). During the lockdown, local citizens were not allowed to go out of their homes. In the context of the massive outbreak of the pandemic, especially during the fourth wave, people from these social groups have been the hardest hit. These are the most powerless social groups in the society and share some demographic and education characteristics: many of them are from ethnic minorities; they have secondary school education or less; they are often migrating from provinces such as Cao Bang, Thanh Hoa and Lang Son in the North and Dak Lak, Gia Lai and Dak Nong in the Central Highlands. They come to Vietnam's major southern economic centres—Ho Chi Minh City (HCMC), Binh Duong, Dong Nai and Long An—for employment opportunities. These are the provinces and cities that have undergone rapid social and economic development in the past decades, and there are jobs here for a wide range of social groups with national and international enterprises. These provinces and cities have become preferred migration locations for many people, both nationally and internationally (Minh et al. 2021).

People from these social groups were already highly vulnerable even before the outbreak of the COVID-19 pandemic (Sugishita 2021). Most of them participate in the informal economy, while many do manual labour jobs in enterprises and factories that are often associated with low salaries, long working hours, no work contracts or health insurance, huge work pressures and often abuse in different forms (Nguyen T.C.Y. et al. 2021). Their increased vulnerability due to the pandemic, which was predictable (Sugishita 2021), is fundamentally associated with their lack of necessary power to respond and adapt to the fast-changing context over time as a result of the rapid escalation of the pandemic (Le et al. 2020).

In addition, people from these vulnerable groups often live in small houses with limited access to safe drinking water, hygienic latrines, healthcare and counselling services (Le et al. 2020). Many of them, for example factory workers and labourers, live in small, shared rooms. The cramped housing conditions significantly added to the stress they experienced. Their housing conditions are also associated with numerous adverse emotional outcomes such as depression, boredom, irritability, and stigma related to quarantine requirements (Duong et al. 2020). Many of them have experienced depressive thoughts or nightmares as a result of the strict imposition of the national COVID containment strategy (Duong et al. 2020).

When the pandemic escalated further into a health crisis, many lost their livelihoods due to the closure of their workplaces. According to the General Statistics Office (GSO) of Vietnam, as of mid-April 2020, nearly five million people lost their jobs because of the pandemic (Tran P.B. et al. 2020). As a result, many were not able to provide for their families or to cover basic living costs, such as rent, water or electricity bills. They had to survive on their small savings before they were able to access limited financial support, healthcare and basic materials from the government.

As a response to the hardship many people were experiencing, the Vietnamese government provided short-term economic support for local populations, including for many types of household businesses and for individuals who became unemployed. This policy response strategy aimed to help mitigate the pandemic's economic impacts. Vietnam was able to roll out a 62 trillion VND (US$2.6 billion) financial relief package that aimed to target certain social groups—such as the poor, near-poor, furloughed workers or those on unpaid leave—in the form of a three-month cash transfer scheme (Tran P.B. et al. 2020).

The country prioritised only six categories of individuals and businesses that were eligible to access the package (Tran P.B. et al. 2020). Under this interim financial package, individuals who lost their jobs due to the COVID-19 crisis for 14 days or more were provided with a monthly allowance of VND1.8 million ($77), while part-time workers who were made unemployed were provided with a monthly allowance of VND1 million ($43). Poor and near-poor households were provided with VND250,000 ($10) per month, and those with a record of meritorious services to the nation would get VND500,000 ($21) per month. Household businesses with revenues below VND100 million ($4,300) a year that had to suspend operations from 1 April 2020 due to the COVID-19 pandemic would also be supported with VND1 million per month ($43). This raft of economic support served to ensure that people were able to maintain a basic standard of living for food and housing costs whilst unemployed due to the pandemic. This was especially important for the most vulnerable groups who were a part of the mass out-migration from city centres and back to the provinces, and who had little chance of earning a subsistence income (Tran P.B. et al. 2020).

This short-term economic support helped ease the material hardships of the pandemic; however, there were significant impacts on individual and social mental health (Tran P.B. et al. 2020). Economic confidence plummeted and mental health impacts escalated without positive signs of the economy re-opening in the near future (Nguyen T.C.Y. et al. 2021). This emotional distress was compounded by the loss of livelihoods. Many felt insecure about their ability to survive as they did not know how long the lockdown would last or when they could get back to work. With over 50% of the labour force employed in the informal job markets, the pandemic had a significant impact on vulnerable workers and further highlighted social inequalities (Dabla-Norris and Zhang 2021).

Moreover, as a result of the prolonged lockdown, local populations lost many of the basic social and cultural connections that are meaningful to them. For example, children were not able to go to school to meet their teachers and friends due to school closures, workers were unable to go to their factories and enterprises, and the elderly were not able to gather with their peers in their clubs (Le et al. 2020). In many parts of the country, churches and pagodas were closed to break the transmission of the virus, meaning that public worship was impossible. This alongside the difficulty in accessing safe medical care of the elderly also increased the risk of psychiatric illness attributed to COVID-19 as people felt increasingly isolated (Le et al. 2020).

When vulnerability peaked during the prolonged application of the preventive methods, especially the strict compulsory lockdown, most migrants to the cities and provinces, such as HCMC, Binh Duong, Dong Nai and Long An, decided to leave their livelihoods behind to return to their home provinces, causing the largest return migration by motorcycle since the country's reunification in 1975. It was estimated that 1.3 million people left the cities and provinces that had once been their dream destinations. Many of the returning migrants were alarmed by the rapid exponential increase in the number of positive cases, as well as the number of deaths every day, lower income levels and a lack of social and familial support networks (Tran P. B. et al. 2020).

Sacrifice of individual rights for the community's safety

The rapid dangerous escalation of the COVID virus required rapid and effective responses from the Vietnamese government (Le et al. 2020). In the context of the rapid escalation of the fourth 'Delta' wave in Vietnam, the government called for national unity and invited the entire community to participate in the fight against the pandemic. It was the first time since the country's unification in 1975 that the whole Vietnamese community, including military, scholars, businessmen and many different classes in Vietnamese society, had participated in a common fight, making different contributions. For example, soldiers became public servants, while ordinary citizens and businessmen across the country donated financial incentives and basic goods, such as rice, vegetables, meat and fish. At the same time, the government continued to tighten its preventive non-pharmaceutical measures, such as social distancing and partial and full lockdowns, believing that they would help to quickly break the transmission of the virus in communities (Duong et al. 2020).

Many felt the infringement of their personal freedoms and basic rights, such as restrictions on freedom of movement and the right to gather in public places (Le et al. 2020). If judged through the Western lens of human rights, individual rights and freedoms are often prioritised over collective well-being. However, as the Vietnamese government saw it, in the context of a global pandemic, individual rights had to be considered in terms of societal well-being. There is thus a difference between Western and non-Western societies in how human rights are understood. While the former highlight individuality and promote liberal values such as personal rights and freedoms, the latter emphasise and embrace collectivity (Ivic 2020). The community is valued over the individual. Individuals are rather seen as members of a certain group, such as family, society or nation. So, individuals can be prevented from exercising their rights and freedoms at the same time as they contribute to the preservation of collective health and the realisation of the right to life (Ivic 2020). The prevention of the spread of the virus was seen by government as a legal and moral responsibility.

As an Eastern society influenced by Confucianism, Vietnamese society emphasises core values that embrace concepts of social obligation, freedom and political organisation (Ivic 2020). These values, which differ from Western liberal understanding of the concepts in many ways, include collectivism, personal sacrifice for others, respect for the elderly, respect for authority, loyalty, social harmony, and so forth. The measures that Vietnam applied in response to the pandemic were more aggressive and tougher than those in other countries such as the United States and the United Kingdom (Ivic 2020). However, it is suggested that any judgement of Vietnam's response strategy should take into account its contextual specificities such as culture, healthcare and economic infrastructure. As an Eastern society with a low-middle income background and a weak public healthcare system, the response was culturally appropriate.

Based on its perceptions of human rights that put local people's safety first and foremost, Vietnam further tightened its non-pharmaceutical measures, such as compulsory lockdown in any communities where the likelihood of the virus mutating was high. During the strict prolonged lockdown period, no one was allowed to go out of their homes for fear that public gatherings would add to the rapid widespread transmission of the virus in a community. The government considered that by stopping individuals from breaking the lockdown, it was protecting their right to life and protecting the lives of the entire community. Achieving this goal required the sacrifice of individual personal rights. So, while the Vietnamese government agrees that rights are interrelated and interdependent, they are also hierarchical and depend on the actual context. For example, in a non-pandemic context, rights to assemble in a public place are encouraged and protected, while these rights may be forbidden in a context of a pandemic. The aim of the latter is to better ensure the ability of individuals to enjoy the former.

Perspectives regarding rights, even among people sharing the same culture, are sometimes hostile. There were moments when the hostility turned into conflicts on a small scale between local residents and local authorities. The Vietnamese government considered itself as having a legal and moral obligation to protect and care for its citizens in the crisis, especially the most socially vulnerable and marginalised such as the poor, women and children. The slogan "no one is left behind" has been used throughout the fight against the pandemic, and in the context of the pandemic reflects the government's political and moral commitments to protect its citizens. It has argued that, in the context of life and death, any sacrifices or trade-offs that lead to saving more human lives are necessary, right and worth trying. This further reinforces the perception that, while all rights are important, they are hierarchical, with the community first.

Assessment

Vietnam has responded to a deadly pandemic that has dramatically disrupted its health system and economy. There are basically two different approaches to understanding this experience. Some tend to argue that the government-imposed non-pharmaceutical methods, such as strict prolonged lockdown, can be understood as an act of limiting or even violating basic human rights that local people are entitled to, such as the right to enjoy their freedoms, right to go to school for children, right to gather in public places and right to freely engage in the economy to earn a living. In Western countries, this focus on individual rights and freedoms was the source of many public protests and rallies across the world (BBC 2021). The restriction of individual rights versus utilitarian concepts was a problem faced by many governments worldwide.

When it specifically comes to the issue of human rights, the Government of Vietnam's strategy can be linked to the third generation of human rights, known as Collective Rights or Peoples' Rights, of the universal framework that also puts collective and solidarity rights above individuals' rights (Ivic 2020). Third-generation or 'solidarity' rights are the most recently recognised category of human rights. This grouping has been distinguished from the other two categories of human rights in that its realisation is predicated not only upon both the affirmative and negative duties of the state but also upon the behaviour of each individual (Ruppel 2008). Rights in this category include the right to development (Hawksley and Georgeou 2020), the right to peace, the right to a healthy environment, the right to benefit from the common heritage of mankind, the right to humanitarian assistance and the right to intergenerational equity (Ruppel 2008). Rights of this grouping emerge from post-colonial discourses, drawing on the newly decolonised states' mosaic of imperial experiences (Freedman 2014) and their desire to achieve the elusive state of 'development'.

In Vietnam, there were little to no protests at the infringement of personal rights and freedoms because the population held that the government had acted in accordance with cultural and societal norms of communitarianism. The government itself argued that the country's COVID-19 prevention strategy should be viewed as altruistic, implemented to protect lives and community well-being over economic activity. The multi-layered strategies can be understood as the product of the government's intention to benefit its citizens in the context of a serious health crisis, one for which the country had little experience or expertise (Ivic 2020). The way the government responded to the pandemic ultimately aimed to protect citizens' lives at all costs, including sacrifice of other things, such as economic activity, rather than being intended to violate human rights, as was sometimes depicted in media reports. However, as of 17 February 2022, 91.5% of the entire population, some 74,805,128 million people, have been fully (double) vaccinated, and 32,849,000 people have received booster doses, accounting for 34.0%. Despite its initial low death rate, by mid-February 2022, Vietnam had recorded 39,188 deaths (Doan et al. 2023). From a statistical perspective in relation to the size of the population, the strategy that Vietnam has applied in response to the pandemic can be seen as successful as compared to many other countries in the region and beyond (Yen et al 2021; WHO 2021). Combined with unexpectedly strong economic growth in 2020, this means that the future development outlook for Vietnam is positive (Dabla-Norris and Zhang 2021).

It is evident that the way that Vietnam responded to the pandemic enjoyed public support, consensus and trust (Ivic 2020). Some readers may find this surprising, especially those in the Western world, where citizens often have a low level of trust in their governments. Vietnam was however ranked second of 23 states for the level at which participants trust their country's government to take care of its citizens in an international survey of public opinion with a sample of over 12,500 respondents conducted in May 2020: China placed first with 85% approval and Vietnam second with 77% (Blackbox 2020). The finding of this study can be aligned with another independent study that shows that 94% of Vietnamese interviewed expressed their full trust in the government-led strategy against COVID-19 (Nguyen T.C.Y. et al. 2021).

Conclusion

The global pandemic has shone a light on many of the complexities and nuances of public health strategies which have aimed to disrupt the spread of the COVID virus. This chapter has outlined the way that the Vietnamese government developed a set of principles that were entirely appropriate for the population it serves. The various groups and levels of community were enlisted in non-pharmaceutical measures through unifying discourses which emphasised nationalistic duty, community well-being and citizen responsibility. The Vietnamese population was not entirely without agency in how the pandemic was addressed. This is illustrated in the way that strong cultural and historical values provoked many to avoid vaccines that were made in China. Future government health strategies need to recognise that in order to be successful, they will need to pay attention to such cultural nuances in order to continue to be held in a position of trust by the population and to forge a pathway towards sustained, inclusive and greener growth.

References

BBC. (2021, November 21). Covid: Huge Protests across Europe over New Restrictions, https://www.bbc.com/news/world-europe-59363256.

BlackBox. (2020, May). *The World in Crisis: A Global Public Opinion Survey Across 23 Countries (Summary Report)*, https://issuu.com/blackbox4/docs/world_in_crisis_final_report?fr=sZTM1ODEyNzA0Nzc.

Bouchnita, A., Chekroun, A., and Jebrane, A. (2021). Mathematical Modeling Predicts That Strict Social Distancing Measures Would Be Needed to Shorten the Duration of Waves of COVID-19 Infections in Vietnam. *Frontiers In Public Health*, https://doi.org/10.3389/fpubh.2020.559693.

Dabla-Norris, E. and Zhang, Y.S. (2021, March 10). Vietnam: Successfully Navigating the Pandemic. IMF, https://www.imf.org/en/News/Articles/2021/03/09/na031021-vietnam-successfully-navigating-the-pandemic.

Do, B.N., Tran, T.V., Phan, D.T., Nguyen, H.C., Nguyen, T.T.P., Nguyen, H.C., Ha, T.H., Dao, H.K., Trinh, M.V., Do, T.V., Nguyen, H.Q., Vo, T.T., Nguyen, N.P.T., Tran, C.Q., Tran, K.V., Duong, T.T., Pham, H.X., Nguyen, L.V., Nguyen, K.T., Chang, P.W.S., and Duong, T.V. (2020, November 12). Health Literacy, eHealth Literacy, Adherence to Infection Prevention and Control Procedures, Lifestyle Changes, and Suspected COVID-19 Symptoms Among Health Care Workers During Lockdown: Online Survey. *Journal of Medical Internet Research*, 22(11): e22894, https://doi.org/10.2196/22894. PMID: 33122164; PMCID: PMC7674138.

Doan, L.P., Dao, N.G., Nguyen, D.C., Dang, T.H.T., Vu, G.T., Nguyen, L.H., Vu, L.G., Le, H.T., Latkin, C.A., Ho, C.S.H., and Ho, R.C.M. (2023). "Having vaccines is good but not enough": Requirements for optimal COVID-19 immunization program in Vietnam. *Frontiers in Public Health*, 11, https://www.frontiersin.org/articles/10.3389/fpubh.2023.1137401.

Duong, M.D., Le, T.V., and Bui, T.T.H. (2020). Controlling the COVID-19 Pandemic in Vietnam: Lessons From a Limited Resource Country. *Asia Pacific Journal of Public Health*, 32(4), 161–162, https://doi.org/10.1177/1010539520927290.

Freedman, R. (2014). Third Generation Rights: Is There Room for Hybrid Constructs within International Human Rights Law. *Cambridge Journal of International and Comparative Law*, 2(4), 935–959.

Hawksley, C. and Georgeou, N. (2020). Right to Development: Theory, Practice, and Articulation with SDGs. In W. Leal Filho, A. Azul, L. Brandli, A. Lange Salvia, P. Özuyar, and T. Wall (eds) *No Poverty. Encyclopedia of the UN Sustainable Development Goals*. Springer, Cham, https://doi.org/10.1007/978-3-319-69625-6_47-1.

Hoang, T.D., Colebunders, R., Fodjo, J.N.S., Nguyen, N.P.T., Tran, T.D., and Vo, T.V. (2021). Well-Being of Healthcare Workers and the General Public during the COVID-19 Pandemic in Vietnam: An Online Survey. *International Journal of Environmental Research and Public Health*, 18(9), https://www.mdpi.com/1660-4601/18/9/4737.

Ivic, S. (2020). Vietnam's Response to the COVID-19 Outbreak. *Asian Bioethics Review*, 12, 341–347. https://doi.org/10.1007/s41649-020-00134-2.

Lam, M.H. and Nam, A.T. (2021). 'The 5k Message in the Context of Covid-19 Pandemic at Vietnam: A Case Study', *Proceedings of the 4th International European Conference On Interdisciplinary Scientific Research at Warsaw*, Poland, https://www.researchgate.net/publication/354600099_THE_5K_MESSAGE_IN_THE_CONTEXT_OF_COVID-19_PANDEMIC_AT_VIETNAM_A_CASE_STUDY

Le, X.T.T., Dang, A.K., Toweh, J., Nguyen, Q.N., Le, H.T., Do, T.T.T., Phan, H.B.T., Nguyen, T.T., Pham, Q.T., Ta, N.K.T., Nguyen, Q.T., Nguyen, A.N., Duong, Q. Van, Hoang, M.T., Pham, H.Q., Vu, L.G., Tran, B.X., Latkin, C.A., Ho, C.S.H., and Ho, R.C.M. (2020). Evaluating the Psychological Impacts Related to COVID-19 of Vietnamese People Under the First Nationwide Partial Lockdown in Vietnam. *Frontiers in Psychiatry*, *11*, 824.

Minh, L.H.N., Khoi Quan, N., Le, T.N., Khanh, P.N.Q., and Huy, N.T. (2021, November 24). COVID-19 Timeline of Vietnam: Important Milestones Through Four Waves of the Pandemic and Lesson Learned. *Frontiers in Public Health.*, *9*, 709067, https://doi.org/10.3389/fpubh.2021.709067.   PMID: 34900885;   PMCID: PMC8651614.

Nguyen, L.H., Hoang, M.T., Nguyen, L.D., Ninh, L.T., Nguyen, H.T.T., Nguyen, A.D., Vu, L.G., Vu, G.T., Doan, L.P., Latkin, C.A., Tran, B.X., Ho, C.S.H., and Ho, R.C.M. (2021). Acceptance and Willingness to Pay for COVID-19 Vaccines Among Pregnant Women in Vietnam. *Tropical Medicine & International Health*, *26*(10), 1303–1313.

Nguyen, T.C.Y., Hermoso, C., Laguilles, E.M., Castro, L.E. De, Camposano, S.M., Jalmasco, N., Cua, K.A., Isa, M.A. Akpan, E.F., Ly, T.P. Budhathoki, S.S., Ahmadi, A., and Lucero-Prisno, D.E. (2021). Vietnam's Success Story Against COVID-19. *Public Health in Practice*, *2*, https://doi.org/10.1016/j.puhip.2021.100132.

Nguyen, T.V., Tran, Q.D. Phan, L.T., and Vu, L.N. (2021). In the Interest of Public Safety: Rapid Response to the COVID-19 Epidemic in Vietnam. *British Medical Journal Global Health*, *6*(1), https://doi.org/10.1136/bmjgh-2020-004100.

Pham, N.N. (2021). Basic Solutions to Develop Human Resources for Responding Covid-19 in Ho Chi Minh City Health Department, Vietnam. *European Journal of Public Health Studies*, *4*(2), 565153.

Quach, L. and Hoang, N.-A. (2020). COVID-19 in Vietnam: A Lesson of Pre-Preparation. *Journal of Clinical Virology*, *127*, https://www.sciencedirect.com/science/article/pii/S1386653220301219.

Ruppel, O.C. (2008). Third-Generation Human Rights and the Protection of the Environment in Namibia. In *Human Rights and the Rule of Law in Namibia*. Macmillan Education Namibia, Windhoek.

Sugishita, T. (2021). Epidemiological Situation and Social Vulnerability in the Era of the COVID-19 Pandemic. *Tokyo Women's Medical University Journal*, *5*, 10–18.

Tran, B.X., Nguyen, H.T., Le, H.T., Latkin, C.A., Pham, H.Q., Vu, L.G., Le, X.T. Nguyen, T.T., Pham, Q.T., Ta, N.T.K., Nguyen, Q.T., Ho, C.S.H., and Ho, R.C.M. (2020). Impact of COVID-19 on Economic Well-Being and Quality of Life of the Vietnamese During the National Social Distancing. *Frontiers in Psychology*, *11*, 151–157.

Tran, L.T.T., Manuama, E.O., Vo, D.P., Nguyen, H.V., Cassim, R., Pham, M., and Bui, D.S. (2021). The COVID-19 Global Pandemic: A Review of the Vietnamese Government Response. *Journal of Global Health Reports*, *5*, e2021030.

Tran, P.B., Hensing, G., Wingfield, T., et al. (2020). Income Security During Public Health Emergencies: The COVID-19 Poverty Trap in Vietnam. *BMJ Global Health*, *5*, e002504.

Vuong, M.N., Nguyen, T.L.Q., Doan, T.T., Do, V.T., Nguyen, Q.T., Dao, X.C., Nguyen, T.H.T., and Do, D.C. (2021). The Second Wave of COVID-19 in A Tourist Hotspot in Vietnam. *Journal of Travel Medicine*, *28*(2).https://doi.org/10.1093/jtm/taaa174

WHO. (2021). Viet Nam COVID-19 Situation Report #74, Epidemiological report as of 26 December 2021, 18:00, https://www.who.int/docs/default-source/wpro---documents/countries/viet-nam/covid-19/viet-nam-moh-who-covid-19-sitrep_26dec2021.pdf?sfvrsn=e1240a3f_5.

Yen, C.N.T., Hermoso, C., Laguilles, E.M., De Castro, L.E., Camposano, S.M., Jalmasco, N., Cua, K.A., Isa, M.A., Akpan, E.F., Ly, T.P., Budhathoki, S.S., Ahmadi, A., and Lucero-Prisno, D.E. (2021). Vietnam's success story against COVID-19. *Public Health in Practice*, 2, 100132, https://doi.org/10.1016/j.puhip.2021.100132.

Zaini, K. and Hoang, T.H. (2021). Understanding the Selective Hesitancy towards Chinese Vaccines in Southeast Asia. *Yusof Ishak Institute*, 115, 2335–6677.

7 Nepal

Pandemic and unusual state response

Uddhab Pyakurel and Supriya Gurung

Introduction

Nepal, like many other states, adopted a wait-and-see approach for at least the first five months after the discovery of its first COVID-19 case. Failure to expeditiously activate the state's preparedness and response systems resulted in an inability to avert the full impact of COVID-19, and the disease spread rapidly. Economically, Nepal's economic growth declined from a targeted 8.5% in 2019–2020 to just 2.3% in the fiscal year of 2020/2021 (ADB 2022). Lockdowns led to between 1.6 and 2 million jobs lost due to the COVID-19 crisis in Nepal (Pyakurel 2020a). The socio-economic situation was exacerbated by political tensions, which distracted from the public health emergency and had a detrimental impact on the country's timely response to the pandemic (Pyakurel, Khakurel and Singh 2022: 213–228).

This chapter details the Nepali government's delayed response to the surge of COVID-19 cases, and its use of measures such as travel restrictions, snap lockdowns and a national vaccine rollout to control the virus. It assesses the success or failure of those measures, as well as assessing some unusual government activities that occurred during the pandemic, some of which raised questions of corruption. This chapter will also address several opportunities on which the Nepali state failed to capitalise, measures that would have aided in its fight against the spread of COVID-19.

Background

Nepal recorded its first COVID-19 case on 24 January 2020. At the time of writing (25 May 2022), almost one million Nepalis (979,076) with cases of COVID-19 have been recorded, and 11,952 coronavirus-related deaths (Reuters 2022). COVID-19 remains a significant public health threat as a result of Nepal's low vaccination coverage, as well as the increasing prevalence of COVID variants that have higher transmissibility. The socio-economic impacts of COVID-19 are also considerable and have resulted in widespread job losses, the disruption of education and food insecurity.

DOI: 10.4324/9781003311522-7

Governments across the world were unprepared to deal with the COVID-19 pandemic, but the Nepali state was particularly ill-equipped, largely due to the fragility of its governance systems. The Federal Democratic Republic of Nepal was formed in 2006 following a lengthy ten-year conflict (1996–2006) between the state and Communist Party of Nepal (Maoist) rebel forces. As part of a Comprehensive Peace Process, the state embarked on the preparation of the Constitution of Nepal, adopting an interim constitution in 2007; however, political disagreements meant that there were extensive delays in ratification, even leaving Nepal in a legal vacuum. The 2013 Constituent Assembly had a timeline of January 2015 to resolve the deadlock, but could not deliver. As a result, there was still general administrative confusion on 25 April 2015 when Nepal was hit by the massive Gorkha earthquakes that resulted in the deaths of 9,000 people. The tragic events spurred legislators into action, 90% of whom supported the proposed new constitution on 20 September 2015 with its three-tier system of governance (federal, provincial and local) where each tier has the constitutional power to enact laws and mobilise its own resources. Nepal's powerful southern neighbour India effectively then blockaded Nepal for six months from 25 September, in protest at what it saw as measures in the constitution that were discriminatory towards ethnic groups along the Indian border with separatist demands, as well as because of allegations of human rights abuses by the Nepali state against these groups. The blockade severely affected landlocked Nepal, which relied completely on fuel transports from India to keep its economy going. India was also critical of Nepal's policy of closer engagement with its other powerful neighbour, China.

By the time the COVID pandemic hit in early 2020, Nepal was besieged by economic, social and humanitarian crises within its borders. The federal government and the local governments that managed the 7 federal provinces and 753 municipalities, all still in their administrative infancy, were not prepared to act independently to curtail the spread of the virus, and they had neither the resources nor the experience to do so. The result was a generalised failure of governance.

Initial response

By the first week of February 2020, the COVID-19 virus had spread from Wuhan to all 22 provinces of China (Zhu et al. 2020). According to the surveillance statistics reported by the Chinese government, by 19 February, 2020, the number of confirmed infection cases increased to 44,412 for Wuhan and 74,280 for the whole of China, with 1,497 and 2,009 deaths, respectively. Even though the Nepali embassy in China communicated to its government in Kathmandu that 180 Nepali students were situated in Wuhan, the Health Ministry ruled out the evacuation of any Nepali from China, stating that there was "hardly any difference between staying in China or returning back to the country". Further confusing the situation were the rumours that alleged that the United States was responsible for the COVID-19 outbreak, with Narayan

Man Bijukchhe, chair of the Nepal Workers and Peasants' Party, just one of several figures who expressed such suspicions in public. As governments across the world began to formulate responses, Nepal's national government did not hold any serious discussions on how to handle the situation.

On 6 February 2020, the government finally ceded to mounting public pressure and declared that it would bring back the Nepali students from China; however, when this announcement was made, the Chinese Ambassador to Nepal, Hou Yanqi, in an interview with Nepali media, expressed her concerns that evacuating Nepali nationals from Wuhan would only facilitate the spread of the disease. She further questioned Nepal's ability to execute its decision:

> If the Nepali side insists on evacuating its nationals, it is advised that the relevant departments of the Nepali side be fully prepared in terms of airport quarantine, epidemic prevention and control, and seek the advice of the WHO representative in Nepal to prevent the epidemic from spreading.
>
> (My Republica 2020a)

The Nepali government proceeded with the evacuation and, on 16 February, successfully repatriated 175 Nepali citizens from Wuhan. Nepal-China relations were not affected, and Ambassador Hou Yanqi took to Twitter on 15 February to say, "The fundamentals of China's long-term economic development remain unchanged. And the pace of China-Nepal friendly cooperation will not be delayed" (Pyakurel 2020b). The Nepali government followed up the evacuation with a donation of 100,000 protective masks to China as a gesture of friendship and solidarity (My Republica 2020b).

By 6 February 2020, more than 50 states had imposed travel restrictions or tightened visa requirements for Chinese nationals, and some took more severe measures. Australia prohibited the entry of passengers who had either been in or even transited through mainland China after 1 February 2020 (Prasain and Shrestha 2020). Similarly, India invalidated visas issued to mainland China nationals and also denied entry to passengers who had been in China after mid-January. On 2 March 2021, Nepal followed suit, with the government suspending the issuing of on-arrival visas for Chinese nationals entering Nepal. Ten days later, Nepal's government made the decision to stop issuing tourist visas to all international travellers. The Supreme Court also issued an interim order that flights to and from countries affected by the COVID-19 pandemic be suspended to protect public health. This court ruling was challenged, and in response, the Supreme Court's order was retracted. The government instead issued a travel advisory that cautioned Nepali residents against non-essential travel to countries that were severely affected by COVID-19—China, South Korea, Iran, Japan and Italy. The government also faced heavy criticism for its indecision on the matter of prohibiting incoming flights from China. Pre-pandemic, Chinese airlines had operated an average of 48 weekly flights into Nepal; however, Nepal Airlines, the national flag carrier, did not have a permit to fly to China. Five prominent Chinese air carriers—Air China, China Southern, China Eastern, Sichuan Airlines and Tibet Airlines—as well as one Nepal-China joint venture (Himalaya Airlines) continued to operate flights between Nepal and the Chinese cities of Chongqing, Beijing, Changsha, Guiyang and Shenzhen (Prasain 2020).

As the global COVID-19 situation escalated rapidly, on 18 March 2020, Nepal announced that it was planning to ban all incoming passengers, including returning Nepalis, from entering Nepal from territories within the European Union, the United Kingdom, West Asia, the Gulf States and from Iran, Turkey, Malaysia, South Korea and Japan (Pyakurel 2020b). The restrictions came into effect at midnight on 20 March 2020. Five days later, on 25 March 2020, the government took aggressive action and issued a nationwide lockdown (Rayamajhee et al. 2021: 9).

The government's response, however, was strangely conflicted. Nationally, the government was pushing the country into lockdown; however, domestically, it offered differing advice. Prime Minister K. P. Sharma Oli, in his address to the National Assembly, said that there was no need to panic, emphasising to Nepalis the importance of strong willpower and a positive mindset: "Corona is like the flu," he said. "If contracted, one should sneeze, drink hot water and drive the virus away". Appearing before Parliament on 10 June 2020 to respond to questions from lawmakers, Oli stated that Nepalis have a "stronger immune system" than others and that "a majority of Nepalis breathe fresh air and have ginger, garlic and turmeric as integral parts of their daily diet. Those who eat such medicines every day definitely have better immunity" (Ghimire 2020). Prime Minister Oli issued these questionable statements at a time when the entire country was under lockdown, thus promoting general confusion and eroding public awareness of the dangers of COVID-19. The 25 March lockdown was initially intended to last for a week, but it was only lifted on 21 July 2020, almost four months after it was first announced (Thapa M. 2021). When the measure was first imposed, Nepal had only two confirmed cases of COVID-19 and no fatalities. By the last date of the nationwide lockdown, Nepal had reported a total of 17,994 positive cases and 40 deaths (Sharma, Banstola and Parajuli, 2021).

Government controversies

A lockdown is an aggressive measure, and it heavily affected socio-economic activities across Nepal. All national and international flights ceased, preventing all tourism, and all public and private vehicles were banned, except those with prior permission from local authorities, those belonging to security forces, health workers and ambulances. Any who defied the government mandate were arrested under the *Infectious Disease Control Act*. The impacts of the lockdown were multidimensional, causing the loss of jobs, impacting numerous businesses, disrupting supply chains and pushing the most vulnerable further into poverty. The government drew considerable criticism for its snap decision to lockdown, especially as the prime minister of Nepal, KP Sharma Oli, who publicly denied the lockdown was having any adverse effects on Nepali society, described such allegations as part of a "media conspiracy" (Ghimire, 2020), but the lockdown was not the only controversial aspect of Nepal's pandemic management.

The government was already facing considerable criticism for instituting the lockdown while saying its effects were not serious and for claiming Nepalis were uniquely physiologically able to survive COVID's effects when it became embroiled in a number of controversies. The government signed a contract worth NRs1.24 billion (USD$10 million)[1] with Omni Business Corporate International (OBCI) Pty. Ltd (hereinafter the Omni Group) to supply pandemic-related medical equipment and logistics to control COVID-19. However, the government failed to follow the procurement procedure, citing the urgency of the situation as a reason for this action (Sharma B. 2020). The Omni Group not only failed to deliver the amount of goods they had promised to procure from China, but the price for medical equipment procured by the Omni Group was almost three times higher than the usual market price. It was also revealed that the deal came about as a result of an informal agreement established between those in the inner circles of PM KP Oli's office and the Omni Group.

To make matters worse, the quality of the materials that the Omni Group provided was sub-par. The rapid testing kits, for example, were said to be unreliable and showed false negative results. Doctors questioned the quality of the personal protective equipment sets and the portable PCR machines. The Omni Group flew in an initial 10 tonnes of specialist medical goods from China on 29 March 2020 and chartered another flight for 2 April 2020 with the aim of flying in the second consignment when the government, which had initially stood by its procurement decision, scrapped the deal under mounting pressure from the public and the media. However, the controversy did not end there.

The government, instead of taking responsibility and following the *Public Procurement Act*—which clearly states that the authorities should award contracts to the lowest bidder or choose the second lowest bidder if the lower bidder's quote compromises quality—decided to hand the task of procurement over to the Nepal Army. This decision drew criticism from all parties across the political spectrum. Many believed that the national defence force was getting increasingly politicised and was losing its identity as a neutral national institution. The ability of the army to import medical equipment was also questioned, as this was considered far beyond the remit of a defence force. People also wondered exactly why the government had chosen to give the army responsibility for the task of procurement. Further media coverage indicated that this move was not discussed at the cabinet meeting and that even ministers were unaware of the plan. The decision, according to the media, was taken solely at the behest of Prime Minister Oli.

Many suspected that this move was another attempt at self-enrichment, with those in government enlisting the army to assist in their plans to embezzle public money in the name of purchasing medical equipment. Former prime minister Baburam Bhattarai even took to social media and voiced strong opposition to this decision, saying,

> The virus cannot be killed by guns or bullets. So why did the government move the Army forward to bring medical equipment from China? Aren't there civilian bodies that work in the field of commerce and supplies? Why wasn't a G2G [Government to Government] deal instituted earlier? Is this because the Army does not come under the purview of the CIAA [Commission for the Investigation of Abuse of Authority]?

Indeed, the Nepal Army does not even fall under the purview of the Commission for the Investigation of Abuse of Authority (CIAA), and it has constitutional immunity even in cases of financial irregularities. The government has still not released the details about the procurement process.

More controversies followed at the height of the pandemic when the Nepali government issued two irrelevant ordinances, both unrelated to the fight against the virus. On 20 April 2020, the government declared its intention to pass the *Political Party Act*, which if approved would allow a party to split if 40% of either its central committee members or parliamentary party members wished to register for a new party. This was an important shift, as previously a party could split only if 40% of the members of *both* the central committee and parliamentary party voted in favour of doing so. The prime minister voiced his support for the ordinance at the Party Secretariat, claiming that it was introduced to ease the split of one of the opposition parties in Parliament. The Council of Ministers also recommended the endorsement of a second ordinance that would make it possible to convene a meeting of the Constitutional Council—a body headed by the prime minister that makes decisions on constitutional appointments—even in the absence of the leader of the main opposition party (Giri and Pradhan 2020).

Nepal's president, Bidya Devi Bhandari, approved these controversial ordinances within hours of their issuance, leading to consternation that the Office of the President had in fact become an arm of the executive. The common belief was that Prime Minister Oli had urged the changes to secure his political position amidst talk of unease and instability within his own party. Critics maintained that by issuing and approving these ordinances in the manner they were, the government "was subverting the constitutional spirit and bypassing the Parliament". Rajendra Mahato, the leader of the six-member praesidium of the Janata Party went on to say that "this is the most inhumane drama by Oli at this time of crisis when the world is fighting the pandemic" (Giri and Pradhan 2020). Just five days later, however, the government bowed to massive criticism and rescinded both ordinances (My Republica 2020c).

The political controversy continued as Prime Minister Oli became involved in a feud with his co-chair in the Nepal Community Party (NCP), Pushpa Kamal Dahal, and, facing rebellion from those within his own party, dissolved Parliament in December 2020 in a bid to consolidate power. In February 2021, the Supreme Court invalidated Oli's move as unconstitutional and reinstated Parliament (Al Jazeera 2021). The NCP also split into a Maoist Centre, led by Dahal, and a United Marxist Leninist (UML) Party, led by Oli. In May 2021, Oli lost a vote of confidence in Parliament, with many within his own faction of his party withholding their votes for him (Gill 2021). Despite losing the no-confidence vote, Oli maintained his position as prime minister, as no other party had a clear majority; however, in July 2021, the Supreme Court ordered that Nepali Congress president, Sher Bahadur Deuba, be appointed prime minister, which was the fifth time that Deuba had held the post of prime minister of Nepal (Thapa G.S. 2021).[2]

The aforementioned dealings are offered to demonstrate that at a time of a global health emergency—when the elected government should have been focusing on arranging the provision of medication and other required logistics, such as quarantine, isolation centres, testing strategies, public information, awareness campaigns and economic support packages—it was instead embroiled in political machinations and entirely avoidable controversies. Political wrangling and infighting clearly took precedence amongst those in government, resulting in a thorough neglect of the containment and control of COVID-19. As a result, the Nepali people had to contend with both the COVID-19 virus and an ineffective, undemocratic and opaque system of governance.

Foreign players

Nepal is landlocked, and shares long borders with India to the south and China to the north. While there is a great level of interconnectedness between these three countries through Nepal, there is also a geopolitical rivalry between India and China that long predates the onset of the COVID-19 pandemic. Both countries see the solidification of their relationship with Nepal as a key strategy to assert dominance in the region. The economy of Nepal depends heavily on foreign assistance from its two powerful neighbours, as well as from European and other donors. As a result, there was rivalry even in the provision of medical and logistical assistance to Nepal. When Nepal identified its very first case of COVID-19, the Chinese Embassy in Kathmandu wrote a formal letter to Nepal, expressing support and readiness to assist. The letter, quoted by various media outlets read, "Does Nepal want any support and aid from China? For example, in energy? Do we need to send a medical team with masks and other medical supplies? We are ready" (Onlinekhabar 2020).

India's tactic was different, and it called for solidarity and concerted efforts between nations in the region. In a video conference on 15 March 2020, the Indian prime minister, Narendra Modi, requested that leaders and representatives in the eight-member states of the South Asian Association for Regional

Cooperation (SAARC)[3] stand together to tackle the COVID-19 virus. He also proposed the creation of a "COVID-19 Emergency Fund" that would be funded by voluntary contributions from SAARC member nations. Prime Minister Modi also offered $10 million as an initial contribution from India, along with the assistance of a Rapid Response Team of doctors and specialists, testing kits and equipment from SAARC member states to be placed in Nepal specifically to assist with the control of the COVID-19 virus (Chaudhury 2020). The Nepali government, struggling with a lack of medical equipment, however, stressed that it required medical equipment, not personnel, and so this proposal was not adopted.

The Chinese government's response to Nepal's needs was to claim that it would ensure the provision of medical equipment as per a checklist provided by the Nepali government. This response started out with a promising donation. On 26 March 2020, Chinese company Beijing Savanta Biotechnology handed over 2,000 COVID-19 test kits to the Nepali Ambassador to China, a move that was lauded by the Nepali Embassy in Beijing as "an excellent example of friendly age-old ties between Nepal and China" (Khabarhub 2020a). The kits, however, worth $4,700, never made it to Nepal. They were stopped after questions were raised over their quality, as they were not on China's National Medical Products Administration's list of approved kits (Khabarhub 2020b). Following this incident, the Nepali government embarked on the independent procurement of medical equipment, resulting in the previously discussed controversy with the Omni Group.

Owing to Nepal's limited resources, the country's fragile healthcare system and a government preoccupied with political wrangling, the situation was growing increasingly dire when on 11 December 2020, the world's first vaccine to treat COVID-19, produced by Pfizer-BioNTech, was approved for emergency use in the US (FDA 2020). In January, Nepal was the grateful recipient of one million doses of the AstraZeneca-Covishield vaccine, produced in India. Nepal received these doses just days after India launched its own nationwide inoculation programme (Pasricha 2020). India's gesture has been construed as one aimed to expand its influence in South Asia as part of its 'neighbourhood first' policy. The provision of these vaccines also assisted in bridging the divide between the Nepali and Indian governments, which had widened during the 2015–2016 border blockade, and which was exacerbated by a subsequent border dispute in early 2020 over the Limpiyadhura triangle in the northwest corner of Nepal (Dixit and Dhakal 2020). The Nepali government then signed a deal to purchase an additional two million vaccine doses from the Serum Institute of India, the manufacturer of the AstraZeneca-Covishield vaccine.

In early 2021, the incidence of COVID-19 in India increased sharply as the population, hurrying to regain a sense of normalcy after months of being in lockdown, ignored social distancing measures, the use of masks and sanitation (Ethirajan 2020). This second wave of COVID-19 in India had numerous effects that filtered through to Nepal. Heavily dependent on India for the majority of its supplies, particularly medical equipment and liquid oxygen,

Nepal was left struggling to find alternative supplies as India's supplies were diverted to equipment within its own borders (Gill 2021). Thousands of Nepali and Indian migrant workers, many of whom were carrying the COVID virus, moved through the porous border between India and Nepal, returning illegally in a bid to avoid quarantine (Ethirajan 2020). This situation was worsened by political rallies and religious festivals that had been held unchecked in Nepal in the months before, allowing further proliferation of the virus. India, struggling to deal with its own health crisis, was unable to deliver the expected number of vaccines to Nepal; of the two million doses initially ordered and paid for, only half of the doses were delivered as vaccine exports were halted in late March 2021. Kathmandu made repeated appeals to New Delhi to send the remaining one million doses; however, the government was told that the Serum Institute of India was unable to supply the vaccines, as the Indian government had restricted their export when India experienced a second wave of the COVID virus (Ethirajan 2020).

In late March, China stepped in and donated 800,000 doses of the Sinopharm vaccine to Nepal, with another one million doses delivered in early June 2021 (Gill 2021). Political ties between Nepal and China had grown stronger following the election of the NCP in 2017 and have been further strengthened by such shows of support.

As cases of COVID-19 increased sharply in India, the disease followed a similar trajectory in Nepal. By May 2021, the situation in Nepal was dire, with daily infection rates averaging around 9,000, and with over 4,000 people dead. Vaccine shortage meant that by June 2021, only 1.4 million Nepalis, mostly vulnerable and elderly Nepalis,[4] had received their first dose of the vaccine. These elderly Nepalis then waited over 12 weeks for their second doses, and concerns were raised that their immunity would run out.

With the assistance of its neighbours and other international donors, by the end of 2021, Nepal had received a total of 13,357,590 vaccine doses from various producers, including AstraZeneca (4,422,740 doses), Sinopharm (7,400,000 doses) and the Janssen vaccine (1,534,850 doses) (Hayat et al. 2022). The COVID-19 Vaccines Global Access programme provided 348,000 doses of the Covishield vaccine; Bhutan and Japan provided 230,000 and 1,614,740 doses of the AstraZeneca vaccine, respectively; the United Kingdom supplied 130,000 doses of the AstraZeneca vaccine; and the United States provided 1,534,850 doses of the Janssen single-shot vaccine (Hayat et al. 2022). All these vaccines were made available for free by the respective governments and organisations.

With the help of the World Bank Group, WHO, UNICEF and GAVI, the government of Nepal also developed plans to implement its COVID-19 vaccination programme for up to 71.6% of its population. By late 2021, the government's plans had not however been achieved, as by November 2021, only 26.2% of Nepal's population had been fully (two doses) vaccinated (Hayat et al. 2022). By 26 May 2022, this figure had however reached 67.8%, with a booster shot given to 13.2% of the population (Reuters COVID-19 Tracker 2022).

Assessment

The Nepali government was thoroughly lackadaisical and complacent in its dealings to control the spread of the COVID-19 pandemic within the country's borders. The government missed several opportunities to manage the spread of the virus, of which we discuss five main issues.

Firstly, Nepali society is still largely rural and unindustrialised, and most people have their roots in the countryside, only travelling into urban cities for job opportunities. Once the government imposed the lockdown, many returned to these villages. Thus, given their rural dwellings and the isolation of these villages, it should have been possible to maintain adequate COVID-19 protocols, such as social distancing. In fact, according to WHO's COVID-19 protocols, crowded places must be avoided, people must stick to a small and consistent social circle and avoid gathering in large groups, there must be limited contact with outsiders and a distance of two metres must be kept between individuals in public settings. Such protocols are eminently feasible in a rural setting, and the government should have capitalised on the natural isolation of those rural villages and worked with those people in semi-urban and rural areas to spread awareness and maintain COVID-19 protocols such as social distancing.

Secondly, the government should have prioritised budget allocation for those who wished to regenerate the rural economy, helping them create a conducive economic environment through measures that supported small farming activities, initiatives for micro-irrigation, promotion of connectivity of those villages through maintenance of postal ways which are shorter than roadways and hassle-free loan subsidies if villagers ran a small business in certain rural localities. Instead, the government refused to readjust its budget and existing priority programmes. Instead, those individuals who had returned to their villages when the lockdown was first announced flocked back to the congested urban areas where they had been living, as they did not see a sustainable future by remaining in their rural locale.

Thirdly, due to the lockdown and the COVID-19 pandemic, the Nepali government was unable to spend the budget allocated for the fiscal year of 2019/2020, and ultimately it only spent 74% of what had been approved. This raised the risk of future budget shrinkages, and so the government in power rushed to allocate money to new budgetary headings, essentially wasting money on useless, non-transparent development programmes and plans instead of reorientating the budget and existing programmes towards the fight against COVID-19. Road construction projects using heavy mechanisms, for example, were a popular way to divert such unspent money. Though this was viewed as helping locals gain connectivity through road networks, and such activity does contribute to a sustainable economy, it should not have been an immediate priority, and arguably the money could have been much better spent, as during the pandemic, the health sector was woefully underfunded, under-resourced and in great need of a budget injection. In the fiscal year of

2020/2021, the government allocated NRs90.69 billion to the health sector, a 32% increase from the NRs68 billion it had allocated the year before (Poudel 2020). However, though the budget had increased by over NRs20 billion, even this amount proved insufficient. The government planned too many programmes and had not balanced funding proportionally, thus while roads were being built, healthcare and the provision of public health remained under-funded and under-equipped.

Fourthly, the government started and then halted a key initiative that would have assisted those who caught COVID. The Nepali state does not provide universal health coverage, so the scheme issued by *Beema Samiti* (Insurance Regulatory Authority of Nepal), titled the COVID-19 Insurance Policy, was a promising and welcome initiative (Sharma B.R. 2020). On 19 April 2020, Beema Samiti introduced a policy that provided insurance for those who tested positive for COVID-19. Insurers offered upwards of NRs50,000 depending on the premium chosen. However, five months on, as the number of COVID-19 cases increased, the regulatory authority amended the policy and reduced the benefit to 25% of the insured amount. On 4 June 2020, the insurance policy that had been included in the budget for the fiscal year 2020/2021 was suspended by the Nepali government until further notice.

Finally, the government was criticised for its harsh treatment of campaigns that were organised to support and feed the less fortunate within the city. Immediately after the lockdown was imposed, volunteers mobilised and began the distribution of free food to people who had been rendered jobless by the government's lockdown mandate. Many within the capital live on daily wages and exist hand-to-mouth, so the provision of food was an initiative many welcomed. However, the government voiced its concern that by feeding people in open spaces around the city, the capital would be seen as a city of beggars. The government also claimed that the campaigners had not sought or received permission from the Kathmandu Metropolitan City to initiate such campaigns. Ultimately, the government mobilised the police force to stop this charitable movement, and so the 'free food for the poor' campaign ended abruptly. Instead of seeing this as an opportunity for valuable collaboration the Nepali society, the government was openly critical and obstructive to attempts to ameliorate the worst effects of its own inept response.

Conclusion

By late May 2022, there were 979,091 confirmed cases of COVID-19, with 11,952 coronavirus-related deaths reported in Nepal since the pandemic began. As getting tested in Nepal is a costly and challenging process, it is believed that the number of COVID-19 cases is actually much higher. Also, by late May 2022, at least 42,560,157 doses of COVID-19 vaccines had been administered, enough to have vaccinated about 74.4% of the country's population. As the daily infection rates of COVID-19 cases decline, it seems Nepal has now weathered the worst of the virus, but at the cost of considerable casualties. Nepal's economic growth declined from a targeted 8.5% in 2019–2020 to just 2.3% in fiscal year 2020/2021 (ADB 2020). Between 1.6 and 2 million jobs were lost due to the COVID-19 crisis in Nepal. Households had to deal with food security and vulnerability. Quarantine, social isolation and travel restrictions also affected the mental health of Nepalis, with an increase in anxiety and/or depression (Sharma et al. 2021). In uncertain situations, the population relies on leaders who are in a position to make crucial decisions during challenging times. Perhaps in the future, the Nepali government will heed expert recommendations, implement anti-corruption strategies effectively, collaborate with its citizens and co-produce and implement policies for the proper management of unprecedented pandemic situations.

Notes

1 Nepal Government Announced a Budget of Rs. 1798.83 billion (approximately 142 million USD) for this fiscal year in 2022.
2 https://southasianvoices.org/nepal-in-2021-uncertainty-looms/ (Accessed: 13 May 2022)
3 Initially formed in 1985 by Bangladesh, Bhutan, India, Maldives, Nepal, Pakistan and Sri Lanka, the SAARC expanded to eight members with the admission of Afghanistan in 2007.
4 According to 2011 census data, *Nepal* had a total of 2,154,003 elderly (60+ years and above), which accounts for 8.1% of the total population.

Reference

ADB. (2022). Economic Indicators for Nepal. https://www.adb.org/countries/nepal/economy (Accessed: 13 May 2022).

ADB (Asian Development Bank). (2020, September 15). Nepal's Economy to Slow Further in FY2021. https://www.adb.org/news/nepals-economy-slow-further-fy2021.

Al Jazeera. (2021, May 26). Nepal Plunges into Crisis – Again. Here's What You Need to Know. https://www.aljazeera.com/news/2021/5/26/no-vaccine-novote-why-is-nepal-in-political-crisis-again.

Chaudhury, D.R. (2020). India Extends Covid Assistance Worth $1 Million Under SAARC Emergency Fund. https://economictimes.indiatimes.com/news/politics-and-nation/india-extends-covid-assistance-worth-1-million-under-saarc-emergency-fund/articleshow/74722067.cms?from=mdr.

Dixit, K.M. and Dhakal, T.P. (2020, May 19). Territoriality Amidst Covid-19: A Primer to the Lipu Lek Conflict between India and Nepal. *ScrollIn*, https://amp.scroll.in/article/962226/territoriality-amidst-covid-19-a-primer-to-the-lipu-lek-conflict-between-india-and-nepal.

Ethirajan, A. (2020, May 12). As India Halts Vaccine Exports, Nepal Faces Its Own Covid Crisis. *BBC News* (Asia), https://www.bbc.com/news/world-asia-57055209.

FDA (United States). (2020, December 11). FDA Takes Key Action in Fight Against COVID-19 by Issuing Emergency Use Authorization for First COVID-19 Vaccine. https://www.fda.gov/news-events/press-announcements/fda-takes-key-action-fight-against-covid-19-issuing-emergency-use-authorization-first-covid-19.

Ghimire, B. (2020, June 10). Oli Peddles Mistruths and Sidesteps Criticism before Parliament. *The Kathmandu Post*.

Gill, P. (2021, May 14). Facing a COVID Crisis, Nepal Cries Out for Help. *The Diplomat.*

Giri, A. and Pradhan, T.R. (2020, April 20). Oli's Sudden Issuance of Two Ordinances Raises Concerns of a Party Split in the Making. *Kathmandu Post*, https://kathmandupost.com/national/2020/04/20/oli-s-sudden-issual-of-two-ordinances-raises-concerns-of-a-party-split-in-the-making (Accessed: 13 May 2022).

Hayat, M., Uzair, M., Ali Syed, R., Arshad, M., and Bashir, S. (2022). 'Status of COVID-19 Vaccination around South Asia', *Human Vaccines & Immunotherapeutics*, 18(1), p. 2016010.

Khabarhub. (2020a, March). Chinese Company Provides Nepal 2,000 Coronavirus Kits. https://english.khabarhub.com/2020/26/84696/.

Khabarhub. (2020b, March 28). Chinese Kits Donated to Nepal Stopped Midway Over Quality Concerns. https://english.khabarhub.com/2020/28/85402/.

My Republica. (2020a, February 5). Chinese Envoy Tells Nepal to Make Necessary Preparations before Evacuating Its Citizens. *My República*, https://myrepublica.nagariknetwork.com/news/chinese-envoy-urges-nepal-to-make-necessary-preparations-before-evacuating-nepali-nationals-from-wuhan/ (Accessed: 15 February 2020).

My Republica. (2020b, February 8). Nepalis in Wuhan to Be Evacuated Only After Setting Up Quarantine Facilities: Minister. https://myrepublica.nagariknetwork.com/news/nepalis-in-wuhan-to-be-evacuated-only-after-setting-up-quarantine-facilities-minister/ (Accessed: 19 September 2021).

My Republica. (2020c, April 24). Prez Bhandari Repeals Controversial Ordinances. https://myrepublica.nagariknetwork.com/news/prez-bhandari-repeals-controversial-ordinances/ (Accessed: 13 May 2022).

Onlinekhabar. (2020, March 17). China 'Ready' to Extend Any Needful Support to Nepal to Combat Coronavirus Crisis. Available at https://english.onlinekhabar.com/china-ready-to-extend-any-needful-support-to-nepal-to-combat-coronavirus-crisis.html (Accessed: 18 August 2022).

Pasricha, A. (2020, January 24). India Launches 'Neighborly Vaccine Diplomacy'. *VOA News*, https://www.voanews.com/a/covid-19-pandemic_india-launches-neighborly-vaccine-diplomacy/6201140.html.

Poudel, A. (2020, May 29). Health Sector Gets 32 Percent More Budget Compared to Previous Year. *Kathmandu Post*, https://kathmandupost.com/national/2020/05/29/health-sector-gets-32-percent-more-budget-compared-to-previous-year.

Prasain, S. (2020, February 2). Chinese Carriers Cut Flights to Kathmandu as Passengers Cancel Tickets En Masse. *The Kathmandu Post.*

Prasain, S. and Shrestha, P.M. (2020, March 18). Government Bans Entry of All Passengers, Including Nepalis, from Midnight March 20. *The Kathmandu Post.*

Pyakurel, U. (2020a, May 8). Nationwide Lockdown: For Corona Control or Dirty Politics? *The Himalayan Times.*

Pyakurel, U. (2020b). Nepal: Dealing with the Big Neighbor and Pandemic (online). https://cssame.nchu.edu.tw/2020/03/30/nepal-dealing-with-the-big-neighbor-and-pandemic/?fbclid=IwAR2P0J7fB9kt3yAmB14qDcZ636Dr6TH_tNhZiAxwn1Gj-mHCWuX4H3wSSAk (Accessed: 19 May 2022).

Pyakurel, U., Khakurel, P., and Singh, A.R. (2022). 'Chapter 12 Higher Education in Nepal during COVID-19: Prospects and Challenges'. In F. Netswera, A.A. Woldegiyorgis, and T. Karabchuk, *Higher Education and the COVID-19 Pandemic* (pp. 213–228), https://doi.org/10.1163/9789004520554_013.

Rayamajhee, B., Pokhrel, A., Syangtan, G., Khadka, S., Lama, B., Rawal, L.B., Mehata, S., Mishra, S.K., Pokhrel, R., and Yadav, U.N. (2021). 'How Well the Government of Nepal Is Responding to COVID-19? An Experience from a Resource-Limited Country to Confront Unprecedented Pandemic', *Frontiers in Public Health*, 9, p. 597808.

Reuters COVID-19 Tracker. (2022). Nepal. https://graphics.reuters.com/world-coronavirus-tracker-and-maps/countries-and-territories/nepal/ (Accessed: 13 May 2022).

Sharma, B. (2020, September 29). The OMNI Scandal and Its Impacts. *The Record*, https://www.recordnepal.com/the-omni-scandal-and-its-impacts (Accessed: 13 May 2022).

Sharma, B.R. (2020, October). COVID 19 Regulatory Relief Issuance in Nepal. *Beema Samati (Insurance Regulatory Authority of Nepal)*, https://nib.gov.np/wp-content/uploads/2020/10/COVID-19-Presentation-By-Bhoj-Raj-Sharma.pdf.

Sharma, K., Banstola, A., and Parajuli, R.R. (2021). 'Assessment of COVID-19 Pandemic in Nepal: A Lockdown Scenario Analysis', *Frontiers in Public Health*, 9, p. 599280, https://doi.org/10.3389/fpubh.2021.599280.

Thapa, G.S. (2021, December 27). Nepal in 2021: Uncertainty Follows a Turbulent Year. *South Asian Voices*.

Thapa, M. (2021, November 14). Government's Response During COVID-19 Pandemic in Nepal. *Kathmandu University*. https://mpra.ub.uni-muenchen.de/111666/ (Accessed 20 February 2022).

Zhu, H., Wei, L., and Niu, P. (2020). 'The Novel Coronavirus Outbreak in Wuhan, China', *Global Health Research and Policy*, 5(1), pp. 1–3.

8 Australia and COVID-19

Cracks in the Commonwealth

Charles Hawksley and Nichole Georgeou

Introduction

To prevent COVID-19 infection, illness and deaths, Australia imposed international border controls on aircraft and cruise ships, restricted entry to all but citizens and permanent residents, adopted quarantine, social distancing, implemented lockdowns, contact tracing for those infected, mobile phone apps and free polymerase chain reaction (PCR) testing. Generous stimulus packages meant that people prevented from travelling to their workplaces received financial support during pandemic lockdown periods, and those out of work received increased social security payments. These measures were temporary and were wound back as widespread public compliance with a national vaccine rollout meant that by the end of December 2021 in a total population of 25.7 million, 42.5 million doses of vaccine had been administered, and 18.8 million people over 16 years of age (73.1% of all Australians) had received two vaccine doses (ANAO 2022).

Despite being an island continent, Australia was not immune from COVID; however, throughout 2020 and up until the end of 2021, the overall result was very successful. Up to 31 December 2021, there had been just over 500,000 total cases in a population of almost 26 million, with 2,279 COVID deaths. On 17 November 2021, Australia had a rate of 211 COVID average excess deaths per million, comparatively better than the Organisation of Economic Co-operation and Development (OECD) average of 1,495, with only Denmark (195), Iceland (188), Republic of Korea (52) and Norway (−277) recording lower figures (OECD 2021).

This success was not however due to strong central government action, and indeed the federal structure of Australia led to part of the problems in pandemic management. One of the more interesting features of the COVID experience in Australia is that the day-to-day management of the COVID pandemic was conducted at a state and territory level, and not by the national ('Commonwealth') government. While there was cooperation between different levels of government, the national COVID response over 2020 and 2021 in the Commonwealth was largely sidelined as the state premiers of New South Wates (NSW), Victoria (Vic), Queensland (Qld), Western Australia (WA),

DOI: 10.4324/9781003311522-8

South Australia (SA), Tasmania (Tas), and the chief administrators of the Australian Capital Territory (ACT) and the Northern Territory (NT) implemented lockdowns and border closures when they chose to do so, and often against the express wishes of the Australian prime minister.

Between 2020 and 2021, there were four main 'waves' of COVID in Australia: (1) initial infections largely from overseas returnees in March 2020, (2) community transmission infections during April 2020, (3) community transmission (Delta variant) from July to November 2021 and (4) the very steep rise in cases from late 2021, when the Omicron variant became dominant in the community. The following graphs show comparatively low levels of deaths and infections during 2020–2021 with a very large increase in daily COVID cases once states lifted restrictions. With the late 2021 Omicron wave, the total number of Australians with COVID went from under 400,000 at the end of 2021 to over 10 million by August 2022 (Our World in Data 2022). Unlike many other states, as Figures 8.1 and 8.2 show, Australia had far more cases and deaths in 2022 than it had in the entire first two years of the pandemic.

This chapter argues that even though the general picture for Australia in 2020–2021 appears successful there were some "cracks in the Commonwealth" that led to a large number of preventable deaths, particularly in aged care facilities. State and territory practical leadership of the national COVID response led to some unusual outcomes, including the Commonwealth government openly supporting a challenge to the validity of WA's state border closures (Brennan 2021) and the truly baffling secret arrogation of the sweeping powers of five federal ministries, including health, by the then prime minister Scott Morrison during 2020 and 2021, a matter kept from even his closest cabinet colleagues (Karp 2022a).

This chapter has two parts. It first outlines why Australia's 'pandemic politics' resulted in the states and territories managing the COVID response while the Commonwealth's role was largely reduced to the control of international borders, regulating quarantine, economic support and securing sufficient doses of COVID vaccines. Shared responsibilities between the Commonwealth and the states in areas such as aged care led to preventable deaths and blame shifting. The second part details the 'national' health and economic responses, concentrating on the effects of Commonwealth fiscal stimulus on the economy, and the social effects of lockdowns on the population. Differential enforcement of stay-at-home orders and lockdowns in lower-socioeconomic and largely migrant parts of Australia's two largest cities, Melbourne and Sydney, raised allegations of racism in the management of the pandemic, while the national vaccination rollout was affected by delays.

Part I: Emergency powers and pandemic politics

In the period under consideration, January 2020 and December 2021, the Commonwealth was governed by a coalition of the Liberal Party of Australia and the smaller National Party. The Liberals as the larger coalition partner had

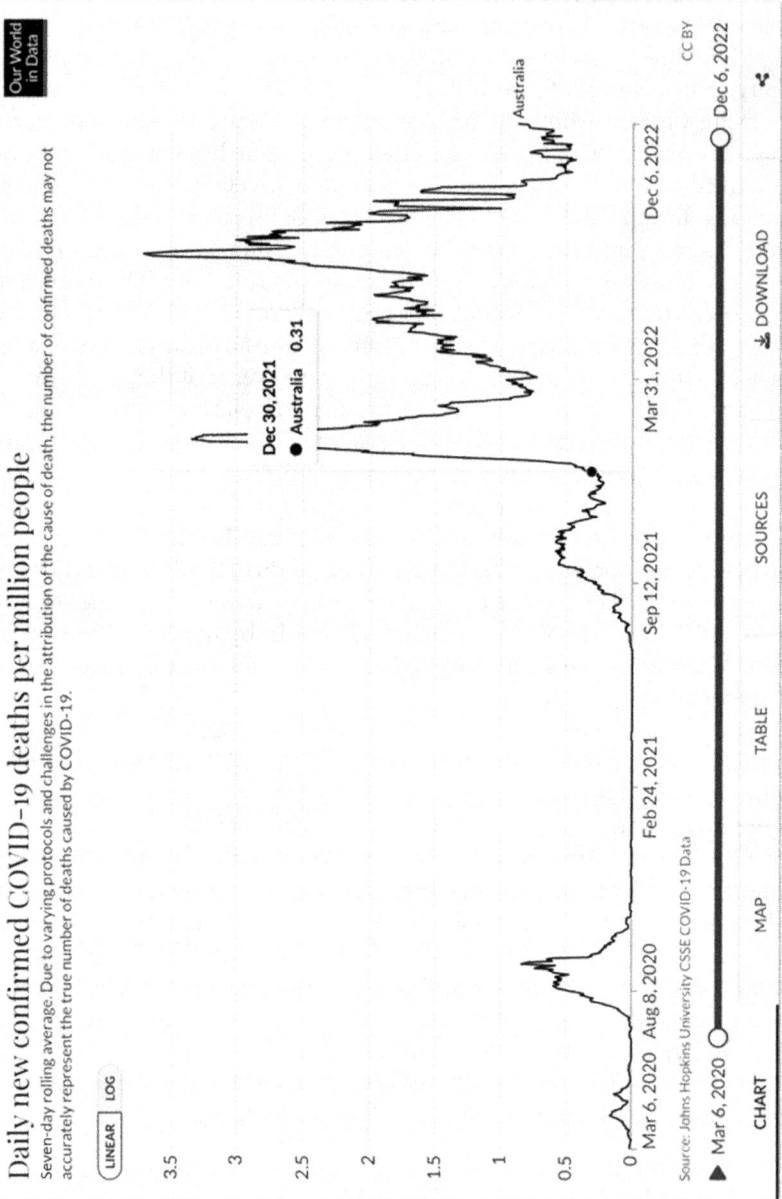

Figure 8.1 Australia—COVID deaths per million March 2020–December 2022.

Source: Johns Hopkin University CSSE COVID-19 Data.

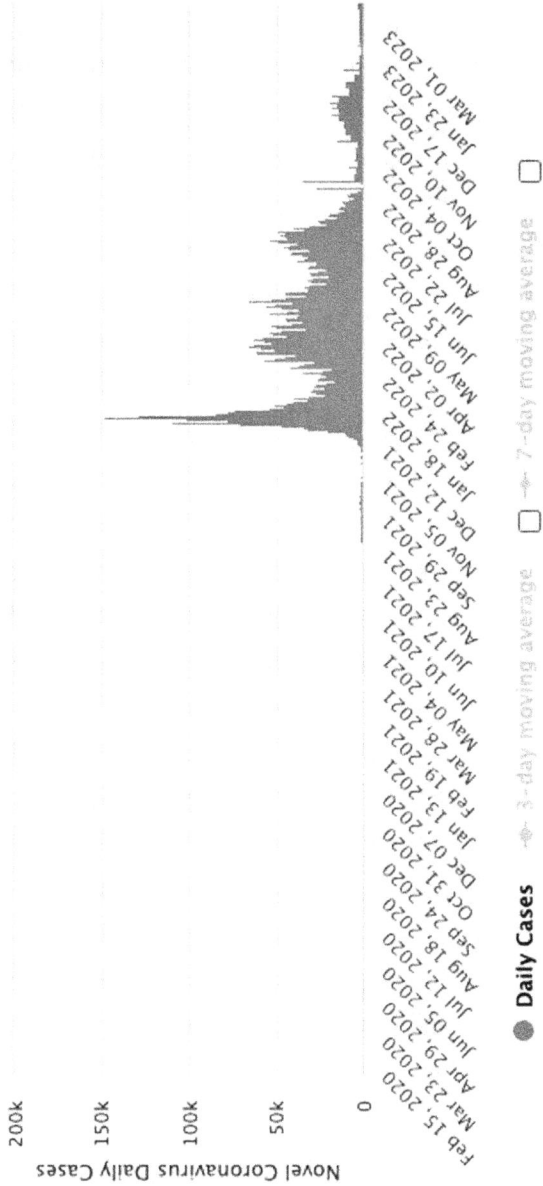

Figure 8.2 Daily COVID cases in Australia February 2020–March 2023.

elected as party leader and Prime Minister Scott Morrison to succeed Malcolm Turnbull after internal infighting in August 2018, and in September 2019, Morrison led the coalition to a federal election victory against its main opposition the Australian Labor Party ('Labor') (PoA 2022). Across Australia, there were state and territory governments of different political persuasions that often found themselves acting together, and even together against the Commonwealth. As Phillip Coorey (2021) noted, "At the onset of the pandemic, Morrison fought the states, be it on school or border closures, and lost. Frequent attempts to force a nationally uniform series of hot-spot definitions, border rules and other responses proved fruitless". During 2020–2021, there were Liberal Premiers in South Australia (SA) (Steve Marshall) and Tasmania (Tas) (Peter Gutwein); however, there were Labor premiers in Queensland (Qld) (Annastacia Palaszczuk) and Western Australia (WA) (Mark McGowan) and Labor chief ministers in both the Australian Capital Territory (ACT) (Andrew Barr) and the Northern Territory (NT) (Michael Gunnar). Victoria (Vic) (pop. 6.5 million) was led by Premier Daniel Andrews (Labor), and New South Wales (NSW) (pop. 8.1 million) by Premier Gladys Berejiklian (Liberal). On 5 October 2021, Berejiklian resigned due to a corruption inquiry (McGowan and Davies 2021); her NSW Liberal party room colleagues then elected Dominic Perrottet as premier.

Under Section 51 (s.51) of the *Commonwealth of Australia Constitution Act* (hereinafter 'the Constitution') the Commonwealth has clearly defined powers in specific areas of activity, including *inter alia*: currency, defence, postage stamps, immigration, quarantine, foreign affairs, lighthouses, taxation and banking. Australia supported the COVID-19 Vaccines Global Access (COVAX) initiative and committed AUD$350 million to the $8 billion global fund to seek a vaccine (Hawksley 2020). Much to the annoyance of Australian exporters, in May 2020, Morrison chose to support then-US President Donald Trump's calls for an enquiry into the origins of COVID, which triggered a dispute with Australia's largest trading partner, China. This attempt to curry favour with the Trump administration led to the imposition of Chinese tariffs of 80.5% on Australian barley (Osborne 2022), while Chinese imports of Australian wine, which had been valued at over AUD$1 billion in 2018–2019, were halted as a Chinese enquiry into 'dumping' into its domestic market was announced; beef was also affected, as China suspended imports due to 'irregularities' in Australian labelling (Sullivan 2020).

Under s.107 and s.108 of the Constitution, all powers previously held by the governments of the British colonies in Australia that were not transferred to the Commonwealth in 1901 remained with what then became the six states of the Commonwealth of Australia (NSW, Vic, Qld, WA, SA and Tas).[1] Over time, a sort of 'creeping federalism' has meant that there are now several areas in which both the Commonwealth and the states have joint responsibility. Education is one such area where there are concurrent powers; health and aged care are others. For example, in health, the Commonwealth administers the management of the Australia-wide universal healthcare system (Medicare) that controls payments to doctors and rebates to patients. As part of the Commonwealth budget, moneys are distributed to state and territory governments to fund their health services to staff and manage hospitals (PEO 2022).

When it came to COVID, the federal structure of the state meant that the management of what was a national public health emergency became politically messy. While many expected national leadership in the COVID response, the Commonwealth lacked effective emergency powers for disaster management. This fact was however known. During 2019, a series of devastating bushfires raged across eastern Australia. Commencing in late July 2019 in NSW, by November and December 2019, there was catastrophic damage to forests and fauna in SA, Vic, NSW and Qld, with smaller fires in WA and Tas. As Eburn (2019) argued in the context of the bushfires: "There is no legislation to allow the Prime Minister or the Governor-General to declare a National Emergency. In the absence of that legislation the only value of such a declaration is symbolism".

In December 2019, at the height of the bushfire emergency, Morrison travelled with his family to Hawaii for a holiday, a fact that was kept from the Australian public. Trenchant public and media criticism of Morrison ensued, and the public castigation no doubt affected his desire to be seen to be 'managing' the COVID pandemic that emerged shortly afterwards. By late January 2020, there were reports Morrison was exploring having the Commonwealth obtain emergency powers (Lawson 2020); however, the Constitution can only be amended through a referendum. The Commonwealth government eventually passed the *National Emergency Declaration Act* in December 2020, which notes in Section 3 (italics added),

(1) The object of this Act is to recognise and enhance the role of the Commonwealth in preparing for, responding to and recovering from emergencies that cause, or are likely to cause, nationally significant harm.

(2) This object is achieved by providing for the making of national emergency declarations, which will allow the Commonwealth *to mobilise resources to prepare for, respond to, and recover from such emergencies.*

Thus, both before and after COVID, the Commonwealth could only really play a financial and supporting role, while states and territories carry out relief operations during emergencies.

The use of the Australian Defence Force is within the purview of the national government, and the resources and personnel of the defence forces were on occasion offered by the Commonwealth to the states and sometimes were accepted.

There were other areas where responsibility was more contested. By August 2020, Morrison was arguing that the failure to properly protect aged care residents in the state of Victoria—over 80 of whom had died of COVID in the previous week—was largely the fault of the government of Victoria, and by inference its Labor Party Premier Daniel Andrews. As political commentator Kathryn Murphy (2020a) noted, this claim conveniently overlooked the fact that the funding and regulation of the aged care sector is in fact a federal responsibility.

In a move that completely baffled all sides of politics, during the pandemic, Morrison asked Australia's governor-general to appoint him to an additional five government ministries, all of which had existing ministers. While technically legal, bizarrely Morrison (except in the case of health) did not even inform his own ministers, and neither were the new appointments gazetted, as is usual practice. After Labor formed the government following the May 2022 federal election, incoming Prime Minister Antony Albanese commissioned the former High Court justice, the Hon Virginia Bell, to head an inquiry into the legality of Morrison's actions. The November 2022 *Report of the Inquiry into the Appointment of the Former Prime Minister to Administer Multiple Departments* found (Bell 2022: 1) that Morrison had himself appointed

> to administer the Department of Health on 14 March 2020, the Department of Finance on 30 March 2020, the Department of Industry, Science, Energy and Resources ("DISER") on 15 April 2021, and the Departments of the Treasury and Home Affairs on 6 May 2021. In other words, Mr Morrison had been appointed to administer six of the 14 departments of State. These appointments had not previously been disclosed to the Parliament or to the public.

Morrison assuming co-control of these ministries was found to be legal; however, his actions in not informing his own ministers fundamentally undermined all known conventions of cabinet government. As the COVID pandemic deepened Morrison's attorney general, Christian Porter, had first suggested that the prime minister also become minister for health, with the rationale that under the *Biosecurity Act 2015* (Cth), Health Minister Greg Hunt could wield extraordinary power, and in some way, Morrison's appointment could act as a check on this power. Other members of the government understood Morrisons's co-appointment to the Health Ministry as precautionary—for example, it might even be sensible to have a senior government minister act as a 'backup' if the health minister became too ill to perform his duties. Such logic may explain why Morrison assumed co-control of the Ministry of Health, with the knowledge of Health Minister Greg Hunt and some other senior ministers, but Morrison's co-appointment to the Ministry for Finance was without the knowledge of Minister Mathias Corman, and the same lack of transparency occurred with three other ministries in 2021. Former Justice Bell found all these appointments were "unnecessary" as if either Hunt or Corman had been unable to discharge their functions due to COVID illness, Morrison, or any other senior government figure, could have been appointed to those posts "in a matter of minutes" (Bell 2022: 1). Arguably the most flagrant violation was in the case of Treasury, as Morrison did not inform Treasurer and Deputy

Liberal Leader Josh Frydenberg, of the co-appointment, even though they had worked together on crafting budgets and had shared a period of lockdown at the prime minister's residence in Canberra, the Lodge during August of 2021 (7 News 2021).[2]

Political cooperation

In a system that denied the Commonwealth government the opportunity to play a leading role in combatting the COVID pandemic, the levels of articulation in health policy required to manage COVID-19 nationally ushered in a new semi-regular political meeting known as 'National Cabinet'.[3] While consensus was sought for major initiatives, the decisions of National Cabinet were not binding:

> National Cabinet was established on 13 March 2020 and is chaired by the Prime Minister. The Commonwealth and state and territory governments individually have flexibility to determine the best way to achieve any agreed outcomes made by National Cabinet in their jurisdiction.
>
> (PM&C 2020)

National Cabinet stressed the notion that the response to the COVID pandemic required high levels of goodwill, coordination and cooperation to make it nationally effective. Premiers and chief administrators took the lead on communicating with the public, providing daily news briefings alongside their chief health officers; the Commonwealth did likewise. They initiated or relaxed measures of economic shutdown and social distancing as they saw fit to best manage COVID-19 in their jurisdictions, often in spite of what the Commonwealth wanted. To help control the spread of COVID, the state premiers moved to protect their 'internal' borders. From 19 to 24 March 2020, led by the offshore state of Tasmania, Australian states restricted movement into their jurisdictions (PoA 2021). While Morrison was calling for the Australian economy to remain open, the premiers of the two most populous states NSW (Beriljkian) and Victoria (Andrews) both moved to implement lockdown measures (Needham 2020). From April to June/July 2020, Australia was under a generalised lockdown, after which the different jurisdictions locked down when necessary. Figure 8.3 shows the timeline of when Australian states and territories went in and out of lockdown during the eight quarters of 2020–2021 from the March, June, September and December quarters of 2020 (i.e. MQ 2020) to the March quarter of 2022 (MQ 2022). It also notes when the rather more lethal Delta and Omicron strains were first detected in Australia.

Restrictions on movement included closing previously open state borders, a move that disrupted internal travel and commerce, as well as causing enormous economic and social disruption. Preventing people from moving across borders was a complicated exercise that required border checks to enforce COVID restrictions. When they were available, passenger flights and interstate

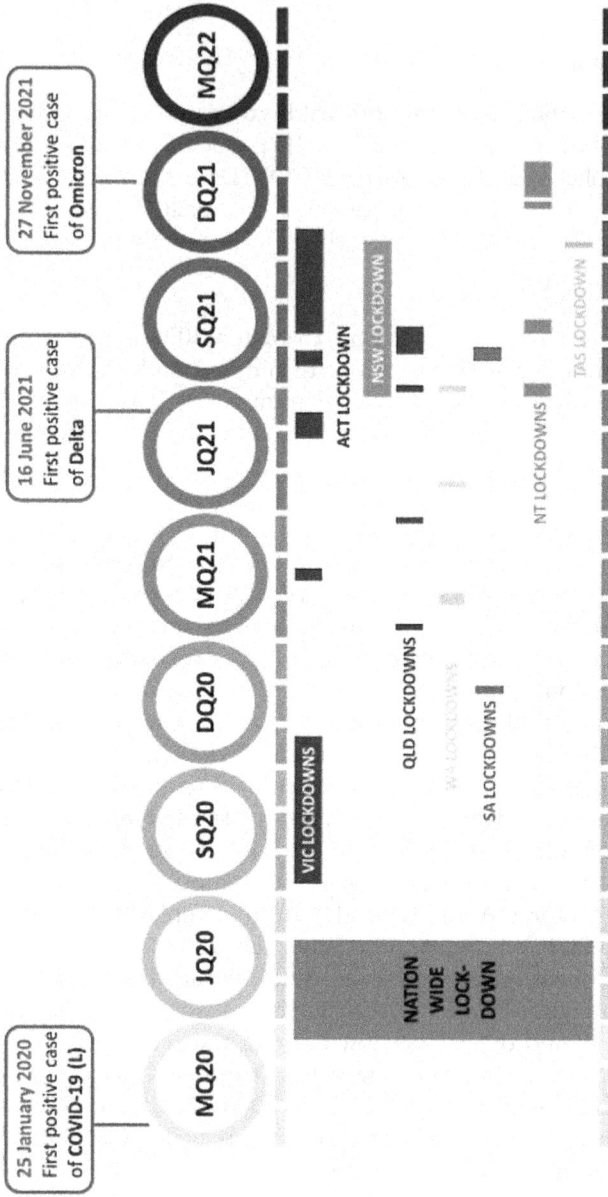

Figure 8.3 Timeline of Australian states and territories in and out of lockdown 2020–2021 (by quarters).

Source: https://www.abs.gov.au/articles/effects-covid-19-strains-australian-economy.

Note: The lockdowns shown in the above timeline are for metropolition areas only

trains required proof of abode documentation and pre-approval for travel (through online forms).

Western Australia's 'hard border' policy promoted a legal challenge from Queensland mining tycoon and sometime politician Clive Palmer on the basis that "interstate trade, commerce and intercourse should be 'absolutely free'". In a politically 'courageous' move, Morrison openly supported Palmer's challenge to the validity of Western Australia's border closure (Brennan 2021). The case went to the High Court, which in November 2020 ruled that there were no grounds for Palmer's challenge, as the emergency powers of states complied with the Constitution of Australia. Western Australia kept its borders sealed until March of 2022, a 697-day isolation from all other Australian states (Marcus 2022), and during this time, its government allowed in only authorised Fly-in-Fly-out (known as 'FIFO') mining workers. West Australians took offence at Morrison's 2021 comments, which had accused them of wanting to 'stay in the cave' of hard borders when other states were looking to lift border restrictions (9 News 2021). WA voters carried the resentment to the ballot box at the May 2022 federal election in which the Liberal primary vote in WA declined by over 10%, and the number of WA seats held by the Liberal party halved from 10 to 5. Four of these WA seats went to Labor, and that provided half of the eight seats it needed to form a new national government (ABC 2022).

Aged care

The cracks in the Commonwealth were perhaps clearest in the aged care sector, which is operated by a mix of federal government, state government and private providers. The Senate Select Committee on COVID-19, which reported in April 2022, found that by December 2020, COVID deaths in aged care facilities accounted for 74% of Australia's COVID dead. The Federal Ministry of Health and Aged Care has responsibility for the licensing and regulation of aged care facilities. Despite this being a Commonwealth responsibility, the Committee found the federal aged care minister, the Hon Senator Richard Colbeck,[4] "sought to minimise the government's responsibilities for the continually poor outcomes in the aged care sector" (COA 2022: 59). Privately run facilities Newmarch House and Dorothy Henderson Lodge (both in Sydney NSW) had early aged care COVID casualties (Hawksley 2020), and were the subjects of independent reviews, as were Melbourne's aged care facilities St Basil's Home for the Aged in Fawkner, and Heritage Care's Epping Gardens in Epping. A review of the Melbourne homes found the second 'wave' of COVID infections in July and August 2020 resulted in over 200 separate COVID outbreaks in aged care facilities that affected over 2,000 residents and over 2,200 staff. St Basil's infections totalled 94 residents and 95 staff (with 45 resident deaths), while at Epping Gardens, there were 103 residents and 86 staff infected (with 38 resident deaths) (Gilbert and Lilley 2020: 6). Aged care homes are licensed by the Commonwealth and are meant to adhere to Commonwealth guidelines. A special report of the 2000 Royal Commission into Aged Care Quality and Safety, 'Aged Care and COVID-19' (RC 2020) found that in relation to deaths in Victorian aged care,

> [t]here were no active cases of COVID-19 in residential aged care before 7 July 2020 but by 13 July 2020 there were 28 cases. By 9 August 2020, the day before our hearing commenced, this figure exceeded 1000. The first recorded death of an aged care resident from COVID-19 in Victoria was on 11 July 2020. As at 13 September 2020, there have been 563 deaths.
>
> During this period, both the Australian Department of Health and the Aged Care Quality and Safety Commission were active in providing advice. However, this did not extend to mandating, or recommending, the use of face masks in aged care facilities. This is despite the fact that … masks are 'a very cheap and effective method' of slowing the spread of COVID-19.

Both the Senate Committee and the Royal Commission concluded that Australia's experience of COVID revealed significant gaps in the capacity of the aged care system to function under stress. One of the main issues was that the aged care sector workforce was generally underpaid, understaffed and often took shifts at different facilities. While facilities worked tirelessly to prevent their residents from being infected, aged care staff often worked in precarious casual or part-time employment, and so were often holding down up to three jobs across different facilities to pay the bills. A worker who had acquired COVID in one facility might then have worked at a different facility the next day, before any symptoms were obvious, and may have unknowingly infected patients at both. Once a COVID infection was detected in a staff member, there was a requirement of at least two weeks of recuperative leave, but this led to widespread staffing shortages. The COVID pandemic exposed the very poor working conditions of aged care workers, many of whom are migrants to Australia working for minimum wages.

Part II: The health and economic responses

As a result of the Constitutional Framework, the states and territories, and not the Commonwealth, were on the front line of combatting COVID-19; however, the issue of quarantine was clearly understood as a federal power, as specified in the Constitution under Section 51 (xxix) (Tingle 2021). As a large and continental island state, most people come in or out of Australia by air (99%) and most goods (99.93% by volume) by sea. Implementing quarantine measures to prevent COVID cases from reaching Australia was straightforward: the Commonwealth government could deny permission for planes to land or cruise ships to dock. Container ships are vital for Australian trade and were permitted to dock as long as they had been at sea for 14 days and had no

COVID cases. Ships captains were required to certify there were no cases. In Western Australian ports, this caused concerns and later crews were only allowed to disembark to carry out essential vessel functions (9 News, 2020).

In the first six months of 2020, the Commonwealth announced several measures to protect the public from COVID as it enhanced screening measures for passengers on direct flights from Wuhan (21 January), aimed to evacuate Australian nationals from Wuhan and Hubei provinces of China (29 January), imposed entry bans of 14 days on foreign nationals who had visited mainland China (1 February) and then extended that ban for a further week, implemented the Australian Health Sector Emergency Response Plan for Novel Coronavirus (COVID-19) (Feb 29), increased travel restrictions on Iran (1 March), imposed restrictions on Italy and South Korea (5 March), banned cruise ships from entry (15 March) and declared all international arrivals in Australia had to isolate for 14 days (15 March). Finally, on 20 March, the borders of Australia were closed to all except Australian citizens and residents (POA 2021).

Air travel restrictions for all other countries remained, and they prevented tourists, migrant workers and international students from coming to Australia. The bans on travel to Australia led to a massive decline in short-term visits, which fell by 99.2% between January 2020 (1.16 million) and June 2020 (14,020) (ABS 2020). This decline led to labour shortages, especially in the agricultural sector—which had historically relied on backpackers for seasonal work such as fruit picking—as well as hospitality, retail and the tourism sectors. In April 2021, Australia and New Zealand introduced a 'travel bubble' that did not require passengers to isolate.[5]

While Australian citizens and permanent residents were permitted to return to Australia, there were fewer flights, and they were more expensive. Those citizens or permanent residents who were able to secure a flight to Australia faced 14 days of isolation. The Commonwealth initially intended its immigration detention processing centre on Christmas Island in the Indian Ocean for quarantine but decided on the Howard Springs Accommodation Facility, a former mining camp outside Darwin in the Northern Territory.[6] Howard Springs was used initially for 266 evacuations from Wuhan in February 2020 quarantining for 14 days (Hunt 2020). By March 2021, Howard Springs could take 850 people a fortnight, and by August 2021, this had increased to 2,000 (Shams 2021).

The cracks in the Commonwealth quarantine system were clear early when the *Ruby Princess* cruise ship was allowed to dock in Sydney on 18–19 March and all 2,700 passengers, including over 100 suspect COVID cases (Walker 2020: 200), were permitted to disembark without testing. Some 900 people later tested positive, and 28 died (BBC News 2020). A NSW Special Commission of Inquiry noted that allowing all passengers off the ship was "not rational" (Walker 2020: 201) and that despite what should have been a workable system and an exercise in cooperative federalism, the interlocking responsibilities of multiple agencies—both Commonwealth (Australian Border Force,

Department of Agriculture, Water and Environment) and State (NSW Ambulance, the Port Authority, the NSW Police Force and NSW Health) resulted in an outcome that "did not work as intended" (Walker 2020: 25–28).

Elsewhere, the number of returning Australians was much larger than could be accommodated at the Commonwealth's Howard Springs facility, and on 27 March 2020, National Cabinet agreed on the 'hotel quarantine programme'. This solution dovetailed with the state and territory-led strategy to support the tourism sector as returnees were transported from the airport to quarantine for 14 days in otherwise empty four- and five-star hotels in capital cities (Hawksley, 2020). The unusual aspect of this agreement was that while quarantine was a Commonwealth responsibility, the states and territories agreed to manage arrivals and initially to pay quarantine costs.[7] One of the reasons later given for this decision was that state and territory leaders lacked confidence in the Commonwealth's capacity to manage quarantine, a suspicion later borne out by its mismanagement of the aged care sector (Tingle 2021).

State variation

Between the January 2020 outbreak of the pandemic and the end of 2021, each Australian jurisdiction managed its own COVID response within a broad national objective of attempting to eradicate COVID. The highest COVID case numbers and the highest number of COVID deaths were in the two largest states by population, NSW and Victoria, which also had the most severe COVID outbreaks. As Table 8.1 shows, by 31 December 2021, Victoria had recorded 1,525 COVID deaths, which was 68% of all Australian COVID deaths, and NSW 663 COVID deaths (29.6%). The combined populations of Qld, WA, SA, Tas, the ACT and the NT, which represent around 45% of the population, had registered just 7.6% of COVID cases, and 2.2% of all Australian COVID deaths.

Australian state leadership and COVID statistics (2020–2021)

As Figure 8.4 shows, Australia was like many other states across the world in that COVID deaths were mostly among older people. To the end of 2021, for all age cohorts except those over 90 years, more men died from COVID than women.

Whatever their political persuasion, all Australian jurisdictions managed COVID outbreaks with utmost caution, aiming to restrict the spread of the virus from any known clusters. In Melbourne and Sydney (the two most affected Australian cities), there were different levels of enforcement, with robust policing of lower socio-economic areas, while more affluent areas were largely unaffected. In Melbourne, police services were used to enforce restrictions with COVID-affected populations in the Flemington Public Housing Estate (colloquially known as the 'Flemington flats') a complex of nine tower

Table 8.1 National, state and territory populations, government leaders, total COVID cases and COVID deaths to 31 December 2021

	Population (March 2022)	National and state leaders (and party)	Total COVID cases to 31 Dec 2021	Total COVID deaths to 31 Dec 2021
Australia	25,978,773	Scott Morrison (Liberal)	399,514	2,239
NSW	8,130,115	Gladys Berejiklian/ Dominic Perrottet (Oct 2021) (Liberal)	187,504	663
Victoria	6,593,314	Daniel Andrews (Labor)	176,534	1,525
Queensland	5,296,098	Annastacia Palaszczuk (Labor)	13,863	7
WA	2,773,435	Mark McGowan (Labor)	1,158	9
SA	1,815,485	Steve Marshall (Liberal)	11,078	6
Tasmania	571,165	Peter Gutwein (Liberal)	785	13
ACT	455,869	Andrew Barr (Australian Labor Party)	4010	15
NT	250,398	Michael Gunnar (Labor)	572	1

Source: Authors—adapted from: https://www.abs.gov.au/statistics/people/population/national-state-and-territory-population/latest-release and https://www.health.gov.au/resources/publications/coronavirus-covid-19-at-a-glance-31-december-2021#

blocks. These flats experienced severe lockdown restrictions from 4 July 2020, imposed with no notice. A report by Victoria's Ombudsman Commission (Victorian Ombudsman 2020) found a heavy police presence was stationed on each floor of the tower blocks. Residents of most towers were let out for air and exercise after five days; however, those of the tower at 33 Alfred St were kept inside for another nine days and were only allowed out for air and exercise after 16 days. The Flemington flats residents were largely migrants from culturally and linguistically diverse (CALD) and refugee backgrounds. Although most politicians who spoke on this event regarded it as necessary from a health perspective, some news articles conveyed how residents of the 'Flemington

DEATHS BY AGE GROUP AND SEX

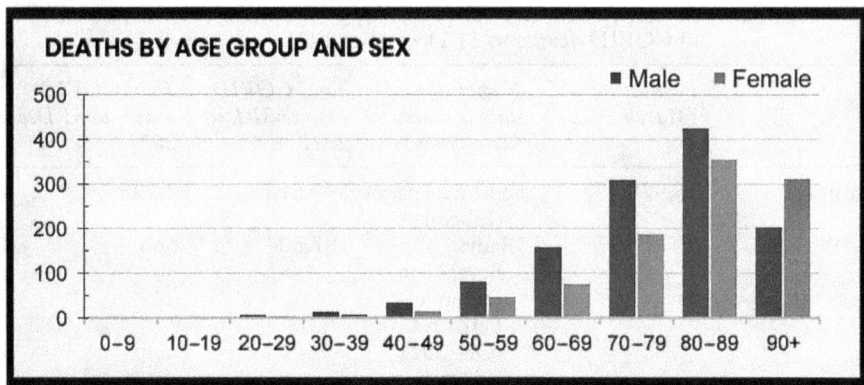

Figure 8.4 COVID deaths to 31 December 2021 by age cohort (Australia).

Source: Department of Health (https://www.health.gov.au/sites/default/files/documents/2022/01/coronavirus-covid-19-at-a-glance-31-december-2021.pdf)

flats' were also stereotyped due to their ethnic backgrounds and the languages spoken at home, as well as being labelled as 'alcoholics' and 'drug addicts' (Georgeou et al. 2023). The intense invigilation and scrutiny of lower-class and predominantly migrant areas did not occur in other areas of Melbourne that were wealthier and more demographically 'white'.

In Sydney between July to September, residents of 12 local government areas in Western and South-western Sydney were singled out for harsh lockdown conditions during a Delta outbreak (SBS 2021). A highly visible police presence, including police helicopters, was mobilised to enforce the curfew in Western Sydney, and the Australian Defence Force (ADF) was brought in to ensure compliance. There was a public outcry when no restrictions were required for residents of Sydney's affluent eastern suburbs, the original source of the same Delta outbreak, and the heavy-handed presence in Western Sydney led to reports of some communities being traumatised. Lockdowns in Sydney's West and Southwest contrasted also with lockdowns in Sydney's affluent Northern Beaches in late 2020, which were not as stringent.

Analysis of COVID-related media articles throughout 2020–2021 revealed that the media initially worked to promote public health messaging, but became more critical of government responses over time. As Georgeou et al. argued (2023), the pandemic caused a form of 'slow violence' in which people were stigmatised for breaching public health orders, or for the perception that they had breached public health orders. Healthcare workers (i.e. nurses, doctors, pharmacists, aged care workers, and disability workers) experienced stigma due to the fear that they were carrying and spreading the COVID-19 virus through their close proximity to COVID-positive patients. Australian media reported incidents of abuse where healthcare workers were coughed at or spat on in public spaces, or where they were being advised to avoid wearing their uniforms in public. There were reports of healthcare workers being refused service in retail spaces, or being denied or forced to leave accommodation. Apart from the irrationality of stigmatising a group of people who were on the forefront of controlling COVID transmission (and who usually had the protective gear to assist them), such incidents demonstrated intersections of race and stigma experienced by healthcare workers of 'Asian' descent/appearance who were described as 'dirty' and as 'bat-eaters' (Georgeou et al. 2023).

Vaccination

By mid-late 2020, there were a number of vaccine candidates emerging. In August 2020, the Commonwealth announced its vaccine and treatment strategy, committing to securing vaccines internationally, and to using local manufacturing where possible (ANAO 2022), with Morrison announcing the Commonwealth would work with Oxford University on an Australian-made AstraZeneca vaccine (Murphy 2020b). Some 50 million doses of AstraZeneca were manufactured by the pharmaceutical company CSL in Melbourne by February 2021 (DHAC 2022a), with doses donated to the Pacific Islands as part of Australia's aid programme. As the emphasis shifted to vaccine delivery, the distribution of vaccines was initially handled through local general practitioners across Australia before larger cities introduced mass vaccination hubs in 2021. Vaccines were available free of charge for everyone (DHAC 2023).

Elderly people in the aged care sector were among the first to be offered vaccines, which became mandatory for healthcare workers and for teachers in state school education systems. As the vaccination programme progressed the target cohorts became progressively younger. By 31 December 2021, 90.2% of all people over 12 in Australia had received two doses of a COVID vaccine (ANAO 2022).

While this was an excellent eventual result, not everything had gone to plan. An August 2022 audit of the national vaccine rollout concluded,

> Initial planning was not timely, with detailed planning with states and territories not completed before the rollout commenced, and Health underestimated the complexity of administering in-reach services to the aged care and disability sectors. Further, it did not incorporate the government's targets for the rollout into its planning until a later stage.
>
> (Karp 2022b)

Prime Minister Morrison had insisted from early March 2021 that the COVID vaccine response was 'not a race' (Taylor 2021); however, by May 2021, the delays in rolling out vaccination, and the constant shifts in vaccine timeline implementation, led Australian Council of Trades Unions president Sally McManus to criticise the slow pace of the Commonwealth's efforts, dubbing it the 'vaccine strollout', a word that captured the *zeitgeist* and which in November 2021 was named 'word of the year' (Burnside 2021). To counter public criticism and reclaim the narrative, in July 2021, the Commonwealth appointed senior Australian Defence Force officer Li eutenant General John (JJ) Frewen as the coordinator general of what was called 'Operation COVID Shield' (ANAO 2022), which imparted more rigour into the response.

While a response of over 90% of those over 12 years being double vaccinated was commendable, there was vaccine hesitancy in some parts of the Australian population. The Australian media and social media carried reports that some people in the United Kingdom had developed side effects from the AstraZeneca vaccine (Baron and Adhikari 2022: 9–10), which helped establish the popular wisdom that the Pfizer vaccine was preferable to others. The Commonwealth's Australian Technical Advisory Group on Immunisation (ATAGI) tried to assuage concern, noting in July 2021 that there were no substantive differences between any of the vaccines approved in Australia and that the benefits of vaccination outweighed any risks (ATAGI 2021).

A broad collection of disaffected groups formed a protest movement that challenged mask wearing, restrictions and the national vaccination programme. Protestors included those opposed to vaccination on the grounds it was in some way unsafe or would lead to allergic reactions (dubbed 'anti-vaxers'), as well as so-called 'sovereign citizens' who did not accept the right of governments to restrict their movements, mandate mask wearing, encourage vaccination or even levy taxation or issue driver's licenses (McMahon 2022). More extreme political elements also attended the protest marches held in capital cities, both during and after lockdown periods, with protests in Melbourne in August 2021 turning violent after the crowd of over 4,000 turned on police (AAP 2021).

With the vaccination programme proceeding, from early July 2021, National Cabinet considered how to emerge from the pandemic, and it used complex modelling from the Doherty Institute to chart a path back to a 'new normal' through a four-phase plan (PM&C 2020) that relied on lifting restrictions in response to higher levels of vaccination. NSW Premier Dominic Perrottet championed this plan claiming, "We can't stay closed. We need to learn to live alongside the virus", even while acknowledging that lifting all restrictions would lead to an increase in cases (Wu 2021). The lifting of restrictions in NSW coincided with the onset of the Omicron variant after November 2021, which quickly overtook all previous COVID strains. The massive increases in COVID transmission and deaths from December 2021 (McGowan 2021) caused the NSW public to dub its premier 'Domicron' (Dominic + Omicron) for his 'Let it rip' COVID strategy (Davies 2021).

On the last day of 2021, the total number of COVID infections in Australia was recorded as 395,504, but half of these had come in just the last six weeks of the year (Our World in Data 2022). The relaxation of restrictions led to sizeable increases in COVID cases and deaths in 2022. Despite high vaccination rates, by 31 December 2022, over 10 million Australians had contracted

COVID. By the end of 2022, the number of Australians had who died from COVID had increased almost six times, from the 2,139 at the end of 2021 to 15,361 (WHO 2022).

The economic response

The Commonwealth has powers over taxation and distributes funds to the states and territories. With the resources of the national state at its disposal, the Commonwealth was able to support the states and territories through the national social security system. Ideologically, this required the centre-right Liberal/National coalition government to drop its neoliberal fixation with balanced budgets, and to adopt Keynesian stimulus policies that "inaugurated the golden age of entitlement" (Cooke 2020). The Commonwealth moved quickly to create payments to those people the states and territories were putting out of work through the enforcement of social distancing, and to mitigate the effects of preventing people from working, it provided stimulus spending, especially for casual workers who had been laid off (Verrender 2020).

The first package on 12 March 2022 provided AUD $17.6 billion (c. $12 billion US) to assist six million welfare recipients with a $750 cash payment. Small- and medium-sized businesses received between $2000-$25,000 to pay wages or hire extra staff. On 22 March another package of $66 billion was announced, providing another $750 cash grant to welfare recipients, and doubling the amount of money available to the unemployed, with new fortnightly payments to those looking for work ('Job Seeker' $750). Those prohibited from going to work received 'Job Keeper' ($1,500 a fortnight), with payments made to employers to then pay to staff (Hawksley 2020). Despite these measures, the restrictions on movement meant the hospitality sector was severely affected; some 272,000 jobs were lost in hospitality, and over 120,000 workers stood down (Statista 2022). By mid-2020, the economic cost of COVID restrictions to Australia was estimated at around $4 billion per week (Hawksley 2020).

Victoria and New South Wales both endured prolonged lockdowns, with Melbourne in particular frequently cited as the city that had the world's longest lockdown (here understood as enforced 'stay-at-home' orders) of 262 days, including one stretch of 111 days and another of 77 days in the period 31 March 2020 to 21 October 2021 (ABC 2022).[8]

There was a general recognition during the pandemic that levels of unemployment benefits were too low and that they were trending well below the poverty line, with calls for the increased Job Seeker payment (which had almost doubled the unemployment benefit) to be retained into the future as some form of universal basic income (Wade 2021). The Morrison government, however, had not entirely shed its ideological prejudices and was working consistently to 'snapback' to the pre-COVID economic growth that Australia had enjoyed in the early 2000s, largely on the back of commodity prices for iron ore, copper and other minerals (Cooke 2020).

While the government bailed out most companies, it drew the line at supporting the university sector, which along with sex workers, was excluded from support payments. Australian universities are publicly funded, but they rely heavily on international student fees, particularly from China and India. The ban on travel meant that international students did not come to study, so universities faced a cash shortfall. Despite the fact that education was Australia's third largest export industry (valued at over 80 billion per year) the Commonwealth refused to extend Job Keeper to the tertiary sector, prompting large-scale (27,000) job losses (Hare 2022). One explanation for this stance was that government opposition was essentially ideological: the Morrison government "just hates universities" (Megalogenis 2021), as they believed they were breeding grounds of that mythical political bloc, 'the left'. Nor was support offered to the around 90,000 international students who stayed in Australia during the pandemic, even though education effectively went online for two years, and they did not attend campus. Morrison, in fact, strongly encouraged international students to return home.

International students were neither citizens nor residents, so were not eligible for government relief payments. Some had limited casual employment, but without means of support, it was up to states and the community to assist this cohort. The NSW state government worked with civil society organisations, and the staff and management of universities, to organise food baskets and other assistance for international (and domestic) students (NSW gov 2021). Domestic undergraduates who commenced studies in 2020 had a couple of weeks of normal campus life before retreating to their bedrooms to undertake the first two years of their three-year degrees online. Mental health services in Australia were already failing to provide adequate treatment for those who needed it before the pandemic (Krasnostein 2022: 5), and pandemic learning conditions added to the strain.

By the end of April 2020, the Commonwealth had provided around $194bn in stimulus. This figure was almost 40% of the total pre-COVID 2019 budget and around 9.5% of gross domestic product. By mid-2020, a further $15 billion in stimulus had come from the states and territories (Hawksley 2020). The Commonwealth provided billions in support from money it did not have, and in an effort to calm inflationary concerns the independent Reserve Bank of Australia, which implements monetary policy, reduced the official bank lending rate to an historic low of 0.25%. It also guaranteed AUS$90 billion in funding for banks to lend to businesses to keep economic activity ticking over. With panic buying and occasional food shortages during 2020 and 2021, stores placed limits on the purchase of essentials (Hawksley 2020), while governments implemented various schemes to promote consumption. For example, NSW ran a range of free voucher systems to get people to travel, eat at restaurants and attend cinemas (NSW gov 2022). The high rate of vaccine take-up by the end of 2021 was perhaps boosted by businesses adopting policies that restricted entry to restaurants, entertainment centres, shopping centres and supermarkets to those with proof of vaccination.

The Commonwealth attempted a national phone app for managing COVID. By late April 2020, its COVIDSafe app had been downloaded by one million people, but the government argued it would need ten million users (40% of the population) to make COVID-19 monitoring more effective. The federal government then held out the promise of relaxations in social distancing with a higher rate of COVIDSafe downloads, but the public failed to get behind the national app. With just two positive COVID tests detected that were not picked up through contact tracing, the $21 million app was generally considered a massive waste of taxpayer money (DHAC 2022b).

Individual states instead developed their own apps for managing COVID. For example in NSW, during 2020, widespread use of the New South Wales government's COVID app and its QR codes ensured that those who checked into a location that was later declared a 'COVID hotspot' were texted and encouraged to get a PCR test, which was also free to the public and established in numerous locations as case numbers increased. While case numbers were low, this system worked well; however, by late 2021, the system broke down under overwhelming case numbers.

COVID testing was at first conducted by PCR test, which "detects genetic material of the virus using a lab technique called reverse transcription polymerase chain reaction (RT-PCR)" (Mayo Clinic 2021). A PCR test was the 'Gold Standard', as Australians were told, and PCR testing was free to the public during the pandemic; however, each test cost the government around $80–$85. The cost of these tests was borne by the Commonwealth, which provided private pathology companies with a subsidy through universal health (Medicare) of $85 per test while public laboratories received $42.50 (Alexander and Carrol 2021). Rapid Antigen Tests (RATs) were less exact, but are much cheaper than PCR tests. During 2021, the Commonwealth proclaimed the use of RAT tests as an acceptable alternative to PCRs, but without securing a sufficient supply. Some Australian companies made RATs, but they sold their entire production to American companies and American states. Australia was thus forced to import RATs from China and Europe (AU Manufacturing 2021). Profiteering on the limited stock meant a $10 RAT was initially being sold for up to $50. States and territories purchased stocks for schoolchildren (free to all pupils), but even by the end of December 2021 as lockdown restrictions were being lifted, RAT tests were still difficult to obtain. A perfect storm of spiking COVID case numbers, long lines at PRC testing and no available RATs ensured widespread community transmission into 2022.

The Commonwealth provided extensive economic support for those affected by restrictions on movement, and it ended up spending over three times in COVID fiscal stimulus as it had during the Global Financial Crisis of 2008 (Megalogenis 2021). During 2020–2021, many Australian workers spent at least some period of time at home, with their pay covered or subsidised by government benefits. The rather extraordinary thing about this financial support was that it came from a government that for over a decade had been championing the notion of balanced budgets, smaller government and getting rid of welfare rorts. The ideological conversion did not however last, and most support measures were wound back by early 2021.

Conclusions

With an increasingly vaccinated population from the end of 2021, Australia moved into a 'living with COVID' mentality; however, the pandemic is far from over. The difference for Australia was that by the end of 2022, 96% of the population over 16 years had been double vaccinated and 72.4% had received a booster shot (DHAC 2022c). Vaccination does not however prevent one from contracting COVID. As the editors of this book can attest, even triple vaccination does not prevent COVID infections; however, the effects of COVID do appear to be less serious for those vaccinated. As noted, despite spite high vaccination rates nationally, the number of COVID infections and deaths in Australia climbed rapidly during 2022. The vast majority of COVID deaths continue to be among those aged 70 years and over.

Overall, Australia's COVID experience during 2020–2021 compares favourably with other states on both a total cases per million and a deaths per million basis. Part of this success is no doubt due to the natural defences of Australia as an island continent. Another explanation is that early and incisive government interventions isolated Australia from the rest of the world, and then Australian states and territories isolated themselves from each other. Australia was fortunate in that it could afford massive economic stimulus that sustained people financially when they were not permitted to attend a physical workplace. Credit must go to the state premiers and territory chief ministers who took unpopular lockdown and restriction decisions early, and who closed borders and kept them closed, usually against the Commonwealth government's wishes. Rather than coordinate and manage the national response, the Commonwealth experienced an uneven record on the procurement and delivery of vaccines, and in areas like healthcare, it often attempted to shift the blame to the states. Scott Morrison's performance as prime minister was not the only thing that led to his party's defeat in the May 2022 federal election, but his denial of responsibility, buck-passing and arrogation of sweeping powers during the COVID pandemic were certainly factors.

Notes

1 The Commonwealth of Australia entered into force in January 1901 and is the result of three constitutional conventions (held in 1981, 1983 and 1897) by the six colonies of the Australian continent—New South Wales, Tasmania, Victoria, Queensland, South Australia and Western Australia. By 1890, all colonies had powers of self-government, and they met to discuss the formation of one national government. The proposal to federate—the Commonwealth Constitution Bill—was put to referendum in 1898 (in Vic, NSW, SA and Tas), then again in 1989 (in Vic, NSW, SA, Tas and Qld). The proposal was put to a vote in WA in 1900 after the *Commonwealth of Australia Constitution Act* had been passed by the British parliament in July 1900 (for full details, see AEC 2022). The ACT is an administrative territory centred around Australia's capital city Canberra. It was chosen as it was

roughly half-way between Melbourne and Sydney, Australia's two largest cities. Created in 1909 as a gift to the Commonwealth from NSW, the federal government moved to Canberra in 1927 from its original home of Melbourne. The region officially became the Australian Capital Territory in 1938. The Northern Territory was administered by South Australia from 1863 to 1911) when it was transferred to Commonwealth control. In 1978, the Northern Territory was given self-government. Both territories have unicameral parliaments and are run by chief ministers rather than premiers. Australian states elect 12 senators each to the federal parliament and each of the territories selects two. The Commonwealth Parliament has the power to override some territory laws.

2 After the election loss Frydenberg commented that Morrison's additional secret ministerial appointments were "wrong", "profoundly disappointing" and "extreme overreach" (SBS 2022).

3 National Cabinet officially replaced the more formal, and usually annual, Council of Australian Governments (COAG), which had functioned mostly to discuss budget allocations, on 29 May 2020.

4 In January 2022, Minister Colbeck was lampooned for spending more time at a cricket test match than at his ministerial aged care duties. Colbeck cited his other important ministerial responsibilities, as minister for sport (attending three days of the Australia v England Test in Hobart in Jan 2022 when the rest of the country was battling outbreaks of Omicron), as the reason why he could not front the Senate Select Committee on COVID-19, which sought to explore the Australian government's response to COVID-19 (Karp, 2022b).

5 At various times during the discussion, the Pacific Islands were considered for inclusion in this bubble, but this did not eventuate. The Pacific Islands remained closed to international visitors until mid-2022.

6 Howard Springs outside the Northern Territory capital of Darwin is an open-air facility which was regarded as a quarantine success and was later used as a model for three Centres for National Resilience (in Melbourne, Brisbane and Perth): "purpose-built quarantine facilities that will support overseas travel and ensure the safety of the Australian community." Memoranda of Understanding with Victoria, Queensland and Western Australia were signed, and the first beds at the Centre for National Resilience Melbourne were expected to open by the end of 2021 (DoF 2021).

7 After 18 July 2020, incoming passengers had to pay for the costs of their quarantine (NSW gov 2020).

8 Buenos Aires, Argentina, had a longer continuous lockdown of 234 days between March and November 2020. The Chilean city of Iqueque had 287 days of lockdown (ABC 2022).

Bibliography

7 News. (2021, August 25). *Sunrise*, https://7news.com.au/sunrise/on-the-show/josh-frydenberg-explains-what-its-like-living-at-the-lodge-with-prime-minister-scott-morrison-c-3773898.

9 News. (2020, November 9). *A Current Affair*. 'Whistle Blower Concerned Seaports Are a Coronavirus Corridor into Australia', https://9now.nine.com.au/a-current-affair/coronavirus-corridor-through-carrier-ship-ports-exposed/190aa204-bf8f-433e-80f1-bddbddb6168c.

AAP (Australian Associated Press). (2021, August 22). 'Police Say Melbourne Anti-Lockdown Protest "Most Violent in Nearly 20 Years"', *The Guardian*, https://www.theguardian.com/australia-news/2021/aug/22/police-say-melbourne-anti-lockdown-protest-most-violent-in-nearly-20-years.

ABC. (2022). 'Fact Check: Matthew Guy Says Melbourne Was the World's Most Locked-Down City. Is That Correct?', https://www.abc.net.au/news/2022-11-21/fact-check-is-melbourne-world-s-most-locked-down-city/101659926.

ABS (Australian Bureau of Statistics). (2020). 'Overseas Travel Statistics, Provisional', https://www.abs.gov.au/statistics/industry/tourism-and-transport/overseas-travel-statistics-provisional/jun-2020.

AEC (Australian Electoral Commission). (2022). 'The Referendums 1898–1900', https://education.aec.gov.au/teacher-resources/federation/the-referendums.html.

Alexander, H. and L. Carrol. (2021, July 27). 'Taxpayers Spend More than $580 Million on COVID-19 Testing in NSW', https://www.smh.com.au/national/nsw/taxpayers-spend-more-than-580-million-on-covid-19-testing-in-nsw-20210726-p58d1b.html.

ANAO (Australian National Audit Office). (2022). 'Australia's COVID-19 Vaccine Rollout',https://www.anao.gov.au/work/performance-audit/australia-covid-19-vaccine-rollout.

ATAGI (Australian Technical Advisory Group on Immunisation). (2021). 'ATAGI Update Following Weekly COVID-19 Meeting – 14 July 2021', https://www.health.gov.au/news/atagi-update-following-weekly-covid-19-meeting-14-july-2021.

AU Manufacturing. (2021). '$60 Million for Imported Rats, No Order for Brisbane's Ellume',https://www.aumanufacturing.com.au/60m-for-imported-rats-no-order-for-brisbanes-ellume.

Baron, S. and N. Adhikari. (2022). *Challenging COVID-19 "Infodemic": A Six-Country Comparison 2021*, Humanitarian and Development Research Initiative (HADRI), Western Sydney University, https://doi.org/10.26183/0t1b-ry67.

BBC News. (2020, August 17). 'Coronavirus: 'Serious Mistakes' Made over Ruby Princess Outbreak', https://www.bbc.com/news/world-australia-53776285.

Bell, V. (2022). 'Report of the Inquiry into the Appointment of the Former Prime Minister to Administer Multiple Departments', https://www.ministriesinquiry.gov.au/publications/report-inquiry.

Brennan, F. (2021). 'Clive Palmer, COVID, and the WA Border', https://www.eurekastreet.com.au/article/clive-palmer--covid--and-the-wa-border.

Burnside, N. (2021). 'In Choosing 'Strollout' As Its Word of the Year, the National Dictionary Centre Alludes to a Uniquely Australian Problem', *ABC News*, https://www.abc.net.au/news/2021-11-17/australian-word-of-the-year-is-strollout-referencing-vaccines/100626698.

COA (Commonwealth of Australia). (2022). 'Senate Select Committee on COVID-19 Final Report', https://www.aph.gov.au/Parliamentary_Business/Committees/Senate/COVID-19/COVID19/Report.

Cooke, R. (2020, May). 'The Ministry of Pandemics: How the Virus Revealed Our Leaders to Us', *The Monthly*, pp. 19–25 at 21.

Coorey, P. (2021, September 24). 'Morrison Has Been Unseated by the Premiers', *Australian Financial Review*,https://www.afr.com/politics/federal/morrison-has-been-unseated-by-the-premiers-20210824-p58le8.

Davies, A. (2021, December 23). 'Dominic Perrottet Has Finally Realised That 'Letting It Rip' Comes at too High a Cost – For All of Us', *The Guardian*, https://www.theguardian.com/australia-news/2021/dec/23/dominic-perrottet-has-finally-realised-that-letting-it-rip-comes-at-too-a-high-cost-for-all-of-us.

DHAC (Department of Health and Aged Care). (2022a). 'Australia's Vaccine Agreements', https://www.health.gov.au/our-work/covid-19-vaccines/about-rollout/vaccine-agreements.

DHAC (Department of Health and Aged Care). (2022b). 'Failed COVIDSafe App Deleted',health.gov.au/ministers/the-hon-mark-butler-mp/media/failed-covidsafe-app-deleted.

DHAC (Department of Health and Aged Care). (2022c). 'Vaccination Numbers and Statistics', https://www.health.gov.au/our-work/covid-19-vaccines/vaccination-numbers-and-statistics.

DHAC (Department of Health and Aged Care). (2023). 'Getting Vaccintated', https://www.health.gov.au/topics/immunisation/getting-vaccinated.

DoF (Department of Finance). (2021). 'Centres for National Resilience', https://www.finance.gov.au/government/property-and-construction/centres-national-resilience.

Eburn, M. (2019). 'What Is a 'National Emergency?'', https://australianemergencylaw.com/2019/12/25/what-is-a-national-emergency/.

Georgeou, N., Buhler King, C., Tame, L., Ergler, C., and Huish, R. (2023). 'COVID-19 Stigma, Australia and Slow Violence: An Analysis of 21 Months of COVID News Reporting', *Australian Journal of Social Issues*. https://doi.org/10.1002/ajs4.273

Gilbert, L. and Lilley, A. (2020, November 30). 'Independent Review: St Basil's and Epping Gardens', https://www.health.gov.au/sites/default/files/documents/2020/12/coronavirus-covid-19-independent-review-of-covid-19-outbreaks-at-st-basil-s-and-epping-gardens-aged-care-facilities.pdf.

Hare, J. (2022, February 13). 'Pandemic-Hit Unis Cut Up to 27,000 Jobs in a Year', *Australian Financial Review*, https://www.afr.com/work-and-careers/education/university-jobs-slashed-as-pandemic-forces-students-away-20220211-p59vqn.

Hawksley, C. (2020). 'Australia', in N. Georgeou and C. Hawksley (eds.), *State Responses to COVID-19: A Global Snapshot at 1 June 2020*, Western Sydney University.

Hunt, G. (2020). 'Interview about Novel Coronavirus with Katie Woolf on Mix1049 Darwin', https://www.health.gov.au/ministers/the-hon-greg-hunt-mp/media/interview-about-novel-coronavirus-with-katie-woolf-on-mix1049-darwin.

Karp, P. (2022a). 'Scott Morrison's Secret Ministries 'Fundamentally Undermined' Responsible Government, Advice Shows', https://www.theguardian.com/australia-news/2022/aug/23/scott-morrison-secret-ministries-minister-portfolios-fundamentally-undermined-responsible-government-advice-shows.

Karp, P. (2022b). 'Aged Care Minister Richard Colbeck Went to Ashes Test on Same Day He Declined to appear at Covid Committee', https://www.theguardian.com/australia-news/2022/jan/25/aged-care-minister-richard-colbeck-went-to-ashes-test-on-same-day-he-declined-to-appear-at-covid-committee.

Krasnostein S. (2022). 'Not Drowning Waving', *Quarterly Essay*, 85, Black Inc. Sydney.

Lawson, K. (2020, February 2). 'Scott Morrison Wants National Emergency Powers', *Canberra Times*, https://www.canberratimes.com.au/story/6603176/pm-setting-out-much-bigger-role-for-feds-in-managing-fire-risk/.

Marcus, L. (2022, March 3). 'Western Australia Ends One of the World's Longest Border Closures', *CNN*, https://edition.cnn.com/travel/article/western-australia-border-reopening-intl-hnk/index.html.

Mayo Clinic. (2021). 'COVID-19 Diagnostic Testing', https://www.mayoclinic.org/tests-procedures/covid-19-diagnostic-test/about/pac-20488900.

McGowan, M. (2021, December 29). 'Perrottet Stands by Decision to Ease Restrictions as NSW Records 11,201 Covid Cases and Omicron Surges around Australia', *The Guardian*, https://www.theguardian.com/world/2021/dec/29/

nsw-daily-covid-cases-surge-to-11201-as-perrottet-stands-by-decision-to-ease-restrictions.

McGowan, M. and Davies, L. (2021). 'NSW Premier Gladys Berejiklian Resigns after Icac Announces Investigation', https://www.theguardian.com/australia-news/2021/oct/01/nsw-premier-gladys-berejiklian-resigns-after-icac-announces-investigation.

McMahon, M. (2022). 'The Flawed Logic Behind the Sovereign Citizen Movement', https://www.thesaturdaypaper.com.au/news/law-crime/2022/02/19/the-flawed-logic-behind-the-sovereign-citizen-movement/164518920013362#hrd.

Megalogenis, G. (2021). 'Exit Strategy: Politics After the Pandemic', *Quarterly Essay 82*, Black Inc. Sydney.

Murphy, K. (2020a). 'Scott Morrison's Coronavirus Mea Culpa Was Barely Disguised Score-Settling with Daniel Andrews', https://www.theguardian.com/australia-news/2020/aug/15/scott-morrisons-coronavirus-mea-culpa-was-barely-disguised-score-settling-with-daniel-andrews.

Murphy, K. (2020b, August 18). 'Australian Government Does Deal to Secure Potential Oxford University Covid Vaccine', *The Guardian*, https://www.theguardian.com/australia-news/2020/aug/18/australian-government-does-deal-to-secure-potential-oxford-university-covid-vaccine-for-free.

Needham, K. (2020, March 27). 'Australia's Fight Against Coronavirus Sees Confusing Mixed Messages', *Reuters*, https://www.reuters.com/article/us-health-coronavirus-australia-politics-idUSKBN21E0YH.

NSW gov. (2021, February 11). 'NSW Rolls Out Food Hampers to support International Students', https://www.study.nsw.gov.au/news/news/nsw-rolls-out-food-hampers-to-support-international-students.

NSW gov. (2022). 'NSW Vouchers for People', https://www.nsw.gov.au/money-and-taxes/vouchers-and-support/voucher-for-people.

NSW gov (NSW government). (2020). 'Revenue', https://www.revenue.nsw.gov.au/news-media-releases/covid-19-tax-relief-measures/quarantine-fees.

OECD (Organisation for Economic Cooperation and Development). (2021, November 17). 'Excess Mortality since 2020', https://www.oecd.org/coronavirus/en/data-insights/excess-mortality-since-january-2020.

Ombudsman, V. (2020). 'Tower Lockdown Breached Human Rights, Ombudsman Finds', https://www.ombudsman.vic.gov.au/our-impact/news/public-housing-tower-lockdown/.

Osborne, Z. (2022, August 5). 'Stung by China's Tariffs, Australian Growers Embrace New Markets', *Al Jazeera*, Stung by China's Tariffs, Australian Growers Embrace New Markets', https://www.aljazeera.com/economy/2022/8/5/stung-by-chinas-tariffs-australian-growers-embrace-new-markets.

Our World in Data. (2022). 'Australia', https://ourworldindata.org/coronavirus/country/australia.

PEO (Parliamentary Education Office). (2022). 'Three Levels of Government: Governing Australia', https://peo.gov.au/understand-our-parliament/how-parliament-works/three-levels-of-government/three-levels-of-government-governing-australia/.

PM&C (Department of Prime Minister and Cabinet). (2020, June 2). 'COAG becomes National Cabinet', https://www.pmc.gov.au/news-centre/government/coag-becomes-national-cabinet.

PoA. (2022). 'Scott Morrison, Member for Cook', https://www.aph.gov.au/Senators_and_Members/Parliamentarian?MPID=E3L.

PoA (Parliament of Australia). (2021). 'COVID-19: A Chronology of Australian Government Announcements (up until 30 June 2020)', https://www.aph.gov.au/About_Parliament/Parliamentary_Departments/Parliamentary_Library/pubs/rp/rp2021/Chronologies/COVID-19AustralianGovernmentAnnouncements.

RC (Royal Commission). (2020). 'Aged Care and COVID-19: A Special Report', https://agedcare.royalcommission.gov.au/sites/default/files/2020-10/aged-care-and-covid-19-a-special-report.pdf.

SBS. (2021). 'Western Sydney Residents Felt 'Punished' by the COVID-19 Lockdowns. Here's Why', https://www.sbs.com.au/news/article/western-sydney-residents-felt-punished-by-the-covid-19-lockdowns-heres-why/8nk2906hf.

SBS (2022). 'Josh Frydenberg breaks his silence on Scott Morrison's 'extreme overreach' in secret ministerial appointments', https://www.sbs.com.au/news/article/extreme-overreach-josh-frydenberg-breaks-his-silence-to-criticise-scott-morrisons-secret-ministeries/u0t77lo8p.

Shams, H. (2021, August 7). 'Howard Springs Quarantine Facility Expected to Reach Capacity for Overseas Arrivals for the First Time', https://www.abc.net.au/news/2021-08-07/nt-howard-springs-set-to-reach-capacity-quarantine/100358058.

Statista. (2022). 'Number of Job Losses and Suspensions during the COVID-19 Crisis in Australia in 2020, by Industry', https://www.statista.com/statistics/1113718/australia-job-losses-and-suspensions-during-coronavirus-crisis-by-industry/.

Sullivan, K. (2020). 'How China Hit Australian Barley, then Beef and Now Eyes Our Wine', *ABC News*, https://www.abc.net.au/news/2020-08-19/china-eyes-australian-wine-export-in-latest-trade-move/12571672.

Taylor, J. (2021). 'From 'It's Not a Race' to 'Go for Gold': How Scott Morrison Pivoted on Australia's Covid Vaccine Rollout', https://www.theguardian.com/society/2021/jul/29/from-its-not-a-race-to-go-for-gold-how-scott-morrison-pivoted-on-australias-covid-vaccine-rollout.

Tingle, L. (2021, January 19). 'Who Is Responsible for Quarantine in Australia?', *ABC News*, https://www.abc.net.au/news/2021-01-19/who-is-responsible-for-quarantine-in-australia/130701080.

Verrender, I. (2020, April 27). 'COVID-19 Stimulus May Not Provide the Hoped-For Boost as JobKeeper Tensions Mount', *ABC News*, https://www.abc.net.au/news/2020-04-27/jobkeeper-coronavirus-payments-begin-balancing-act-economy/12187664.

Wade, M. (2021, August 14). 'Pandemic a 'Natural Experiment' for Universal Basic Income Proposals', *Sydney Morning Herald*, https://www.smh.com.au/business/the-economy/pandemic-a-natural-experiment-for-universal-basic-income-proposals-20210812-p58i9v.html.

Walker, B. (2020). 'Special Commission of Inquiry into the Ruby Princess', *NSW Government*. https://www.dpc.nsw.gov.au/assets/dpc-nsw-gov-au/publications/The-Special-Commission-of-Inquiry-into-the-Ruby-Princess-Listing-1628/Report-of-the-Special-Commission-of-Inquiry-into-the-Ruby-Princess.pdf.

WHO. (2022). 'Australia Situation', https://covid19.who.int/region/wpro/country/au.

Wu, C. (2021, October 11). 'Dominic Perrottet Says We've Got to "Live Alongside the Virus" as NSW Celebrates the Easing Of Restrictions', *Sky News*, https://www.skynews.com.au/australia-news/coronavirus/dominic-perrottet-says-weve-got-to-live-alongside-the-virus-as-nsw-celebrates-the-easing-of-restrictions/news-story/8c3a7f47ba335e8d2c80cd9274edf337.

9 Taiwan

How COVID-19 sharpens Taiwanese identity

Tse-Min Hung

Introduction

Taiwan's response to COVID-19 is widely accepted as one of the most successful examples in the world since the World Health Organization (WHO) announced its first alert on 31 December 2019 (Summers et al. 2020; World Health Organization 2020). By the end of 2021, Taiwan had navigated two periods of COVID-19 community transmission outbreak and was ranked as having the lowest number of COVID-19 cases among Organisation for Economic Co-operation and Development (OECD) countries. According to the data on 22 October 2021, Taiwan had only 69 COVID-19 cases reported per 100,000 population (Cheng 2021a). From April 2022, COVID-19 broke out in Taiwan again due to the highly contagious Omicron variant, which spread much faster than the previous Delta variant of 2021. The number of confirmed cases in a single day quickly exceeded the peak of the pandemic in May 2021. The confirmed cases reached their peak in late May 2022, with more than 90,000 cases registered per day (Reuters 2022). The number slowly descended to around 30,000 cases per day by the end of June 2022. While many countries experienced the Omicron variant earlier than Taiwan and entered the phase of co-existing with COVID-19, Taiwan is following the path of what other countries have learnt, with the hope being that this knowledge could reduce the damage to a minimum.

One of the key factors for Taiwan's success is that it learnt a hard lesson from the Severe Acute Respiratory Syndrome (SARS) outbreak of 2003 (Wang et al. 2020). Taiwan's controversial political status[1] has resulted in it being isolated from the international society and left without assistance from the WHO (Tsai 2020). This experience forced Taiwan to reform its long-term institutional flaws in its performance-oriented medical systems. More importantly, Taiwan has realised that it cannot depend on the WHO or other international organisations. Both lessons learnt served to develop a stronger foundation for responding to the current COVID-19 pandemic (Yeh 2020; Lu 2020; Tsai 2020).

DOI: 10.4324/9781003311522-9

The rest of the world views Taiwan as one of the most successful examples of pandemic management as it has very low numbers of COVID-19 confirmed cases with continued economic growth; however, the long-term struggle to assert a Taiwanese identity amidst an anti-China narrative is often overlooked. The narrative and construction of a separate Taiwanese identity are not novel. Ever since its democratic transition in the 1980s, Taiwanese society has continuously undergone the challenge of forming and re-forming its identity discourses (Lee and Jian 2016; Wu 2015). This challenge became acute when COVID-19 began. When incidents of racist behaviour towards Chinese-looking persons increased around the world—a situation worsened after US President Donald Trump referred to COVID-19 as the 'Chinese virus'—Taiwanese people living both on the island and overseas felt even more strongly about differentiating Taiwan from China. More importantly, the current Democratic Progressive Party (DPP) government in Taiwan has also taken many steps to demonstrate the distinction between Taiwan and China in relation to responding to the pandemic. For example, when China rejected to cooperate with WHO's second phase of investigating the origin of COVID-19 in July 2021, DDP initiated a campaign called "Taiwan Can Help" by donating facemasks and contributing to the development of vaccinations to strengthen its connection with other countries (Tiezzi 2021; Dou and Rauhala 2021; Ministry of Health and Welfare 2022). A survey conducted by the Brookings Institution also revealed that despite Taiwan and China both having some of the lowest COVID-19 death rates in the world, the survey shows that Taiwan is not impressed by China's COVID-19 response due to China's authoritarian measures, which is against the value of democracy that sits at the centre of current Taiwan identity (Rigger, Nachman, Mok, and Chan 2022). The re-articulated and re-shaped Taiwanese identity, instead of focusing on the ethnicity, seems to gradually transform to emphasise its democracy (Ruiz Casado 2021).

Since the outbreak of COVID-19 in Taiwan, every Taiwanese citizen has carried the responsibility of preventing the spread of the disease. This feeling of shared responsibility has been transformed into a sense of shared future and identity. The authority of a country seems constructed on its effective control of its borders, public health prevention measures and mobilising the public to cooperate fully with the government's advice (Tsai 2020). The public and the private spheres have become intermingled, and any boundary has become blurred. This dynamic process in Taiwan has gradually formed a narrative of a shared destiny and identity built on confronting the virus while struggling to overturn its unrecognised international status.

This chapter will begin with an overview of how Taiwan managed the pandemic between 2020 and 2021. The discussion will then demonstrate how the Taiwanese government and the Taiwanese public have consciously and strategically moved to be part of the global effort in combatting COVID-19 while emphasising its distinction from China. Since understanding the rising tensions between Taiwan and China needs to consider its dynamic with the United States, the history of Taiwan–China relations will also be briefly explained, as well as how the 'New Cold War' between the United States and China contributes to Taiwan's controversial international identity. Later, this chapter attempts to discuss how the global wave of Sinophobia during the pandemic has become the breeding ground for forming a Taiwanese identity. The chapter concludes by examining this nuanced and emerging Taiwanese identity during COVID-19.

Overview of the COVID-19 situation in Taiwan

Taiwan's COVID experience can be divided into three periods: (1) manageable cases from January 2020 to mid-May 2021, (2) a surge in cases from mid-May 2021 to July 2021 and (3) a return to manageable cases from July 2021 to the end of 2021. There were only two major outbreaks between 2020 and 2021, and even then, Taiwan's confirmed COVID-19 cases and the recorded deaths were much lower than at the same time in the rest of the world. Between 12 April and 21 November 2020, Taiwan recorded no locally acquired COVID-19 cases for 222 days (Dai, Dai, Shen, and Ho 2021). In general, throughout the pandemic Taiwanese society lived a relatively 'normal' life, with schools mostly continuing to open and large gatherings remained, except for the mandatory facemasks wearing and the strict border control.

Period 1: January 2020 to mid-May 2021

During the first period, there were a total of 1,057 confirmed cases and 11 deaths recorded by Taiwan's Centers for Disease Control (CDC). These low infection and death figures sit in stark contrast to other countries that were ravaged by COVID. As of 3 March, 2020, there were only 42 confirmed cases with 1 death reported in Taiwan, compared to 287 confirmed cases and 6 deaths in Japan and 4,812 cases and 28 deaths in Korea (Cheng 2020).

The comparatively very low rates are due to the Taiwanese government's implementation of a set of measures that established a strong base for Taiwan to prevent the entry of the COVID virus into the community (Cheng 2020), measures adopted as soon as it was informed of events in the city of Wuhan at the end of December 2019. On 1 January 2020, flights between Taiwan and China were suspended, except for the return of Taiwanese citizens living in China. From 25 January 2020, all returning travellers needed to follow quarantine measures for a 14-day period (Dai, Dai, Shen, and Ho 2021). The government had implemented strict travel restrictions and entry protocols since 6 February 2020, and foreign nationals, who had entered China, Hong Kong and Macao in the past 14 days, were prohibited from entering Taiwan. By 18 March, all foreign nationals were not allowed to enter Taiwan, and Taiwanese citizens travelling from certain areas required different levels of quarantine measures (Taiwan Ministry of Foreign Affairs 2022). These proactive border control measures were to ensure overseas acquired cases do not initiate local transmissions (Dai, Dai, Shen, and Ho 2021).

The Central Epidemic Command Centre (CECC), which serves to coordinate all COVID-19-related matters, was established by mid-January 2020. CECC works closely with Taiwan's CDC, which is the government organisation administering Taiwan's public health insurance system. CECC hosted daily media conferences to keep the public informed about daily infections and deaths, and any new government measures to manage the spread of COVID-19. Measures that the government implemented included travel restrictions, 14-day quarantines, contact tracing, social distancing, hand hygiene and mandated mask wearing. The measures of contact tracing, quarantine and mask wearing, in particular, are credited with preventing large-scale community transmission. More importantly, Taiwan's Information and Communication Technology (ICT) allowed multiple government organisations to access the real-time data, which enabled the government to respond and adjust to constantly changing circumstances (Cheng 2020; Soon 2021). These measures, however, would not have been successful without a high level of cooperation among Taiwanese residents. By way of contrast, during the SARS outbreak in 2003, Taiwan reported the third largest number of SARS infections and deaths followed by Hong Kong and China (World Health Organization 2004). Lo and Hsieh (2020) used the lens of 'societalisation' to investigate how the SARS pandemic unpreparedness in Taiwan led to reforms of the public health administration and therefore encouraged early response and centralised government coordination 17 years later during the COVID-19 outbreak in Taiwan. Taiwan's failure in managing SARS became a societal crisis, which mobilised the civil society to address related systematic dysfunctions and transform institutional cultures. Taiwan's civil society has contemplated what Lo and Hsieh (2020) describe as its "pandemic unpreparedness", and it has been "reinterpreting the boundaries between personal freedom and civic duties through the lenses of public health crises" (Lo and Hsieh 2020: 385). Therefore, a discourse of societal collaboration and civic interdependence has gradually formed in the aftermath of SARS, and it has demonstrated a strong collective will among Taiwan's society to cooperate during the COVID-19 outbreak.

Period 2: mid-May 2021 to July 2021

After a long period without any large-scale community transmission in Taiwan, when Taiwanese residents were living a fairly 'normal live', a second wave of COVID arrived. In mid-May 2021, a sudden surge of cases appeared, and so the Taiwanese government quickly raised the emergency alert from Level 1 to Level 2 (out of four levels) (Table 9.1). The alert levels of Taipei City and New Taipei City, the two main cities in northern Taiwan, were raised to Level 3 in mid-May 2021.

However, the government officials soon realised that different alert levels across the island not only caused unnecessary confusion but also hindered the effectiveness of the measures implemented. Therefore, by 19 May, the alert of to all Taiwan jurisdictions was increased to Level 3. The new measures meant

Table 9.1 Taiwan's COVID alert levels

Level 1	Level 2	Level 3	Level 4
No community transmission	Unknown source of locally acquired cases	Three community transmission cases per week or more than ten locally acquired cases of unknown source per day	Large-scale community transmission
Facemasks wearing is suggested in public	Mandatory facemasks wearing in public. Penalty applied if not followed	Mandatory facemask wearing in public. Penalty applied if not followed	Mandatory facemask wearing in public with social distancing measure. penalty applied if not followed
Suggested to cancel or postpone unnecessary gatherings and travels	Public gatherings are limited to 500 people and indoor gatherings are limited to 100 people	Public gatherings are limited to ten people and indoor gatherings are limited to five people	All gatherings and travels are banned unless necessary (e.g., medical appointments)
Schools and entertainment venues are suggested to implement social distancing measures	Schools and entertainment venues need to be closed if cannot implement social distancing measures	Schools and entertainment venues are closed; only essential institutions such as hospitals are allowed to open	Schools and entertainment venues are closed; only essential institutions such as hospitals are allowed to open

Source: Taiwan Centers for Disease Control (2021c), 11 May 2021.

the closure of most schools and entertainment venues, no large gatherings or indoor dining, mandated mask wearing both indoors and outdoors, social distancing and a limit on private gatherings to five people indoors and ten people outdoors. Meanwhile, border controls continued to stay in effect.

By 21 May 2021, there was a total of 3,896 confirmed COVID-19 cases and 17 deaths (Reuters 2021). Between May 11 and July 13, there were 14,103 confirmed cases reported, which accounted for 92% of the total cases since January 2020 (Cheng 2021b). Although the overall infection number was still much lower than in most countries at this time, a sense of under-preparedness had emerged among Taiwanese residents and policymakers. There were reports that the patient demand for beds in hospitals exceeded available beds, which resulted in long waits, and of some patients being treated outdoors (Cheng 2021a). A lack of vaccine supply was another major issue causing public concern. Infections peaked at the beginning of June, and by the end of June, the government announced that the situation had stabilised (Central

News Agency 2021). On 13 July, some restrictions were eased, and on 27 July, the alert level applied to all of Taiwan had been downgraded to Level 2.

Period 3: July 2021 to December 2021

After July 2021, community transmission remained low, with either single-digit or zero daily infections. There was a period between 29 September and 8 October when no COVID deaths were reported in Taiwan. In contrast, the average daily deaths during the same period in the United States was about 2,000 or more (Cheng 2021a). Taiwan's educational institutions and daycare centres were reopening, and the number of people allowed to gather in public was increasing. At the same time, 14-day quarantine for confirmed COVID-19 patients and close contacts remained in place, and mask wearing was still required both indoors and outdoors (Cheng 2021a).

The vaccination rate served as an important indicator for the government as to when the alert level would be downgraded to Level 1. The government announced that downgrading to Level 1 would only be possible when the first dose of vaccination reached 70% and 60% for the second dose.

Taiwan's vaccination programme

Taiwan secured a shipment of Oxford-AstraZeneca COVID-19 vaccine on 3 March 2021 (Taiwan Centers for Disease Control 2021a). The COVID-19 vaccination programme commenced on 22 March 2021 after the government approved the emergency use authorisation (EUA) of AstraZeneca on 18 March 2021. This was followed by the EUA approval of Moderna on 5 May 2021 and Pfizer-BioNTech COVID-19 vaccine on 3 August 2021 (Aljazeera 2021; Jiang and Chen 2021; 2021; Taiwan Centers for Disease Control 2021a; Taiwan News 2021). In addition, a locally developed Medigen COVID-19 vaccine also received approval for its vaccine production on 19 July 2021 (Taiwan Centers for Disease Control 2021b; 2021e). These vaccines are free for all people, including non-citizens, living in Taiwan. An electronic and online COVID-19 vaccination booking system designed by a designated minister without portfolio—Audrey Tang—was implemented starting July 2021, and its reliable mechanism has ensured equality and uniformity when administrating the vaccine (Lin et al. 2021). Meanwhile, the database that the National Health Insurance (NHI) has contributed to the ease of rolling out the vaccine registration system, as the administrators can easily access the eligibility of applicants. The vaccine information has been translated by the Ministry of Labor into Vietnamese, English, Thai and Indonesian, which are the major languages commonly used by migrant workers in Taiwan (Lin et al. 2021).

A community pharmacy-based model has been implemented in COVID-19 vaccine distribution in Taiwan due to its accessibility to the public. Three thousand one hundred and one health insurance special pharmacies, equivalent to 80% of all community pharmacies in Taiwan, participate in the vaccine programme (Lin et al. 2021). Community pharmacists have also played a critical role for those who need to travel long distances to access vaccines or were unaware of vaccine availability since they have a relationship developed with the community where they serve (Lin et al. 2021). With all the effort dedicated, the CECC announced that the rate of first-dose vaccination had achieved 70% and 30% for the second-dose vaccination by 28 October 2021 (Taiwan Centers for Diseases Control 2021d).

How to secure vaccine supply was a key challenge, one that later had several implications for Taiwan as it attempted to secure an independent identity in world politics. One of the incidents happened with the supply of the Pfizer-BioNTech vaccine, as President Tsai Ing-Wen said Taiwan had been unable to finalise the contract with Pfizer-BioNTech due to China's intervention. China denied its intention of blocking vaccines for Taiwan and accused Taiwan of setting up political obstacles over the vaccine offer (Blanchard & Lee 2021). Regardless, Taiwan's government continuously used its COVID success as an opportunity to boost its international reputation and to secure support for its ongoing campaign for international statehood.

"Taiwan can help"

An article first published by the Taiwan Ministry of Health and Welfare on 14 May titled "Taiwan Can Help, and Taiwan Is Helping!" (Ministry of Health and Welfare 2022) is written in English. At the time of writing (June 2022), it was last updated on 11 March 2022. The purpose of this article—published under the section on major policies in relation to international cooperation—is demonstrated through four subtitles: "I. Safeguard Taiwan and Help the World"; "II. Intensify the Collaboration with the US, European Union, Australia and Other Countries with regard to Epidemic Prevention"; "III. Promote Participation in the WHO"; and "IV. Strengthening Exchange and Connection with Other Countries".

One of the obvious examples of this Taiwanese 'health diplomacy' was to donate 'Made-In-Taiwan' masks to other countries facing mask shortages. On 27 April 2020, the government announced the campaign—Protect Taiwan and Help the World—which encouraged people to donate their own non-purchased mask quota.[2] Four million masks were successfully collected within a week and then shipped overseas wrapped with banners printed "Taiwan Can Help". The spokesperson of China's foreign ministry Chun-Ying Hua responded to Taiwan's donation of facemasks, "Everyone is happy to see that Taiwan is willing to help, but we suggest the people living on the island think twice if they intend to engage in political manipulation during the pandemic" (BBC News 2020a). Regardless, Taiwan's donation of four million facemasks was portrayed as a demonstration of Taiwan's democracy and of the spirit of the Taiwanese public's intention to be part of global civic society (Ministry of Health and Welfare 2022; Woods 2020).

Taiwan joined the global effort to develop COVID-19 vaccines. The Ministry of Foreign Affairs (Taiwan) and the American Institute in Taiwan issued a joint statement on the partnership against COVID-19 in March 2020. This statement enabled Taiwan and the United States to pool their resources and cooperate on not only developing a vaccine but also on the production of rapid tests (Wu & Christensen 2020). Although Taiwan has excellent research capability, there remains a large gap between vaccine research and market production, which is partly caused by a lack of support from WHO and multinational pharmaceutical companies (Tsai 2020; Chen 2019). As a result, Taiwan's vaccine production is still far off the industrial scale. Nonetheless, the Taiwanese people were anxious that their research institutes would not be left behind. Meanwhile, the scientists in Taiwan have also hoped to leverage its strength in biomedical research and create a narrative for Taiwan to become a glorious biotechnology island on the international stage (Tsai 2020).

An associated incident was a crowdfunding campaign—TaiwanCanHelp. us—that was initiated by a group of ordinary Taiwanese citizens soon after 9 April 2020 when WHO director-general Tedros Adhanom Ghebreyesus said that he had received racist comments from Taiwan (BBC News 2020b; Everington 2020). The origin of the accusation can be traced back to late 2019 when the Taiwanese government tried to warn the WHO of possible human-to-human transmission of the virus detected in China. According to Taiwanese officials, their efforts to alert the WHO were ignored. Taiwan President Tsai Ing-Wen responded to the accusation of Tedros, emphasising Taiwan rejects any form of discrimination and that it completely understood its exclusion from the WHO was due to its inability to participate in the WHO and other international organisations (Aspinwall 2020; Banchard 2020). The crowdfunding campaign's initial step was to raise sufficient funds to place a full-page advertisement in the *New York Times* to increase recognition of Taiwan's contribution to global public health. Approximately 26,000 sponsors contributed a total of one million US dollars within 15 hours. Well-known graphic designer Aaron Neigh worked on the full-page *New York Times* ad (Figures 9.1 and 9.2), published on 14 April 2020, part of which notes:

> In a time of isolation, we choose solidarity. ...We know what you are going through. We know how hard it is. ...Taiwan, having been isolated from the World Health Organisation, knows. ...Who can isolate Taiwan? No one. Because we are here to help.

Thus, an unexpected consequence of international health politics is that a campaign motivated by the accusation of Tedros that Taiwan was being discriminatory has contributed to forging a distinctive Taiwanese identity.

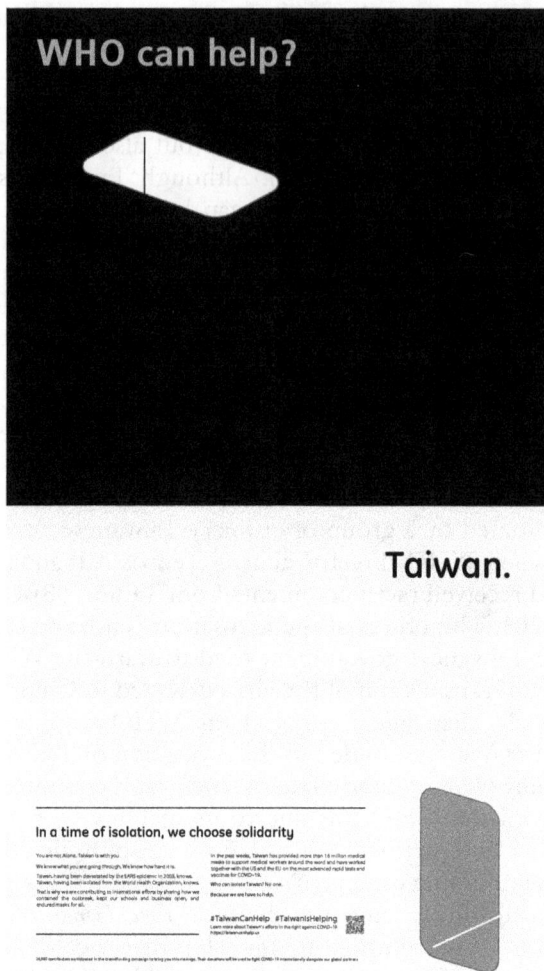

Figure 9.1 The full-page ad in the *New York Times* 15 April 2020.

Taiwan–China relations

Tensions between Taiwan and China date back to the Chinese civil war between 1927 and 1949, which includes a united front period against Japanese occupation between 1937 and 1945. By 1949, Mao Zedong's Chinese Communist Party (CCP) had, however, defeated Chiang Kai Shek's Chinese Nationalist Party (*Kuomintang*; KMT), forcing him to abandon the mainland and relocate his regime to Taiwan, there proclaiming the Republic of China. Around two million mainland KMT-supporting Chinese fled to Taiwan after the civil war, there joining Taiwan's Indigenous peoples, as well as other settlers from the southeast coast of China who had inhabited the island for several centuries.

In a time of isolation, we choose solidarity

You are not Alone. Taiwan is with you

We know what you are going through. We know how hard it is.

Taiwan. having been devastated by the SARS epidemic in 2003, knows. Taiwan, having been isolated from the World Health Organization, knows.

That is why we are contributing to international efforts by sharing how we contained the outbreak, kept our schools and business open, and endured masks for all.

In the past weeks, Taiwan has provided more than 16 million medical masks to support medical workers around the word and have worked together with the US and the EU on the most advanced rapid tests and vaccines for COVID–19.

Who can isolate Taiwan? No one.

Because we are have to help.

#TaiwanCanHelp #TaiwanIsHelping

Learn more about Taiwan's efforts in the right against COVID–19. https//taiwancanhelp.us

26,980 contributors participated in the crowdfunding campaign to bring you this message. Their donations will be used to fight COVID–19 internationally alongside our global partners.

Figure 9.2 Enlarged text of Figure 9.1.

From the seventeenth century onward, Dutch, Spanish, Chinese and Japanese periods of occupation and colonisation have blended cultures and brought different political views from various parts of the world, differences that contribute to a specific 'Taiwanese' identity (Qin and Chien 2022).

Taiwan's claim to be the Republic of China was initially accepted by the United Nations, a status that endured until 1971 when the United Nations formally recognised the Communist government in Beijing. This change of recognition triggered the United States and other countries to follow. At the same time, numerous international organisations began to reject Taiwan's membership or participation. The increasing global diplomatic isolation did not affect the rest of the world's willingness to trade with what was the first of Asia's 'Tiger' economies, and rapid economic growth led to calls for a change to labour relations and democratisation. After a series of political upheavals in the 1990s, Taiwan today is an island with a democratically elected government, governed independently of China.

CCP officials in China view Taiwan as Chinese territory and have vowed to unify Taiwan with the mainland. Despite high levels of trans-Taiwan Strait trade and mobility, tension between Taiwan and China has worsened since the DPP candidate Tsai Ing-Wen was elected to the presidency for the first time in 2016 and then reelected in 2020. Under Xi Jingping, China has increased its attempted intimidation of Taiwan and has attempted to undermine support for Taiwan among other countries which recognise or provide security guarantees to Taiwan. Measures aimed at Taiwan include pointing missiles towards the island, flying military jets near Taiwanese airspace, cyberattacks against Taiwan's government agencies, suspending official communication mechanisms between Taiwan and China, restricting tourism and students going to Taiwan. Such intimidating tactics are also applied to any country which may disrupt China's understanding of its One-China Policy—the principle that there is only one Chinese state and that Taiwan is currently a 'renegade province'. Over the past decade, China has expanded its diplomatic influence across the world, including into the Pacific region, where it has had some success inducing Pacific Island states to switch their recognition of China from Taipei to Beijing (Hawksley and Georgeou 2023). Due to its economic importance, China can push for its view to be accepted across the world, for example in 2021, China suspended its trade with Lithuania due to opening a representative office using the name 'Taiwan' in the Lithuanian capital Vilnius. Tensions over Chinese claims in the South China Sea, and over Taiwan in particular, are frequently cited as an issue that may trigger a war between the United States and China (Maizland 2022).

State recognition and COVID geopolitics

The ongoing clash between the United States and China in relation to regional hegemony in East Asia has intensified since the pandemic (Ruiz Casado 2021; Fukuda 2021) and has been considered by some as a 'New Cold War'. In 2020, US President Donald Trump constantly referred to COVID-19 as the 'Chinese virus', and both countries launched propaganda blaming the other for causing the pandemic (Gaudefroy and Lindaman 2020; Lantier 2020; Ramzy and Chien 2021; Myers 2020; Molter 2020). Additionally, the United States threatened to withdraw its contribution to the WHO due to supposed Chinese influence over the organisation. For its part, China has engaged in an English-language campaign to argue that its effective implementation of high-tech authoritarianism successfully contained the virus (Molter 2020; Kleinfeld 2020). For example, during the beginning of the COVID-19 outbreak in Wuhan, when new cases were reappearing following an easing of the lockdown, the government announced it would test all 11 million residents within 10 days. Although the set target was not met as only six million were tested at the end, this accomplishment seemed to imply that no democratic country could come close to such capability of mobilising social resources (Cooper & Aitchison 2020). Amidst this superpower media tussle, Taiwan's success in managing COVID-19 has become a critical symbol that controlling the pandemic does not require the compromise of freedom and human rights, which are the major characteristics of democracy.

The United States' approach to Taiwan is governed by its One-China Policy (Bush 2017), which is based on multiple documents, including the 'Taiwan Relation Act' in 1972 and 'Six Assurances' in 1982. These documents indicate the United States acknowledges China's position on Taiwan—that there is one China and that Taiwan is part of China. The wording of 'acknowledge', as opposed to 'accept', may imply that the United States does not agree with China's position of considering Taiwan as part of its territory. In 2022, US President Joe Biden said, "Yes" when asked by a journalist if he will defend Taiwan if China invaded, and later he added, "[T]hat is the commitment we made" (Kuhn 2022; Boak, Madhani, and Miller 2022). Similar incidents have occurred since Joe Biden was innaugurated in 2021, but the White House official would later clarify that Biden's comments did not reflect any policy shift (Sanger 2021). Despite not acknowledging it as a state, the United States continues to sell weapons to Taiwan to defend itself. The United States' strategic ambiguity in its Taiwan policy aims to maintain this balance between containment of China and accommodation (or at least public acknowledgement) of Chinese territorial designs.

The debate over democracy and autocracy has escalated as China has continued to highlight how its political system has controlled COVID, and even in mid-2022, it was still aiming for a zero-COVID policy. China criticised other advanced democracies for their high COVID-19 infection rates and deaths. Meanwhile, the Taiwanese government has continuously endorsed the principle of freedom, human rights and democracy in an effort to, not so subtly, demonstrate its distinction from China. At one point, the Chinese government even critisised Taiwan for utilising the pandemic to seek independence (Fukuda 2021). For the United States and its allies, China's pressure on Taiwan appears set on creating a clear enemy (Davis 2021; Lague and Murray 2021).

The long journey to rejoin the WHO as Taiwan

In the list of COVID-19 case numbers published by the WHO, Taiwan's far lower case number has been included under that of China. In other words, there is no option available on the WHO website to choose to only see the Taiwanese data. China has insisted that it is the only state to represent and speak for Taiwan, while the Taiwanese government has stated that the decision of including Taiwan under China made by the WHO has confused other countries and led them to impose the same restriction on Taiwanese travellers, as well as minimalising Taiwan's more successful outcome in controlling the spread of COVID.

Despite being an original member of the United Nations from 1945 and the WHO from 1946, the Republic of China (Taiwan)[3] was expelled from the United Nations on 25 October 1971 when the United Nations General Assembly recognised the People's Republic of China as the official government of China (see Figure 9.3).

As the WHO is one of the many "organisations related to" the United Nations, Taiwan consequently lost its membership, and its international status has been the subject of dispute. With China's strident assertion of the One-China Policy, Taiwan is now recognised as a state by fewer than 24 other states, mostly small island states in the Pacific or Caribbean, or by entities such as Kosovo, itself of dubious international status. Taiwan however maintains an international presence as a member of the Asia Pacific Economic Cooperation (APEC) group (as Taiwan), and competes in the Olympics (as Chinese

---

2758 (XXVI). Restoration of the lawful rights of the People's Republic of China in the United Nations

The General Assembly,

Recalling the principles of the Charter of the United Nations,

Considering that the restoration of the lawful rights of the People's Republic of China is essential both for the protection of the Charter of the United Nations and for the cause that the United Nations must serve under the Charter,

Recognizing that the representatives of the Government of the People's Republic of China are the only lawful representatives of China to the United Nations and that the People's Republic of China is one of the five permanent members of the Security Council,

Decides to restore all its rights to the People's Republic of China and to recognize the representatives of its Government as the only legitimate representatives of China to the United Nations, and to expel forthwith the representatives of Chiang Kai-shek from the place which they unlawfully occupy at the United Nations and in all the organizations related to it.

1976th plenary meeting,
25 October 1971.

Figure 9.3 Text of the United Nations General Assembly Resolution 2758 of 1971 expelling Taiwan from the United Nations.

Taipei), but its efforts to rejoin the WHO and other international health bodies have been blocked.

In 1997, Taiwan's first directly elected president, Lee Teng-Hui (1988–2000), attempted to apply to join the World Health Assembly (WHA) under the name the Republic of China (Taiwan) for five years but was unsuccessful. Since 1997, President Lee Teng-Hui had attempted to use the 'Republic of China (Taiwan)' to become the observer of WHA, but it did not succeed. In 2002, President Chen Shui-bian (2000–2008)[4] applied three times to become the WHA's observer as a 'Health Entity' without involving controversy over Taiwan's sovereignty, but this attempt failed again (Tsai 2020). Between 1997 and 2008, Taiwan tried to gain acceptance to the WHA under various names—Health Authorities of Taiwan, Republic of China (Taiwan) and Taiwan—but none were successful. The only success was between 2009 and 2016:[5] Taiwan was invited to attend the annual WHA in Geneva as an observer under the name 'Chinese Taipei' (van der Wees 2016; Tsai 2020).

In 2003, when the first SARS case appeared in Taiwan, its CDC immediately reported to the WHO Western Pacific Office and sought assistance, such as providing diagnostic reagents to test probable SARS patients, but Taiwan was told by the WHO officials to go to Beijing (Cyranoski 2003). Taiwan instead relied on the CDC of the United States to provide virus strains and related information (Chen 2003; Office of President Republic of China 2020).

After a long period being an 'international orphan', Taiwan has realised that the only way is to establish its own comprehensive infectious diseases control system and disaster prevention mechanism. As the WHO has refused to provide sufficient information regarding Taiwan's unique success in controlling COVID-19 to the international community, the Taiwanese government has made a conscious effort to promote Taiwan's campaign for its continued participation in the WHO, as well as strengthening its information exchange with Japan, the United States, Canada, and other countries.

"We are not China"

Taiwan's successful experience in managing the COVID pandemic has been widely recognised by the international community, despite China's hindering tactics. From the speech of President Tsai Ing-Wen to the exchanges between the Ministry of Foreign Affairs and the WHO, the strategy of "Taiwan Can Help, Taiwan Is Helping" is Taiwan's attempt to revisit its unrecognised status in the international sphere. The international community's general acceptance of the One-China Policy has thus prompted Taiwan to experiment with its name, identity, and international positioning; however, there are also domestic effects. During COVID-19, a sense of solidarity and shared destiny emerged among the Taiwanese people, and the pandemic has inspired a strengthened collective identity of wanting to be seen as Taiwanese—"Taiwan alone"—and not as part of China.

The most drastic and controversial move that the Taiwanese government implemented to distance itself from China is perhaps changing the cover of its passports. The old Taiwanese passports were printed 'Republic of China' on the top of the front cover, with 'Taiwan' written at the bottom. The new passport issued in 2020 has removed 'Republic of China' from the top and enlarged the word 'Taiwan'. The foreign minister of Taiwan announced that the new design of Taiwanese passports was necessary to prevent being mistaken for Chinese passport holders,[6] especially as the mistake led several countries to impose the same border restrictions on Taiwanese citizens as on Chinese citizens during the pandemic (Reuters 2020). The new design of the Taiwanese passport is just one example of the way in which the COVID-19 pandemic focused the spotlight on a specific 'Taiwanese' identity.

More than 60% of Taiwanese citizens identify as 'Taiwanese' alone, a number three times the number recorded in 1992. More importantly, only 2% of the population identified as 'Chinese' alone in 2021 (National Chengchi University 2022). The shift is partly generational, and the change has been accelerated since the Taiwan Sunflower Student Movement in early 2014, followed by the Hong Kong Umbrella Revolution in late 2014 (Rowen 2015). The CCP's brutal crackdown on democracy activists and civil society in Hong Kong, despite promises to maintain Hong Kong's democratic privileges (under the doctrine of "Two Countries One System") has strengthened and reinforced distrust towards China within Taiwanese society. This distance has only grown with the progress of COVID-19, especially as the WHO, due to China's intimidation, has rejected Taiwan's participation and thus hindered its even greater success in battling the pandemic.

Some people living on the Taiwan island have chosen to keep the status quo to avoid possible conflict, while many younger Taiwanese believe the island is already independent without the need to declare this. Identifying as 'Taiwanese' is increasingly understood as supporting democracy or, in other words, standing against autocracy (Qin & Chien 2022) as being Taiwanese also implies a refusal to return to the martial law system initiated by KMT in 1949 and which only ended in 1987. An evolving Taiwanese identity, partly forged by the experience of COVID-19, seems constructed on the discourse of "the enemy", in this case China and its representation. Such an identity construction may pose a challenge to preserving the peace on the island and its liberal democracy due to its populist and nationalist process of identity construction and hegemonic struggle (Ruiz Casado 2021). There is however a note of contradiction in Taiwan's identity formation as it currently appears to require the 'othering' of China within a predominantly ethnically Chinese society. If this trend continues, it may serve as the breeding ground for increased polarisation within Taiwanese society.

Conclusion

The experience of COVID-19 has collated and combined issues of national security and citizenship in Taiwan as people's personal safety and health have become part of the national defence system. Taiwan's unique success in combatting COVID is in many ways due to its international exclusion, and its international charm offensive can be seen as a quest to re-engage with international organisations and to prosecute a case for the abandonment of China-led restrictions on its claims for statehood. The new assertive Taiwanese identity is evidenced both internationally and domestically, and indeed are combined: effective border control, a new national passport, the protection of the public health system and general support for the government's efficient management of the pandemic.

As one of the defining features of sovereignty is the effective management of flows of people and goods over its own borders, the Taiwanese state can clearly differentiate between 'us' and 'them', and its success in pandemic containment shows it is clearly asserting its legal authority over its population. Taken together Taiwan exudes most of the features of a state, lacking only wide international recognition. While this has been the case since the 1970s, the experience of COVID demonstrates how an effective and competent Taiwan government has protected its population from harm, the first duty of the state, while many recognised states have been found wanting.

Notes

1 The question of Taiwan's international status is beyond the scope of this chapter; however, in the sense that Taiwan possesses a recognised government, territory and a permanent population, the word 'state' is used to denote the entity that has previously been called Chinese Taipei and the Republic of China.
2 Every Taiwanese citizen is eligible to purchase 9 masks every 14 days during the first period of the COVID-19 outbreak. This measure is to maintain an affordable price for facemasks for everyone and to ensure sufficient supply.
3 Technically, the United Nations used the term 'the representatives of Chiang Kai Shek' to refer the Republic of China (Taiwan).
4 Chen Shui-Bien (DDP) was elected as the president between 2000 and 2008
5 It happened during the government of President Ma Ying-Jeou (KMT) between 2009 and 2016.
6 According to the data of 2021, Taiwan's passport has 145 visa-free destinations, whereas China's passport has only 79 visa-free destinations.

References

Aljazeera News. (2021, March 18). 'Taiwan Clears Astrazeneca Vaccine, Shots Might Short on Monday', https://www.aljazeera.com/news/2021/3/18/taiwan-clears-astrazeneca-vaccine-shots-might-start-on-monday.
Aspinwall, N. (2020, April 10). 'Tsai Rejects Accusations Taiwan Attacked WHO Chief, Invites Him to Visit', *The Diplomat*, , https://thediplomat.com/2020/04/tsai-rejects-accusations-taiwan-attacked-who-chief-invites-him-to-visit/
Banchard, B. (2020, April 9). 'Taiwan Rebuffs Accusations It Racially Attached WHO Chief', *Reuters,* https://www.reuters.com/article/us-health-coronavirus-taiwan-who-idUSKCN21R04R.
BBC News. (2020a, April 3). 'Taiwan's Version of Mask Diplomacy: 10-Million Government-Aided Masks Are Given to Whom', https://www.bbc.com/zhongwen/trad/chinese-news-52143858.

BBC News. (2020b, April 9). 'WHO Chief and Taiwan in Row over "Racist" Comments', https://www.bbc.com/news/world-asia-52230833.

Blanchard, B. and Lee, Y. (2021, May 6). 'Taiwan Says "China's Intervention" Blocked Vaccine Deal with BioNTech', The Sydney Morning Herald, https://www.smh.com.au/world/asia/taiwan-says-china-s-intervention-blocked-vaccine-deal-with-biontech-20210526-p57vfs.html.

Boak, J., Madhani, A., and Miller, Z. (2022, May 23). 'Biden Says the U.S. Will Defend Taiwan Militarily if China Attacks', *TIME*, 23, https://time.com/6179956/biden-us-defend-taiwan-china/.

Bush, R.C. (2017). 'A One-China Policy Primer', *East Asia Policy Studies Paper 10*, https://www.brookings.edu/wp-content/uploads/2017/03/one-china-policy-primer-web-final.pdf.

Central News Agency. (2021, July 19). 'COVID-19 Global Report on the 19th July 2021', *Central News Agency*, https://www.cna.com.tw/news/firstnews/202107190014.aspx.

Chen, W.X. (2003, June 30). 'Challenges and Opportunities of SARS to Taiwan's Foreign Relations', *New Century Think Tank Forum*, vol. 22, http://www.taiwanncf.org.tw/ttforum/22/22-15.pdf.

Chen, Z.W. (2019). 'Immunising Taiwan in the Post-Genetic Era: Myths and Reflections on Vaccines'. In YY Tsai, ML Pan, and ZW Chen (eds.), *Taiwan's Post-Genetic Era: Paradigm Shifts and Challenges in New Technology*, National Chiao Tung University Press, Hsinchu City, pp.128–150.

Cheng, T.M. (2020). 'Taiwan's Response to the Coronavirus Challenge of 2020', *Taiwan Insight*, University of Nottingham, https://taiwaninsight.org/2020/03/05/taiwans-response-to-the-coronavirus-challenge-of-2020/.

Cheng, T.M. (2021a, December 1). 'How Has Taiwan Navigated the Pandemic?' *Economics Observatory*, https://www.economicsobservatory.com/how-has-taiwan-navigated-the-pandemic

Cheng, T.M. (2021b, July 21). *Taiwan's Ongoing War against COVID-19+ Sixteen Months of Smooth Sailing and One Recent Squall*, Taiwan Studies Programme, University of Nottingham, , https://taiwaninsight.org/2021/07/21/taiwans-ongoing-war-against-covid-19-sixteen-months-of-smooth-sailing-and-one-recent-squall/.

Cooper, L. and Aitchison, G. (2020). *The Dangers and the Answers: Covid-19, Authoritarianism and Democracy*, LSE Conflict and Civil Society Research Unit, http://eprints.lse.ac.uk/105103/4/dangers_ahead.pdf.

Cyranoski, D. (2003). Taiwan Left Isolated in Fight against SARS, *Nature*, vol. 422, no. 652, https://www.nature.com/articles/422652a.

Dai, C.Y., Dai, T.H., Sheng, W.H., and Ho, C.K. (2021). '222 Days without COVID in Taiwan: What Are the Reasons for This Success?' *Journal of Travel Medicine*, vol. 28, no. 2, https://doi.org/10.1093/jtm/taaa225.

Davis, M. (2021, February 11). 'The US and Its Allies Must Ensure Taiwan Doesn't Fall to Beijing', *The Strategist*, Australian Strategic Policy Institute, https://www.aspistrategist.org.au/the-us-and-its-allies-must-ensure-taiwan-doesnt-fall-to-beijing/.

Dou, E. and Rauhala, E. (2021, July 22). 'China Sets Back Search For Covid Origins with Rejection of WHO Investigation Proposal', *The Washington Post*, https://www.washingtonpost.com/world/2021/07/22/china-covid-who-wuhan/.

Everington, K. (2020, April 9). 'WHO Head Accused Taiwan of Racist Attack, Blames MOFA', *Taiwan News*, https://www.taiwannews.com.tw/en/news/3912961.

Fukuda, M. (2021, February 18). 'How the Covid-19 Pandemic Contributes to rising Tensions Across the Taiwan Strait', *Social Science Research Council*, https://items.ssrc. org/covid-19-and-the-social-sciences/covid-19-in-east-asia/how-the-covid-19-pandemic-contributes-to-rising-tensions-across-the-taiwan-strait/.

Gaudefroy, J.V. and Lindaman, D. (2020, April 22). 'Donald Trump's Chinese Virus: The Politics of Naming', *The Conversation*, , https://theconversation.com/donald-trumps-chinese-virus-the-politics-of-naming-136796.

Hawksley, C. and Georgeou, N. (2023). 'Small states In the Pacific: Sovereignty, Vulnerability, and Regionalism', Ch 8 of Thomas Kolnberger and Harlan Koff (eds), *Agency, Security and Governance of Small States: A Global Perspective*, London, Routledge, pp. 139–157.

Jiang, H.J. and Chen, J.L. (2021, August 3). 'Updates on the BNT Vaccine: EUA Approval This Afternoon', *The Central News Agency*, https://www.cna.com.tw/news/firstnews/202108030170.aspx.

Kleinfeld, R. (2020, March 31). Democratic Countries Handle Pandemics Better?, *Carnegie*, https://carnegieendowment.org/2020/03/31/do-authoritarian-or-democratic-countries-handle-pandemics-better-pub-81404.

Kuhn, A. (2022, May 23). 'President Biden Says the U.S. Will Defend Taiwan if China Invades', *NPR*, https://www.npr.org/2022/05/23/1100828744/president-biden-says-the-u-s-will-defend-taiwan-if-china-invades.

Lague, D. and Murray, M. (2021, November 5). 'T-Day: The Battle for Taiwan', *Reuters*, https://www.reuters.com/investigates/special-report/taiwan-china-wargames/.

Lantier, A. (2020, April 24). 'US Propaganda Campaign Promotes Lies Blaming China for COVID-19', *World Socialist Web Site, International Committee of the Forth International*, https://www.wsws.org/en/articles/2020/04/24/chin-a24.html.

Lee, X.L. and Jian, Y.D. (2016, January 29). 'Chinese or Taiwanese? The Identity Problems You and I have Encountered', *The Reporter*, https://www.twreporter.org/a/identity-twstory.

Lin, Y.W., Lin, C.H., and Lin, M.H. (2021). 'Vaccination Distribution by Community Pharmacists under the COVID-19 Vaccine Appoint System in Taiwan', *Cost Effectiveness and Resource Allocation*, vol. 19, no. 76, https://doi.org/10.1186/s12962-021-00331-2.

Lo, M.C.M. and Hsieh, H.Y. (2020). The "Societalization" of Pandemic Unpreparedness: Lessons from Taiwan's COVID Response. *American Journal of Cultural Sociology*, vol. 8, pp. 384–404, https://doi.org/10.1057/s41290-020-00113-y.

Lu, J.W. (2020, January 31). 'SARS Is Not Far Away, Don't Let the Performance-Oriented Medical System Become an "Invisible Virus"', *The Reporter*, https://www.twreporter.org/a/opinion-sars-medical-system-2019-ncov.

Maizland, L. (2022, May 26). 'Why China-Taiwan Relations Are So Tense', *Council on Foreign Relations*, https://www.cfr.org/backgrounder/china-taiwan-relations-tension-us-policy-biden#chapter-title-0-7.

Ministry of Health and Welfare. (2022). 'Taiwan Can Help, and Taiwan Is Helping!', *Ministry of Health and Welfare*, https://covid19.mohw.gov.tw/en/cp-4789-53866-206.html.

Molter, V. (2020, March 19). 'Virality Project (China): Pandemics & Propaganda', Stanford Internet Observatory, Freeman Spogli Institute and Stanford Law School, https://cyber.fsi.stanford.edu/news/chinese-state-media-shapes-coronavirus-convo.

Myers, S.L. (2020, March 13). 'China Spins Tale That the U.S. Army Started the Coronavirus Epidemic', *The New York Times*, https://www.nytimes.com/2020/03/13/world/asia/coronavirus-china-conspiracy-theory.html.

National Chengchi University. (2022, January 10). 'The Distribution of the People's Identity Trends in Taiwan (June 1992–December 2021)', *Election Study Centre, National Chengchi University*, https://esc.nccu.edu.tw/PageDoc/Detail?fid=7804&id=6960.

Office of President Republic of China (Taiwan). (2020, February 27). 'The Vice President Was Interviewed by the Japanese Media Sankei Shimbun', https://www.president.gov.tw/NEWS/25241.

Qin, A. and Chien, A.C. (2022, January 19). 'We Are Taiwanese: China's Growing Menace Hardens Island's Identity', *The New York Times*, https://www.nytimes.com/2022/01/19/world/asia/taiwan-china-identity.html.

Ramzy, A. and Chien, A.C. (2021, August 25). 'Rejecting Covid Inquiry, China Peddles Conspiracy Theories Blaming the U.S.', *The New York Times*, https://www.nytimes.com/2021/08/25/world/asia/china-coronavirus-covid-conspiracy-theory.html.

Reuters. (2020, September 2). 'Taiwan to Change Passport, Fed up with Confusion with China', *Reuters*, https://www.reuters.com/article/us-taiwan-passport-idUSKBN25T0JA.

Reuters. (2021, May 22). 'Taiwan Adds More Domestic COVID Cases but Says Trend Stable', *Reuters*, https://www.reuters.com/world/asia-pacific/taiwan-says-china-is-spreading-fake-news-during-covid-spike-2021-05-22/.

Reuters. (2022, May 27). 'Taiwan's COVID Cases Reach Plateau, Government Says', *Reuters*,https://www.reuters.com/world/asia-pacific/taiwans-covid-19-cases-reach-plateau-government-2022-05-27/.

Rigger, S., Nachman L., Mok, C.W.J., and Chan, N.K.M. (2022, March 11). 'Taiwan's people Are Not Impressed with China's "Zero COVID" Status', *Taiwan-U.S. Quarterly Analysis*, The Brookings Institute, Washington D.C., https://www.brookings.edu/blog/order-from-chaos/2022/03/11/taiwans-people-are-not-impressed-with-chinas-zero-covid-status/.

Rowen, I. (2015). 'Inside Taiwan's Sunflower Movement: Twenty-Four Days in a Student-Occupied Parliament, and the Future of the region', *The Journal of Asian Studies*, vol. 74, no. 1, pp. 5–21, https://www.jstor.org/stable/43553641.

Ruiz Casado, J. (2021). 'The Pandemic and Its Repercussions on Taiwan, Its Identity, and Liberal Democracy', *Open Cultural Studies*, vol. 5, no. 1, pp. 149–160, https://www.degruyter.com/document/doi/10.1515/culture-2020-0123/html.

Sanger, D. (2021, October 25). 'Biden Said the U.S. Would Protect Taiwan. But It's Not That Clear-Cut', *The New York Times*, https://www.nytimes.com/2021/10/22/us/politics/biden-taiwan-defense-china.html?_ga=2.128568458.762101560.1657088969-862092740.1657088969.

Soon, W. (2021, July 29). 'Why Taiwan Is Beating COVID-19 – Again', *The Diplomat*, https://thediplomat.com/2021/07/why-taiwan-is-beating-covid-19-again/.

Summers, J., Cheng, H.Y., Lin, H.H., Barnard, L.T., Kvalsvig, A., Wilson, N. et al. (2020). 'Potential Lessons from the Taiwan and New Zealand Health Responses to the COVID-19 Pandemic', *The Lancet Regional Health*. Western Pacific, vol. 4. http://doi.org/10.1016/j.lanwpc.2020.100044.

Taiwan Centers for Disease Control. (2021a, May 11). 'Epidemic Alert Standards and Responses', https://www.cdc.gov.tw/Uploads/Files/cff51b12-5dfd-4953-86bb-f38027a17175.png.

Taiwan Centers for Disease Control. (2021b, March3). 'First Batch of AstraZeneca's COVID-19 Vaccine Arrives in Taiwan', https://www.cdc.gov.tw/En/Bulletin/Detail/GpdnyWUqMG2cWTJxFsBGjQ?typeid=158.

Taiwan Centers for Disease Control. (2021c, July 19). 'Ministry of Health and Welfare Approves Its Project Manufacturing of Medigen COVID-19 Vaccine', https://www.cdc.gov.tw/Bulletin/Detail/gzkfXTnBuktqDJ3BXhI54w?typeid=9.

Taiwan Centers for Disease Control. (2021d, October 28). 'Taiwan's First-Dose Coverage Reaches 70% and Second-Dose Coverage Reaches 30%, Vaccination Goal for End of October Achieved Ahead of Schedule', https://www.cdc.gov.tw/En/Bulletin/Detail/t2Elj8PuNp0PpCBiP8lnwA?typeid=158.

Taiwan Centers for Diseases Control. (2022e, July 4). 'Weekly Number of Suspected COVID-19 Cases Reported', https://www.cdc.gov.tw/En.

Taiwan Ministry of Foreign Affairs. (2022, June 13). 'Entry Restrictions for Foreigners to Taiwan in Response to COVID-19 Outbreak', https://www.boca.gov.tw/cp-220-5081-c06dc-2.html.

Taiwan News. (2021, May 6). 'Taiwan Clear Modern Vaccine for Emergency Use', https://www.taiwannews.com.tw/en/news/4196247.

Tiezzi, S. (2021, July 20). 'China Rejects WHO Call for More Transparency on Origins Probe', *The Diplomat*, https://thediplomat.com/2021/07/china-rejects-who-call-for-more-transparency-on-origins-probe/.

Tsai, Y.Y. (2020, May 14). 'Imagined Virus Communities: The Battle of Bio-nationalism between the Global and Taiwan', *The Reporter*, https://www.twreporter.org/a/opinion-covid-19-imagined-communities.

Van der Wees, G. (2016, May 10). 'Taiwan and the World Health Assembly', *The Diplomat*, https://thediplomat.com/2016/05/taiwan-and-the-world-health-assembly/ (Viewed 6 May 2022).

Wang, C.J., Ng, C.Y., and Brook, R.H. (2020). 'Response to COVID-19 in Taiwan: Big Data Analytics, New Technology, and Proactive Testing', *JAMA*, vol. 323, no. 14, pp. 1341–1342, https://doi.org/10.1001/jama.2020.3151.

Woods, N. (2020, June 25). 'Taiwan's Mask Diplomacy and the International Responses', Taiwan Studies Programme, University of Nottingham, https://taiwaninsight.org/2020/06/25/taiwans-mask-diplomacy-and-the-international-responses/.

World Health Organization. (2004). 'Summary of Probable SARS Cases with Onset of Illness from 1 November 2002 to 31 July 2003', https://www.who.int/csr/sars/country/table2004_04_21/en/.

World Health Organization. (2020, January 5). 'Pneumonia of Unknown Cause—China. Disease Outbreak News (DONs)', https://www.who.int/csr/don/05-january-2020-pneumonia-of-unkown-cause-china/en/.

Wu, J.S. and Christensen, B. (2020, March 18). 'Taiwan-U.S. Joint Statement on a Partnership against Coronavirus', Ministry of Foreign Affairs & American Institute in Taiwan, https://www.mofa.gov.tw/Upload/RelFile/662/171361/1f9b22e4-365c-4791-8427-58db5ecb5ad6.pdf.

Wu, N.T. (2015). 'Political Competition Framed by the China Factor? – Looking beyond the 2012 Presidential Election'. In G Schubert (ed.), *Taiwan and the 'China impact': Challenges and opportunities*, Routledge, New York, pp.130–148.

Yeh, J.R. (2020). 'Four Legs to Stand On: Taiwan's Fight against COVID 19', *Melbourne Forum on Constitution-Building*, https://law.unimelb.edu.au/__data/assets/pdf_file/0006/3476535/MF20-Web4-Taiwan-Jiunn-rong-FINAL.pdf.

10 Cambodia

The thin line between development and human rights during COVID-19

Natalia Szablewska, Muy Seo Ngouv and Ratana Ly

Introduction

Cambodia's handling of the first two years of COVID-19 has been heralded as a 'success', especially in the context of other countries in the region with much higher rates of infection and deaths. It can be explained partially by Cambodia's relatively small population (16.7 million) and the majority of Cambodian society being under the age of 30 (UNDP, n.d.), thus less likely to have medical pre-existing conditions that can increase the risk of poor outcomes from COVID-19. The relative restraint of the population and following general hygiene measures to avoid the infection spreading also played a role. However, that success has been marked by the introduction of legislation, ostensibly to combat COVID transmission, which in practice limits a number of fundamental freedoms, including freedom of expression, that further restricts critiques of government in its development-orientated policies (ILO 2021).

The Kingdom of Cambodia (Cambodia) has been steadily climbing up the Human Development Index since the 1990s. Following the 1993 general elections (overseen by the United Nations Transitional Authority in Cambodia (UNTAC)), and after decades of war following gaining its independence from France in 1953 (see Szablewska, 2022), Cambodia has been in transition to a full market economy. Between 2010 and 2019, the country had an average annual gross domestic product increase of 7% (WHO, 2021). The key dimensions of human development—income, education, health—have been improving, placing Cambodia in the "medium human development" category among 189 countries and regions according to the 2020 UN Development Programme (UNDP) Human Development Report (UNDP, 2020). However, the Report is based on data before the COVID-19 pandemic and, as the pandemic triggered a global recession, it has impacted Cambodia's development progress as well.

As a result of the outbreak of the pandemic, Cambodia experienced a reduction in both economic activity and overall workforce. It is estimated that in 2020, the economy contracted by 3.1%, but it grew by 2.2% in 2021 (IMF, 2021a). Growth of up to 5.1% in 2022 has been projected by the International Monetary Fund (IMF) (IMF, 2022). However, despite the positive forecasts,

DOI: 10.4324/9781003311522-10

the country is facing new challenges such as the rise in living costs, food, gas and electricity. According to the World Bank, by March 2021, the impact of the pandemic and resultant slower growth had pushed many people below the poverty line and increased inequality (World Bank, 2022).

The example of Cambodia shows the perils of balancing the achievement of universal human rights with development goals, especially when facing global disruptive events such as the COVID-19 pandemic. The relationship between economic development and social progress is complex but mutually reinforcing. Poverty reduction depends, at least partially, on sustained economic growth. But growth that is not equally distributed among the different groups in the society will have less impact on poverty reduction (see Ravallion, 2007). Consequently, respect for human rights plays a key role in ensuring a more equitable society and, in turn, poverty is considered to be one of the greatest obstacles to the universal enjoyment of human rights. Thus, rather than development or human rights being a binary, respect for human rights and development go hand in hand. This, however, is difficult to achieve in practice, as the case of Cambodia demonstrates.

In this chapter, we examine legal developments in Cambodia in response to the COVID-19 pandemic over the past two years. We then provide an analysis of policy and practice implications on the education and business sectors as two areas with a significant long-term impact on Cambodian society. By adopting a human rights lens, we aim to shine a light on the future of Cambodia where prioritising economic growth and recovery has taken place at the expense of, and often by increasingly side-lining, human rights.

First two years of COVID-19 in Cambodia

According to the 2019 Global Health Security Index, in terms of preparedness for infectious diseases, Cambodia ranked 89th out of 195 countries globally and ninth out of 11 countries in the Southeast Asian region. The first COVID-19 case in Cambodia was confirmed on 27 January 2020 by the Ministry of Health (MoH), and as of 10 January 2022, there were 120,636 confirmed cases, including 3,015 deaths, and 117,023 recovered and 16.6% of cases were acquired overseas (WHO, 2022). In mid-2021, the majority of confirmed cases were reported in Phnom Penh, Kandal, Sihanoukville and Banteay Meanchey provinces (Khmer Times, 2021a), and the majority of fatalities were among those not vaccinated against COVID-19, and among those vaccinated but with underlying health problems (MoH, cited in Mom, 2021).

The government introduced a number of non-pharmaceutical interventions, including limiting public gatherings and meetings, cancelling public holidays, closing schools and businesses to lower the risk of the infection spreading (World Vision Cambodia, 2020). The population was required to follow strict procedures of testing and quarantining. During community outbreaks, additional measures were taken, including strict localised lockdowns (Khmer Times

2021b), prohibition on local travel and confinement to households in some areas. The general public in Cambodia reacted early on, with reports of people wearing masks and increasing sanitation measures following the first reported case (Chhut, 2020). This undoubtedly contributed to a relatively slow infection rate in the early days of the pandemic in comparison with other countries in the region (for comparison, see Our World in Data[1]).

In February 2021, the government introduced a nationwide vaccine mandate covering specific public and private locations. Since 6 May 2021, the national vaccination campaign adopted a "flower-blooming" approach and strategy (អភិក្រម"ផ្ការីក"), as declared by Prime Minister (PM) Hun Sen (Press and Quick Reaction Unit, 2021; Ministry of Information, 2021)—that is, a vaccination strategy based on geographical rollout prioritising "vaccination in areas and cities at high risk for transmission, while gradually rolling-out vaccination to the rest of the country" (UN Cambodia, 2021).

As of 10 January 2022, around 82% of the population had been fully (double) vaccinated. Of those who received COVID-19 vaccinations, 66% were given doses of Sinovac and Sinopharm procured from the People's Republic of China (China); 25% received donations doses from China, the United Kingdom and Australia, as well as 9% from the COVAX initiative (including from Japan, Sweden, the United States of America (USA) and the Netherlands) (WHO, 2022). In early January 2022, the Inter-Ministerial Committee to Combat COVID-19 made an announcement that those with confirmed cases of the Omicron variant were not permitted to be treated at home but were required to be treated at a hospital or treatment centre designed by the MoH or capital-provincial committee (WHO, 2022). With these administrative and health measures taken, Cambodia has experienced some positive results in controlling COVID-19 transmission in the medium and long term, which has led to, *inter alia*, lifting of international travel restrictions, a rebound in business and manufacturing and the reopening of schools.

Legal developments

In this section, we provide a brief overview of the legal system in Cambodia to then focus on the legal developments in relation to COVID-19. In particular, the *Law on the Management of the Nation in a State of Emergency 2020* (Emergency Law) and the *Law on Measures to Prevent the Spread of COVID-19 and Other Serious, Dangerous and Contagious Diseases 2021* (COVID-19 Law) are analysed to examine the immediate and long-term implications for human rights in Cambodia.

The Cambodian legal system

Cambodia is a liberal multiparty democracy under a constitutional monarchy (Cambodian Constitution 1993 Preamble, Arts. 1 & 51). The separation of powers between the legislature (represented by the majority-elected Senate and the elected National Assembly), the executive (the PM and government) and the judiciary is codified in the Constitution (Arts. 1 & 51). Cambodia has a civil law system which has been influenced by its former colonial power, France, with some features of common law that have been introduced through the operation of the UNTAC 1992–1993, established to ensure the implementation of the 1991 Paris Peace Accords, as well as multiple foreign legal assistance on legal and judicial reforms that have followed in Cambodia since (Kong, 2012).

The Constitution of Cambodia is the supreme law (Art. 131) and thus all other laws, regulations and decisions made by state institutions must be in conformity with it (Art. 150). Cambodia adopts a monist approach to international human rights law, with the Constitution recognising the direct application of ratified international human rights treaties in Cambodia's domestic system (Art. 31; see also Constitutional Council of Cambodia, 2007).

Legal developments in relation to COVID-19

The COVID-19 pandemic has resulted in an emergency legislative action to control the spread of the pandemic. Since the first case of COVID-19 infection in Cambodia, the most significant legal response to COVID-19 has been the adoption of the Emergency Law (entered into force on 29 April 2020) and the COVID-19 Law (entered into force on 11 March 2021).

Criticisms of these two laws have come from the international community and civil society organisations (CSOs) and focus on their impact on human rights in Cambodia. The adoptions of the Emergency Law and the COVID-19 Law have caused concerns over (a) the drafting process and (b) the use of vague or broadly worded language that could lead to discriminatory practices and abuse of power by the authorities.

Lack of transparency and consultations with stakeholders

Both the Emergency Law and the COVID-19 Law were adopted through a fast-tracked legislative process. In early April 2020, the government forwarded the draft Emergency Law to the National Assembly (Ben, 2020), which approved it on 10 April. A week later, the Senate passed it, followed by the Constitutional Council approving it on 27 April 2020. The Emergency Law entered into force on 29 April 2020 (Emergency Law, p. 1). Similarly, the COVID-19 Law, which was adopted by the National Assembly on 5 March 2021, was approved by the Senate on 11 March 2021 and entered into force immediately, without the review of its constitutionality by the Constitutional Council (COVID-19 Law, p. 1). On both occasions, it took less than a month for the review of the form, legality and constitutionality of these laws by different legislative bodies, and their development occurred without the input of, nor consultation with, relevant stakeholders (Touch, 2020; Sun, 2020; CCHR, 2021; Niem, 2021).

A pandemic might require an expedited legislative process, but emergency legislation should never be an alternative to the government's effective planning for times of crisis. Also, emergency powers should be used within the parameters provided by constitutional rights and standards set up by international human rights laws to avoid abuses of power and causing unintended or otherwise harm, including stigma, discrimination and violence amongst the population (WHO, 2020).

The lack of transparency and any consultation process with relevant stakeholders in relation to both laws is regrettable, especially given their wide-reaching scope and long-term effect on Cambodia's society. Concerns have been raised over the legal standards and measures introduced under the laws. Some of the fears relate to the government widening its powers, which even before the pandemic was a criticism (see Human Rights Watch, 2019; Human Rights Watch, 2020; Reporters Sans Frontieres, 2020). Under the disguise of protecting public health during the COVID-19 pandemic, these laws have been used to restrict and silence critical voices, the formal political opposition parties, rights groups and CSOs (Touch, 2020; Sun, 2020; CCHR, 2021: 2; ICJ, 2021).

Vagueness of the terminology used and the scope of application

The vague wording of certain clauses of the two laws raises concerns about the broad scope of their application, the granting of excessive powers to state authorities and the ambiguity in the wording of the offences that can give rise to their misinterpretation or misapplication (Special Procedures Communication Reports, 2020: 3; Special Procedures Communication Reports, 2021: 4; CCHR, 2021; Niem, 2021; ICJ, 2021).

The Emergency Law consists of 12 articles under five chapters, with Article 1 defining its purpose as the management of the state of emergency to protect the national security, public order and the lives and health of Cambodians, as well as property and the environment. A state of emergency can be declared when the country faces dangers caused by war or foreign invasion, public health emergencies caused by pandemics, tumultuous chaos threatening national security and public order and severe calamities that threaten or cause harm to the nation (Art. 4). Article 5 provides a list of 12 measures the government can take, ranging from a ban or restriction on the rights to freedom of movement, association, peaceful assembly and expression, to giving the authorities permission to confiscate, control and manage properties of legal entities and persons, and to monitor and gather information via all telecommunication systems to introducing any such measures as deemed necessary in the state of emergency.

The scope and application of the law are too broad and arguably incompatible with international human rights law and standards (see also Ly et al., 2021). The broadly worded law does not meet the tests of necessity (providing a basis for pursuing a legitimate objective) and proportionality (that the interference is no more than absolutely necessary to achieve the aims). Even if a state of emergency officially declared by a state is considered a justifiable ground for derogation from derogable rights under Article 4 of the International Covenant on Civil and Political Rights (ICCPR), to which Cambodia is a party (UNGA 1966), international human rights law requires a state to "provide careful justification not only for the decision to proclaim a state of emergency but also for any specific measures based on such a proclamation" (Human Rights Committee, 2001: 2; see also Lebret, 2020).

Article 6 of the Emergency Law imposes an obligation on the government to report to the National Assembly and the Senate on the measures taken, while the COVID-19 Law does not prescribe such a check on the government. Furthermore, the two laws outline the criminal responsibilities of individuals, organised groups and legal entities for violations of the provisions with heavy and excessive penalties, which could jeopardise the work of CSOs and rights-based groups (Special Procedures Communication Reports, 2020; Special Procedures Communication Reports, 2021; CCHR, 2021; Touch, 2020). In particular, Article 5 of the COVID-19 Law grants power to the competent officials to suspend or revoke a business license, certificate or permit, as well as the power to close down a business for infringement of health, administrative or other measures.

The offence of intentional transmission of COVID-19 to other people is subject to imprisonment from 5 to 10 years, and from 10 to 20 years if such an act is committed by an organised group of people or entity (Art. 9). The offences of infringement of administrative measures and of obstruction of measure enforcement are subject to between two to five years of imprisonment (Arts. 10 & 11). Similarly, the Emergency Law imposes imprisonment on individuals or legal entities that obstruct the enforcement measures and infringe the measures taken during the state of emergency (Arts. 7, 8 & 9). The Office of the High Commissioner for Human Rights (OHCHR) provides guidance on emergency measures and COVID-19 and reminds states that the enforcement of measures should comply with the principle of proportionality, including that vulnerable groups—such as people with disabilities and victims of domestic violence—should not be "subjected to penalties should they violate COVID-19 emergency measures to protect themselves" (OHCHR, 2020: n.p.). Cambodia's Emergency Law does not distinguish or provide for mitigating factors in relation to the application of the set penalties. And while COVID-19 Law allows mitigation of criminal liability for offences set in Articles 7, 8, 10 and 11 (Art. 13), it is unclear what would constitute providing "relevant information" to or "necessary cooperation" with health or competent officials, which could lead to an inequitable application of the exemption. Also, while the laws provide for the liability of officials acting in contradiction to the purpose of the laws, they do not specify any penalty, nor provide any remedies for the victims who suffered harm or damage as a consequence of abuse of power (Emergency Law, 2020, Art. 10; COVID-19 Law, Art. 12; see also Special Procedures Communication Reports, 2020: 3).

While the Emergency Law has not yet been invoked, the COVID-19 Law has been used in a number of cases, including to charge people who expressed their views or made critical commentaries through social media on the measures taken to combat the spread of COVID-19, such as lockdown measures (Buth, 2021), treatments during COVID-19 in the red zone and hospital facilities (Khuon, 2021) and the vaccination programme (Finney, 2021; Buth, 2021). Articles 10 and 11 of the COVID-19 Law have been used to charge communities and villagers involved in peaceful demonstrations and protests who have defended their right to compensation in land disputes, including by indigenous communities (Mech et al., 2021).

There are immediate and long-term consequences that derive from both laws. Given their rapid introduction, it is likely that the general public lacks an understanding of the provisions of the laws (Niem, 2021), which not only increases the likelihood of unknowingly breaking their provisions, but it also makes the public vulnerable to self-inflicted censorship due to the fear of violating the provisions relating to preventive measures to combat the spread of COVID-19. Consequently, these laws will have significant social and political ramifications in Cambodia beyond the current pandemic and can impede Cambodia's development and human rights situation.

Education and business sectors

In this section, we focus on the education and business sectors to provide an in-depth analysis of the consequences of the impact of COVID-19 in Cambodia. We start by providing a brief background to both sectors, followed by how they were impacted by the COVID-19 pandemic and the key lessons learnt.

The education sector

The education system in Cambodia offers at least nine years of free public education (Education Law, 2007, Art. 31), and the formal general education comprises 12 years at the primary and secondary levels (Education Law, Art. 17), but informal school fees are still relatively common, which is an obstacle for many children to attend school. Even before the pandemic, Cambodian children faced a number of obstacles to receiving a good quality education, including impeded access to learning devices, the quality of teaching and inadequate funding in particular for the poorest families to be able to send their children to school (UNICEF, n.d.). In terms of tertiary education, in 2019, the enrolment rate was 15% (UNSECO, 2021), which is relatively low for the region. In addition, the majority of higher education institutions are based in major cities, limiting opportunities for those living in rural areas.

In 2018, Cambodia entered the third phase of the Capacity Development Partnership Fund (CDPF), a partnership between the Cambodian Ministry of Education, Youth and Sport (MoEYS) and the European Union (EU); the

Swedish International Development Cooperation Agency (SIDA); the United States Agency for International Development (USAID); the Global Partnership for Education (GPE); and UNICEF. The purpose of the CDPF is capacity building in the education sector, with some US$37 million investment (Van Gerwen et al., 2018). Once the COVID-19 pandemic started and the education system became disrupted, the CDPF engagement plan was adapted, and "emergency assistance was mobilised by the fund to support the MoEYS comprehensive response to the COVID-19 pandemic in the education sector" (Openaid, 2022: n.p.).

COVID-19 impact on education

The education sector was closed early into the pandemic and remained closed for a large part of 2020 and into the year 2021, 250 days in total or almost two-thirds of the combined two school years. The MoEYS established the Centre for Digital and Distance Learning in June 2020 to facilitate remote learning, including television and radio lessons; materials for grades 1 to 12 were streamed on the "Krou Cambodia" Facebook page, in addition to community learning sessions, web-based and paper-based resources. In July 2020, the MoEYS released its digital application (app) for distance learning, allowing students to access resources for grades 9 through 12 via the internet or phone services, free of charge (Sao, 2021).

However, due to Cambodia's unequal technological development and internet access—in 2019, the internet penetration rate was 50%, thus below the world average and the region (Kemp and Moey, 2019)—many students could not, or did not, use the resources (Ly, 2021). This differential access has had a negative impact on many students, and it is seen as a significant contributor to a loss of learning that is predicted to have long-term consequences, including reduced income (estimated at US$783 per person) in purchasing power over these students' lifetime (Ly, 2021). As has been also reported elsewhere, school closures heighten gender-based violence against girls, including sexual harassment and abuse from family members and neighbours (World Vision, 2022).

Limited access to learning technology, as well as the ability of parents and caregivers to provide learning support, have been identified as the main barriers faced during the pandemic. In November 2021, the MoEYS with the support of UNICEF and other partners of the CDPF conducted a national learning assessment. This found that urban schools overall scored higher than rural schools, but urban schools experienced more scores decline than rural schools during the pandemic period (UNICEF and MoEYS, 2022).

Even though schools re-opened in January 2021, a recent study shows that many students were attending school less often, with 8% not attending at all and unlikely to return, while 45% of children were observed to be learning less (UNICEF and the World Food Programme, 2021). The number of children working with or without payment also increased during the study period, which has led to an increase in those who might not be returning to school, either as they could no longer afford schooling or because they had to contribute to support their struggling families.

To address the learning loss attributed to the school closure, it is important that Cambodia increases its spending on and investment in human capital, including new learning technologies and techniques to reduce student dropouts and increase their retention and learning recovery. This is also in line with the recommendation put forward following the national learning assessment in 2021 calling to strengthen the overall access for all students, and in particular for students who are "most vulnerable and farthest behind but who may also have the least amount of access to internet and online learning tools" (UNICEF and MoEYS, 2022: 54).

Higher education institutions returned to face-to-face delivery soon after the secondary schools opened in September 2021, with Minister of Education Hang Chuon Naron prescribing rules on distancing and limitations on class numbers. Universities were required to sign a memorandum of understanding with the Ministry on implementing the Standard Operating Procedures to prevent the spread of COVID-19 (Huaxia, 2021). The Higher Education Improvement Project (2018–2024), which provides US$90 million in financing to support Cambodia's efforts in improving the quality of higher education and research as well as broadening access to higher education for disadvantaged students (World Bank, n.d.), is an important catalyst for improving the overall quality of tertiary education in Cambodia. However, further programmes and investments are needed to facilitate the improvement in the utilisation of information and communication technology (ICT) in education to foster the digital transformation of Cambodia's education system (Heng, 2021).

Increasing digital inclusion is necessary to improve digital equity, in particular between rural and urban areas (Szablewska, 2020), to ensure that students are not disadvantaged in their access to technology and internet as living with COVID-19 becomes normalised. The probability of localised COVID outbreaks continues to be present, along with other natural disasters or emergencies that might lead to the closure of the education sector in the future.

The business sector

The impact of the pandemic, including in relation to the countermeasures introduced by the government, on the business sector in Cambodia must be placed within the wider context of economic and labour affairs in the years leading to and during the pandemic. Under the International Trade Union Confederation's (ITUC) 2018 Global Rights Index, Cambodia ranked as one of the ten worst countries for workers (ITUC, 2018). Land grabbing has been identified as one of the unintended consequences of the increase in profitability of sugar exports linked to the EU trade treatment which has led to increasing land dispositions and other wide human rights abuses (Kijewski, 2018).

Following the introduction of EU Regulation No. 978/2012 on applying a scheme of generalised tariff preferences (European Parliament, 2012), Cambodia enjoyed preferential treatment under the EU's "Everything but Arms (EBA)" trade arrangement for least developed countries. In February 2019, the European Commission announced the introduction of a procedure to withdraw the EBA preferences granted to Cambodia, and on 12 August 2020, Cambodia lost its free access to the EU market on the basis of its unsatisfactory human rights record, in particular in relation to freedom of expression and widespread violations of civil and political rights, labour rights and land disputes in the context of the ongoing reforms (European Commission, 2020). The partial withdrawal of Cambodia's duty-free quota-free to the EU market affected some 20% of Cambodia's exports to the EU. This is not an insignificant amount, as the EU is Cambodia's third trade partner, after China and the USA, accounting for 10.6% of the country's total trade (European Commission, n.d.). Cambodia's export to the EU (mainly shoes and clothing) amount to 39% of the country's total export (European Commission, 2022).

Losing the EU preferential treatment status was a significant blow to the Cambodian economy, especially during the pandemic. The EU's position, however, has been firm in that it recognises the challenges facing the Cambodian economy and employment in times of the pandemic, but considered the respect for human rights and labour rights critical. Some of the demands put forward by the EU to restore EBA preferential treatment included the reinstatement of political rights of opposition parties and revision of some of the laws, in particular the *Law on Political Parties 2017*, the *Law on Associations and Non-Governmental Organisations 2015* and the *Law on Trade Unions 2016*, which aim to curb freedoms of assembly, expression and association.

COVID-19 impact on business activities

The key industries in Cambodia are tourism, hospitality, apparel (textile, garment and footwear), food production and food processing. All of these industries have been hit hard globally and in Cambodia (see UNIDO, 2020; Hardefeldt and Ibrahim, 2021). With the lockdowns in the USA and Europe, along with the disruption of supply chains in China that export raw materials to Cambodia, the scale of orders dropped significantly. In early 2020, there were reports of 256 apparel factories and 169 tourism sector companies suspending their operations, which affected 146,000 workers (Huaxia, 2020). The apparel industry has been hit the hardest, and it is the biggest contributor to Cambodia's economic growth, with around 89% of those working in the industry being women (Care International, 2020).

In 2020, the UNIDO Field Office in Cambodia conducted a survey of the most at-risk industries and businesses in Cambodia to provide recommendations for the recovery of the private sector from the pandemic. Despite some variation in terms of the impact on the different sectors, the research clearly shows that the biggest impact has been on revenue and workers, in particular

in the garment and tourism industries (UNIDO, 2020). The financial challenges faced by many businesses include a general reduction in orders, a drop
in sale prices, ongoing rent costs and salary and social security contributions
(UNIDO, 2020). Household food security deteriorated across Cambodia
(UNICEF and the World Food Programme, 2021), which was further exacerbated by the October 2020 flash floods in many provinces.

As businesses in other countries were also affected, many Cambodian migrant workers wished to return to Cambodia but were met with strict health
restrictions preventing them from entering the country, and when they eventually returned, they struggled with finding employment, with many reporting
food shortages and being destitute (UNAIDS, 2020). Migrant workers returning to Cambodia also affected the level of remittances, a feature on which
many households in Cambodia rely, with a 17% drop in 2020 (May, 2021).

The government introduced a number of measures to respond to the dire
economic situation, including cutting state expenditure in 2020 by a massive
50% (Cambodianess, 2020), as well as introducing tax concessions, credit support and wage subsidies for apparel, tourism and construction sectors (IMF,
2021b). The majority of these measures, however, were directed towards the
formal sector, thus largely not capturing workers in informal employment (in
the formal/informal sectors and in households), which is estimated at 93.1%
in Cambodia. There are further disparities between urban and rural areas, with
95.8% of those in rural areas, *versus* 84.7% in urban areas, being in informal
employment (ILO, 2018).

The UNDP Acceleration Labs in Cambodia conducted a survey with 1,400
informal workers, indicating that in January 2021, a year after the first
COVID-19 case in Cambodia was reported, one in five (18%) of informal workers were still unemployed, a rise from the 14% of October 2020. Unemployment
was higher among women (22%) in comparison to men (13%), while 63% of all
respondents struggled with meeting their daily needs, and 80% had to reduce
their food expenditure (UNDP, 2021). This aligns with the findings in the
UNICEF and World Food Programme Report (2021) that identified three areas of household welfare to be the most affected by COVID-19 outbreaks and
associated measures: income and employment, prices and affordability and long-
term human capital (UNICEF and the World Food Programme, 2021). It
could be argued, therefore, there is a need to enhance food security and nutrition programmes at the level of individual households, along with strengthening
financial literacy and workers' protection, including in the informal economy.

Cambodia holds also one of the fastest-growing microfinance markets in
the world, rising from 300,00 in 2005 (World Bank, 2017) to 2.81 million in
2021 (White, 2021). As the majority of borrowers' households rely on labour
wages to repay the loans (Green and Estes, 2019), the disruptions to the various sectors, in particular the garment industry, have had significant repercussions, leading to over-indebtedness, increasing workers' and their families
sacrifices to meet the repayments. Unsurprisingly, many workers have identified debt to a microfinance institution (MFI) as a bigger immediate threat

than the virus itself (Flynn, 2020), and even before the pandemic, there had been reports of "serious and systematic human rights abuses" in relation to MFI debt (LICADHO, 2019: 1). It is important, therefore, that the National Bank of Cambodia and other banks take into consideration the unprecedented situation and ensure that small-scale borrowers and small-medium enterprises (SMEs) are given support and not penalised extensively (see also Cambodia CSOs, 2020).

In light of these developments, Cambodia's Industrial Development Policy (2015–2025) (RGC, 2015), which aims to maintain sustainable development and inclusive high economic growth, as well as to transform the Cambodian economy from labour-intensive to skills driven, needs to be reviewed carefully to ensure that the lessons of COVID are learnt. This needs to be accompanied by the government offering effective support to the industrial sector to ensure efficient implementation of policies aiming to bolster competitiveness, product and market diversification and capacity building of Cambodian businesses to build better financial and economic resilience to global shocks.

Conclusion

The impact of the measures taken to counteract the immediate health implications of the pandemic must be seen in the wider context of Cambodia's quest for human rights, development, economic growth and prosperity. The laws introduced to address the public health emergency, in particular the Emergency Law and the COVID-19 Law, raise a number of concerns in meeting international human rights law and standards, particularly in relation to the principles of necessity and proportionality, the scope of enforcement during COVID-19 and the penalties for violations of extraordinary measures and their impact on marginalised or vulnerable groups. Any measures introduced in a situation of emergency must be "strictly required by the exigencies of the public health situation", temporary and limited in geographical coverage and scope (Human Rights Committee, 2020: para. 2(b)). Under the veil of COVID, the Cambodian government has curtailed a number of rights, including the rights to freedom of movement, expression, peaceful assembly and association, justifying it on the grounds of protecting public health, life and public order, as well as property and the environment. Even if derogating from these rights is allowed, the scope of limitation needs to be proportionate, and all of these rights also play a significant safeguard in ensuring that the emergency powers are not excessive in scope and abused by the state. Many of the measures introduced do not appear to be sufficiently focused on addressing legitimate public health needs; rather, they seem to aim at further outlawing criticism of the government and repressing opponents of the current regime.

The education sector reacted swiftly and, as elsewhere in the world, moving to online delivery meant that teaching and learning could continue. However, with 80% of the population living in rural areas (UNDP, n.d.), it has intensified the digital divide, leading to digital inequality widening. The drop in the quality of education during the COVID-19 pandemic was also acknowledged by the government, with PM Hun Sen calling on the MoEYS to allow grades 9 to 12 to automatically pass national exams in December 2020 (Sen, 2020). The challenges facing the education sector prior to the pandemic, including quality of teaching, impeded access to learning devices and inadequate funding, were exacerbated by remote learning and are projected to have long-term implications for students. An important lesson learnt for Cambodia has been that better integration between social protection and human capital developments is critical to ensure that education, along with health and economic, programmes can be successfully delivered.

The business sector experienced significant challenges over the past two years. The measures introduced by the government to curb the spread of the virus have had a significant impact on business activities in the country and that, in turn, has had implications for workers. The World Bank's Report "Living with COVID-19" (2021) identifies that the projected growth of 4.5% in 2022 in Cambodia will depend on whether there is a renewal in the spread of the virus, which could jeopardise the economic recovery measures. Recommendations put forward by the World Bank include clarity on regulations around living with COVID-19, fiscal measures to revive the tourist industry, and implementation measures for the new investment law. Given the size of the informal sector in Cambodia, coupled with the government initiatives aiming mainly or exclusively at the formal sector, those in the informal sector in Cambodia have suffered a significant hindrance to their social and economic opportunities. This calls for a better promotion and implementation of the International Labour Organization (ILO) decent work agenda and protection of workers in the informal economy.

Overall, dealing with the health repercussions of the COVID-19 pandemic, including the vaccination campaign response, shows that the government has been responsive to and effective in times of crisis. However, there are reasonable concerns that some of the measures introduced, the legislative actions back burner in particular, have impeded the human rights situation of Cambodians for years to come. There is a danger that prioritising economic development and growth over human rights and social progress in a country with a turbulent history of human rights violations will not only stall its human rights record but also its future economic prosperity and sustainable development.

Note

1 https://ourworldindata.org/coronavirus/country/cambodia.

References

Ben, S. (2020, April 1). 'State of Emergency Law Is Imminent', *Khmer Times*, Available at: https://www.khmertimeskh.com/708017/state-of-emergency-law-is-imminent/ (Accessed: 26 April 2022).

Buth, R.K. (2021, April 13). 'Glass Cutter Arrested for Insulting C-19 Initiatives', *Khmer Times*. Available at: https://www.khmertimeskh.com/50838104/glass-cutter-arrested-for-insulting-c-19-initiatives/ (Accessed: 24 April 2022).

Cambodia CSOs. (2020, April 2). 'Joint Position Paper: Prioritize the Needs of Those at Increased Risk of Gender-Based Violence in Responding to the COVID-19 situation'. Available at: https://media.business-humanrights.org/media/documents/files/documents/CSOs_joint_statement_on_Covid19.pdf (Accessed: 10 May 2022).

Cambodian Constitution [Constitution of the Kingdom of Cambodia]. (1993). Adopted by the Constitutional Assembly on 21 September 1993. As amended in 1999.

Cambodianess. (2020, March 5). 'Hun Sen Announces up to 50 pct Budget Cut Amid COVID-19', *Cambodianess*. Available at: https://cambodianess.com/article/hun-sen-announces-up-to-50-pct-budget-cut-amid-covid-19 (Accessed: 12 May 2022).

Care International. (2020). 'Garment Worker Needs Assessment during COVID-19', *Care International in Cambodia*. Available at: http://www.careevaluations.org/wp-content/uploads/CIC_garment-worker-need-assessment_EN_final_23072020.pdf (Accessed: 10 May 2022).

CCHR [Cambodian Center for Human Rights]. (2021). 'The Human Rights Situation in Cambodia in 2021'. Available at: https://cchrcambodia.org/admin/whatwedo/hrsc/2021-human-rights-situation-in-cambodia-eng.pdf (Accessed: 12 May 2022).

Chhut, B. (2020, January 29). 'Shortage of Masks, Alcohol Gel Amid Fears of Novel Coronavirus Outbreak', *Khmer Times*. Available at: https://www.khmertimeskh.com/684882/shortage-of-masks-alcohol-gel-amid-fears-of-novel-coronavirus-outbreak/ (Accessed: 10 May 2022).

COVID-19 Law [Law on Measures to Prevent the Spread of COVID-19 and other Serious, Dangerous and Contagious Diseases]. (2021). Adopted by the National Assembly on 5 March 2021. Entered into force on 11 March 2021. Cambodia.

Education Law. (2007). Adopted by the National Assembly on 19 October 2007. Entered into force on 8 December 2007. Cambodia.

Emergency Law [Law on the Management of the Nation in a State of Emergency]. (2020). Adopted by the National Assembly on 10 April 2020. Entered into force on 29 April 2020. Cambodia.

European Commission. (2020, August 12). 'Cambodia Loses Duty-Free Access to the EU Market Over Human Rights Concerns'. Available at: https://ec.europa.eu/commission/presscorner/detail/en/IP_20_1469 (Accessed: 11 May 2022).

European Commission. (2022). 'European Union, Trade in Goods with Cambodia', *Directorate-General for Trade*. Available at: https://webgate.ec.europa.eu/isdb_results/factsheets/country/details_cambodia_en.pdf (Accessed: 10 May 2022).

European Commission. (n.d.). 'Cambodia: EU Trade Relations with Cambodia. Facts, Figures and Latest Developments'. Available at: https://ec.europa.eu/trade/policy/countries-and-regions/countries/cambodia/ (Accessed: 10 May 2022).

European Parliament. (2012). Regulation (EU) No 978/2012 of the European Parliament and of the Council of 25 October 2012 Applying a Scheme of Generalised Tariff Preferences and Repealing Council Regulation (EC) No 732/2008.

Finney, R. (2021, March 15). 'Cambodian Activist Arrested for Criticizing Chinese COVID-19 Vaccine', *Radio Free Asia*. Available at: https://www.rfa.org/english/news/cambodia/vaccine-03152021183359.html (Accessed: 24 April 2022).

Flynn, G. (2020, April 16). 'Garment Workers Cornered by Job Loss, Virus Fears and Looming Debt', *VOD*. Available at: https://vodenglish.news/garment-workers-cornered-by-job-loss-virus-fears-and-looming-debt/ (Accessed: 10 May 2022).

Global Health Security Index. (2019). Available at https://www.ghsindex.org/.

Green, W.N. and Estes, J. (2019). 'Precarious Debt: Microfinance Subjects and Intergenerational Dependency in Cambodia', *Antipode*, 51(1), pp. 129–147. https://doi.org/10.1111/anti.12413.

Hardefeldt, S. and Ibrahim, A. (2021). 'Casualties of Fashion: How Garment Workers in Bangladesh and Cambodia Are Wearing the Cost of Covid-19', *ActionAid*. Available at: https://actionaid.org.au/wp-content/uploads/2021/12/CASUALTIES-OF-FASHION-HOW-GARMENT-WORKERS-IN-BANGLADESH-AND-CAMBODIA-ARE-WEARING-THE-COST-OF-COVID-19-Dec2021.pdf (Accessed: 24 April 2022).

Heng, K. (2021, June 25). 'COVID-19: A Catalyst for the Digital Transformation of Cambodian Education', *ISEAS Perspective*, No. 87. Available at: https://www.iseas.edu.sg/articles-commentaries/iseas-perspective/2021-87-covid-19-a-catalyst-for-the-digital-transformation-of-cambodian-education-by-kimkong-heng/ (Accessed: 10 May 2022).

Huaxia. (2020, June 1). 'Cambodian PM Says 256 Factories Suspended Due to COVID-19, Affecting over 130,000 Workers', *Xinhua Net*. Available at: http://www.xinhuanet.com/english/2020-06/01/c_139105722.htm (Accessed: 10 May 2022).

Huaxia. (2021, September 28). 'Cambodia to Reopen Universities after Majority of Population Vaccinated against COVID-19', *Xinhua Net*. Available at: http://www.news.cn/english/2021-09/28/c_1310213298.htm (Accessed: 10 May 2022).

Human Rights Committee. (2001, August 31). 'CCPR General Comment No. 29: Article 4: Derogations during a State of Emergency', CCPR/C/21/Rev.1/Add.11.

Human Rights Committee. (2020, April 24). 'Statement on Derogations from the Covenant in Connection with the COVID-19 Pandemic', CCPR/C/128/2.

Human Rights Watch. (2019). 'Cambodia: Events of 2018', *World Report 2019*. Available at: https://www.hrw.org/world-report/2019/country-chapters/cambodia (Accessed: 1 May 2022).

Human Rights Watch. (2020, March 24). 'Cambodia: COVID-19 Clampdown on Free Speech'. Available at: https://www.hrw.org/news/2020/03/24/cambodia-covid-19-clampdown-free-speech (Accessed: 1 May 2022).

ICJ [International Commission of Jurists]. (2021, May 25). 'Cambodia: Stop Silencing Critical Commentary on COVID-19'. Available at https://www.icj.org/cambodia-stop-silencing-critical-commentary-on-covid-19/.

ILO [International Labour Organization]. (2018). *Women and Men in the Informal Economy: A Statistical Picture*, 3rd Edition, International Labour Office, Geneva.

IMF. (2022). 'Cambodia: At a Glance', *IMF*. Available at: https://www.imf.org/en/Countries/KHM (Accessed: 24 April 2022).

IMF [International Monetary Fund]. (2021a). 'IMF Executive Board Concludes 2021 Article IV Consultation with Cambodia', *IMF*. Available at: https://www.imf.org/en/News/Articles/2021/12/08/pr21365-imf-executive-board-concludes-2021-article-iv-consultation-with-cambodia (Accessed: 24 April 2022).

IMF [International Monetary Fund]. (2021b, May 5). 'Policy Response to Covid-19: Policy Tracker on Cambodia'. Available at: https://www.imf.org/en/Topics/imf-and-covid19/Policy-Responses-to-COVID-19#C (Accessed: 9 May 2022).

ITUC [International Trade Union Confederation]. (2018). 'ITUC Global Rights Index: The World's Worst Countries for Workers'. Available at: https://www.ituc-csi.org/IMG/pdf/ituc-global-rights-index-2018-en-final-2.pdf (Accessed: 10 May 2022).

Kemp, S. and Moey, S. (2019, September 18). 'Digital 2019 Spotlight: Ecommerce in Southeast Asia', *Datareportal.* Available at: https://datareportal.com/reports/digital-2019-spotlight-ecommerce-in-southeast-asia (Accessed: 10 May 2022).

Khmer Times. (2021a, June 28). 'Cambodia Covid-19 Case Breakdown by Province', *Khmer Times.* Available at: https://www.khmertimeskh.com/50881937/cambodia-covid-19-case-breakdown-by-province/#google_vignette (Accessed: 10 May 2022).

Khmer Times. (2021b, April 28). 'List of Yellow, Orange and Red Zones in Phnom Penh', *Khmer Times.* Available at: https://www.khmertimeskh.com/50846770/list-of-yellow-orange-and-red-zones-in-phnom-penh-2/#google_vignette (Accessed: 24 April 2022).

Khuon, N. (2021, May 4). 'Information Ministry Warns Journalists against 'Ambulance Chasing' after Video of Long Waits for COVID-19 Patients Goes Viral', *Camboja News.* Available at: https://cambojanews.com/information-ministry-warns-journalists-against-ambulance-chasing-after-video-of-long-waits-for-covid-19-patients-goes-viral/ (Accessed: 24 April 2022).

Kijewski, L. (2018, July 5). 'Cambodia and the EU: A Farewell to Everything but Arms?', *Globe Media Asia.* Available at: https://southeastasiaglobe.com/a-farewell-to-everything-but-arms/.

Kong, P. (2012). 'Overview of the Cambodian Legal and Judicial System and Recent Efforts at Legal and Judicial Reform'. In Hor, P., Kong, P., and Menzel, J. (Eds), *Introduction to Cambodian Law*, Konrad-Adenauer-Stiftung, Phnom Penh, pp. 7–22.

Lebret, A. (2020). 'COVID-19 Pandemic and Derogation to Human Rights', *Journal of Law and the Biosciences*, 7(1), January–June, lsaa015. https://doi.org/10.1093/jlb/lsaa015 (Accessed: 10 May 2022).

LICADHO [Cambodian League for the Promotion and Defense of Human Rights]. (2019). 'Collateral Damage: Land Loss and Abuses in Cambodia's Microfinance Sector'. Available at: https://www.licadho-cambodia.org/reports/files/228Report_Collateral_Damage_LICADHO_STT_Eng_07082019.pdf (Accessed: 1 May 2022).

Ly, R., Hing, V. and Soy, K. (2021). 'Cambodia: Public Health, Economic, and Political Dimensions'. In V. V. Ramraj (Ed), *Covid-19 in Asia: Law and Policy Contexts*, Oxford University Press, Oxford, pp. 293–306.

Ly, S. (2021, December 3). 'Cambodia Economic Update: Living with COVID—Special Focus: The Impact of the COVID-19 Pandemic on Learning and Earning in Cambodia', *World Bank.* Available at: http://documents.worldbank.org/curated/en/099350012062137172/P1773400f35a770af0b4fa0781dffcd517e (Accessed: 1 May 2022).

May, K. (2021, June 3). 'Remittances Fall 17% to $1.2B in 2020: NBC Data', *The Phnom Penh Post.* Available at: https://www.phnompenhpost.com/business/remittances-fall-17-12b-2020-nbc-data (Accessed: 10 May 2022).

Mech, D., Seng, T. and Khut, S. (2021, August 30). 'Svay Rieng Land Disputants Arrested Under Covid-19 Law', *VOD.* Available at: https://vodenglish.news/svay-rieng-land-disputants-arrested-under-covid-19-law/ (Accessed: 24 April 2022).

Ministry of Information. (2021, June 9). 'Head of the National Covid-19 Vaccination Commission: Vaccination Work Is in Line with Samdech Techo's Flower Strategy'. Available at: https://www.information.gov.kh/articles/45538 (Accessed: 24 April 2022).

Mom, K. (2021, October 12). 'Unvaccinated People the Majority of Covid Fatalities', *The Phnom Penh Post*. Available at: https://www.phnompenhpost.com/national/unvaccinated-people-majority-covid-fatalities (Accessed: 11 May 2022).

Niem, C. (2021, March 11). 'Law on Covid-19 Control Takes Effect', *The Phnom Penh Post*. Available at: https://www.phnompenhpost.com/national/law-covid-19-control-takes-effect (Accessed: 24 April 2022).

OHCHR [Office of the High Commissioner for Human Rights]. (2020, April 27). 'Emergency Measures and COVID-19: Guidance'. Available at: https://www.ohchr.org/sites/default/files/Documents/Events/EmergencyMeasures_COVID19.pdf (Accessed: 12 May 2022).

Openaid. (2022). 'COVID-19 Capacity Development Partnership Fund III 2018–2021'. Available at: https://openaid.se/en/activities/SE-0-SE-6-10524A0101-KHM-11110.

Press and Quick Reaction Unit. (2021, May 6). 'The Royal Government Uses the "Blossom" Strategy as a Vaccination Campaign to Build Socio-Economic Immunity in Cambodia, Starting from the Heart of the Country', *Press OCM*. Available at: https://pressocm.gov.kh/archives/70480 (Accessed: 24 April 2022).

Ravallion, M. (2007). 'Inequality Is Bad for the Poor'. In J. Micklewright and S. Jenkins (Eds), *Inequality and Poverty Re-Examined*, Oxford University Press, Oxford, pp. 37–61.

Reporters Sans Frontieres. (2020, April 9). 'Cambodia: Hun Sen Uses Covid-19 Crisis to Tighten His Grip'. Available at: https://rsf.org/en/news/cambodiahun-sen-uses-covid-19-crisis-tighten-his-grip (Accessed: 10 May 2022).

RGC [Royal Government of Cambodia]. (2015). *Cambodia Industrial Development Policy 2015–2025*. Phnom Penh: Council of the Development of Cambodia.

Sao, P.N. (2021, July 16). 'The Ministry of Education Launches a Digital App for Distance Learning', *Cambodianess*. Available at: https://cambodianess.com/article/the-ministry-of-education-launches-a-digital-app-for-distance-learning (Accessed: 10 May 2022).

Sen, D. (2020, December 16). 'PM Says Grade 12 Exams Cancelled, All Students Pass', *Khmer Times*. Available at: https://www.khmertimeskh.com/50793598/pm-says-grade-12-exams-cancelled-all-students-pass/ (Accessed: 9 May 2022).

Special Procedures Communication Reports. (2020, April 9). 'Information Received Concerning the Plan to Adopt the Draft Law on the Management of the Nation during State of Emergency'. Available at: https://spcommreports.ohchr.org/TMResultsBase/DownLoadPublicCommunicationFile?gId=25186 (Accessed: 10 May 2022).

Special Procedures Communication Reports. (2021, March 31). 'Information Received Concerning the draft Law on the Measures to Prevent the Spread of COVID-19 and Other Serious, Dangerous and Contagious Diseases'. Available at: https://spcommreports.ohchr.org/TMResultsBase/DownLoadPublicCommunicationFile?gId=26266 (Accessed: 10 May 2022).

Sun, N. (2020, April 30). 'Cambodia's Controversial State of Emergency Draft Signed into Law', *VOA Khmer*. Available at: https://www.voacambodia.com/a/cambodia-s-controversial-state-of-emergency-draft-signed-into-law/5398771.html (Accessed: 24 April 2022).

Szablewska, N. (2020). 'Cambodia: Emergency Laws Raise Concerns about Human Rights', in N. Georgeou and C. Hawksley (Eds), *State Responses to COVID-19: A Global Snapshot at 1 June 2020*, Humanitarian and Development Research Initiative (HADRI), Penrith, NSW: Western Sydney University, pp. 31–33. https://doi.org/10.26183/5ed5a2079cabd.

Szablewska, N. (2022). 'Cambodia'. In S. Sayapin, R. Atadjanov, U. Kadam, G. Kemp, N. Zambrana Tévar, and N. Quénivet (Eds), *International Conflict and Security Law: A Research Handbook*, TMC Asser Press/Springer, The Hague, The Netherlands, Springer-Verlag, Berlin-Heidelberg.

The Constitutional Council of Cambodia. (2007, July 10). Case No 131/003/2007 of 26 June 2007, Decision No 092/003/2007 CC.D.

Touch, D. (2020, May 14). 'Cambodia's State of Emergency Law and the Fight Against COVID-19', *Asia Pacific Foundation of Canada*. Available at: https://www.asiapacific.ca/publication/cambodias-state-emergency-law-and-fight-against-covid-19 (Accessed: 24 April 2022).

UN Cambodia. (2021, August 3). 'United Nations Support to Cambodia's National COVID-19 Vaccination Roll-Out, Information Note #11'. Available at: https://reliefweb.int/sites/reliefweb.int/files/resources/UN%20Information%20Note_11_COVID-19%20vaccine%20roll-out_30Jul2021_ENGLISH.pdf (Accessed: 10 May 2022).

UN General Assembly. (1966, December 16). *International Covenant on Civil and Political Rights (ICCPR)*, United Nations: Treaty Series, vol. 999, p. 17.

UNAIDS. (2020, April 27). 'Providing Protection and Support to Returning Migrants in Cambodia'. Available at: https://www.unaids.org/en/20200427_Cambodia_migrants (Accessed: 10 May 2022).

UNDP. (2021, July 14). 'Counting the Cost of COVID-19 to Cambodia's Informal Workers'. Available at: https://www.kh.undp.org/content/cambodia/en/home/blog/2021/counting-the-cost-of-covid-to-cambodias-informal-workers.html (Accessed: 10 May 2022).

UNDP. (n.d.). 'About Cambodia'. Available at: https://www.kh.undp.org/content/cambodia/en/home/countryinfo.html.

UNDP [United Nations Development Programme]. (2020). *Human Development Report 2020: The Next Frontier Human Development and the Anthropocene*. Available at: https://hdr.undp.org/en/2020-report (Accessed: 10 May 2022).

UNESCO [UNESCO Institute for Statistics]. (2021). 'School Enrolment, Tertiary', *The World Bank*, as of September 2021. Available at: https://data.worldbank.org/indicator/SE.TER.ENRR?name_desc=false (Accessed: 9 May 2022).

UNICEF. (n.d.). 'Cambodia. Education'. Available at: https://www.unicef.org/cambodia/education#:~:text=Cambodia%20has%20made%20terrific%20progress,in%20school%20year%202017%2F18.

UNICEF and MoEYS [Cambodian Ministry of Education, Youth and Sport]. (2022). 'Learning Loss in the Covid-19 Pandemic Era: Evidence from the 2016–2021 Grade Six National Learning Assessment in Cambodia: Supplementary Technical Report for the 2021 Grade Six National Learning Assessment', *UNICEF* Cambodia. Available at: https://www.unicef.org/cambodia/sites/unicef.org.cambodia/files/2022-04/Grade%206%20NLA%20Report%20Final%20April%205_clean_Final.pdf.

UNICEF and the World Food Programme. (2021). *COVI-19 Socio-economic Impact Assessment*. Available at: https://www.unicef.org/cambodia/reports/covid-19-socio-economic-impact-assessment (Accessed: 10 May 2022).

UNIDO [United Nations Industrial Development Organization]. (2020). 'Impact Assessment of Covid-19 on Cambodia's Manufacturing Firms: Survey Results May-June'. Available at: https://www.unido.org/sites/default/files/files/2021-03/UNIDO%20COVID19%20Assessment_Cambodia_FINAL.pdf (Accessed: 10 May 2022).

Van Gerwen, F., Bernard, A., Balestrini, M., Ok, A., and Heng, T. (2018). 'Outcome Evaluation of the Education Capacity Development Partnership Fund (CDPF)', *UNICEF*.Availableat:https://www.unicef.org/cambodia/reports/outcome-evaluation-education-capacity-development-partnership-fund-cdpf (Accessed: 10 May 2022).

White, H. (2021, December 9). 'Cambodia Microfinance Association Welcomes Ban on New Deposit-Taking Institutions', *Cambodia Investment Review*. Available at: https://cambodiainvestmentreview.com/2021/12/09/cambodia-microfinance-association-welcomes-ban-on-new-deposit-taking-institutions/ (Accessed: 10 May 2022).

WHO. (2021). 'COVID-19 Joint WHO-MOH Situation Report #33', as of 15 February. Available at: https://www.who.int/cambodia/internal-publications-detail/covid-19-joint-who-moh-situation-report-33 (Accessed: 10 May 2022).

WHO. (2022). 'COVID-19 Joint WHO-MOH Situation Report #78', as of 10 January. Available at: https://www.who.int/cambodia/internal-publications-detail/covid-19-joint-who-moh-situation-report-78 (Accessed: 10 May 2022).

WHO [World Health Organization]. (2020, July 2). 'New COVID-19 Law Lab to Provide Vital Legal Information and Support for the Global COVID-19 Response'. Available at: https://www.who.int/news/item/22-07-2020-new-covid-19-law-lab-to-provide-vital-legal-information-and-support-for-the-global-covid-19-response (Accessed: 24 April 2022).

World Bank. (2017). *Cambodia Economic Update: Staying Competitive through Improving Productivity*, Washington, D.C.: World Bank. Available at: http://documents.worldbank.org/curated/en/780641494510994888/pdf/114938-PUBLIC-may-16-8pm-Cambodia-Economic-report-v2-s.pdf (Accessed: 10 May 2022).

World Bank. (2022). 'The World Bank in Cambodia: Overview', *World Bank*. Available at: https://www.worldbank.org/en/country/cambodia/overview (Accessed: 25 April 2022).

World Bank. (n.d.). 'Cambodia Higher Education Improvement Project'. Available at: https://projects.worldbank.org/en/projects-operations/project-detail/P162971?lang=en (Accessed: 10 May 2022).

World Vision. (2022, February 16). 'Child Protection and COVID-19: Cambodia Case Study', *World Vision International*. Available at: https://www.wvi.org/publications/case-study/child-protection/child-protection-and-covid-19-cambodia-case-study (Accessed: 20 April 2022).

World Vision Cambodia. (2020). 'COVID-19 Emergency Response Situation Report #13', as of 12 August. Available at: https://reliefweb.int/report/cambodia/world-vision-cambodia-covid-19-emergency-response-situation-report-13-12-august-2020?fbclid=IwAR0oPZXs5BwmFKNtsg4kw2tNWIdHw1G9X2RThG7Es4_2NrcB2viiy7QbrSA (Accessed: 10 May 2022).

11 Aotearoa New Zealand

Is the grass really greener here? Social, political, and cultural implications of COVID-19 in New Zealand

Christina Ergler, Nichole Georgeou, Sarah Lovell and Robert Huish

Introduction

We must go hard, and go early, and do everything we can to protect New Zealanders' health.
Prime Minister Jacinda Ardern, 14 March 2020

New Zealand's pandemic journey has been marked by a strong partnership between politicians and public health experts. The government attempted to have clear and accessible messaging to inform, justify and explain the evidence-based pandemic responses. Government communication was led by Prime Minister Jacinda Ardern and Director-General of Health Dr Ashley Bloomfield, a public health physician, who conveyed the rationale for government decisions daily at the height of outbreaks. Government messaging was often supported by strong science communicators such as Siouxsie Wiles and Toby Morris (see Figure 11.1).[1] This partnership between politicians and health experts has so far trod a careful line between "hard and soft pandemic responses" (Freeman et al. 2022)—between rigorous and legally enforced ordinances and empathy—when, for example, the Easter Bunny and Tooth Fairy were declared essential workers. Their communication strategy was meant to be firm, yet kind.

Public health measures such as strictly closing borders and enforcing long-term lockdowns came about quickly when community transmission of the virus was confirmed. These ordinances caused rapid, large-scale disruptions. Yet despite the immediate economic and social disruption, the message of care remained at the forefront. With enforced measures in place and low COVID-19 numbers, buy-in remained high and narratives of teamwork emerged. Amid the celebration of the New Zealand COVID-19 response emerged a subtle disregard for some of the wounds inflicted by the process of implementation of pandemic measures.

As low transmission and case counts continued, so too did public support for the idea that it was such strict measures that kept the virus at bay and that the "team of 5 million" was doing its job. However, the popular support

DOI: 10.4324/9781003311522-11

Level two tips

As New Zealand moved back into alert level two on May 14, Siouxsie and Toby offered some simple rules for playing it safe as we tiptoed back to something like normal life.

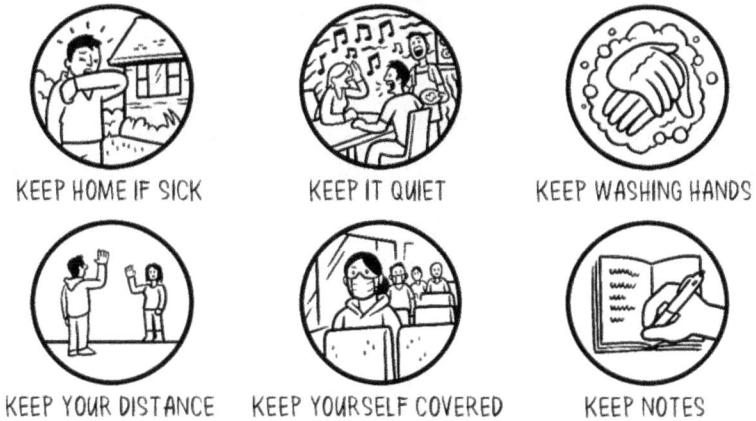

KEEP HOME IF SICK   KEEP IT QUIET   KEEP WASHING HANDS

KEEP YOUR DISTANCE   KEEP YOURSELF COVERED   KEEP NOTES

@SIOUXSIEW @XTOTL thespinoff.co.nz   CC-BY-SA 4.0

Figure 11.1 Clear and simple visual communication of six easy steps to keep people safe after the move to alert level 1 in 2020.

began to wane in October 2021. People's negative experiences, from the loss of social connections, and people's overall physical and mental well-being have not played a major role in looking at the social, economic and political consequences of the pandemic (Appleton et al. 2021). Instead, epidemiological evidence and broader public health concerns masked social, political and economic pandemic consequences. Strong social tension emerged between belief in the public health ordinances, and dealing with personal hardship. We argue in this chapter that despite the hard and soft measures of the government to protect the health of New Zealand's population, visible and invisible wounds were dealt. We conceptualise that these less visible, but still harmful, consequences of the pandemic on experiences, knowledge and bodies are forms of 'slow violence' (Nixon 2013; Ward 2015). In the following, we outline our conceptualisation of how pandemic rhythms and associated government measures and everyday practices have caused harm to some while protecting the health of others as a form a slow violence. We then outline New Zealand's pandemic journey before discussing the social, political, cultural and economic consequences of this journey by focusing on the stigmatisation of particular groups and the invisibility of children and young people at the height of the pandemic. We close this chapter with some optimistic conclusions from these hard lessons learned.

Theoretical embedding: conceptualising pandemic slow violence in New Zealand

Pandemic slow violence remains unseen in New Zealand. To make the pandemic slow violence visible in this chapter, we draw on Nixon's (2013:2) conceptualisation of slow violence as a form of violence that is occurring "gradually and out of sight, a violence of delayed destruction that is dispersed across time and space, an attributed violence that is typically not viewed as violence at all". Slow violence is often invisible to outsiders and less recognisable than physical violence like a cut, but nonetheless, this form of structural violence leaves scars on body and soul, is multi-scalar and has its own temporal rhythms.

Pandemic slow violence in New Zealand has inflicted visible and less visible wounds on diverse groups in the population. Less noticeable wounds are manifold and build on historical practices of silencing and structural inequities. However, these pre-existing slow violence practices are further overlayed and amplified through the often unintended consequences of the regulatory legislation that prioritises government activities and agendas. But, these (mainly invisible) wounds of the pandemic are inflicted and experienced in the everyday pandemic context. Not only is the pandemic slow violence unseen but also people themselves and their material struggles have remained invisible to the wider public as the pandemic continues to unfold. For example, the consequences of extended lockdowns on children and young people have not played a major role in public discourse (Spray, 2020; Freeman et al. 2022). Even when the effects of slow violence can no longer be ignored as the impacts of the felt discrimination and stigmatisation of anti-vaxxers in workplaces show (Breen and Gilliespie 2021), the emotional, physical and intergenerational consequences are ignored. We argue this practice is a tactic to uphold the 'winner narrative' and diminish the corollary of the enactment of public health measures. This practice of public denial of the harmful impacts of the pandemic on different groups within New Zealand society is used to keep the latent landscapes of structural inequality ongoing. Kern (2016) argues this practice is 'stage-managed amnesia' of whose experiences are worthy of recognition and whose are silenced in, for example, news outlets. We conceptualise these less visible, but still harmful, consequences of the pandemic on experiences, knowledge and bodies as a form of 'slow violence' (Nixon 2013; Ward 2015).

Slow violence has its own rhythms spatially and temporally, and therefore we attempt to make visible in this chapter some of "the concerns, knowledge and bodies of those who suffer violence 'unseen,' that have been forgotten, hidden, or otherwise erased" (Cahill and Pain 2019: 1056) among the 'winner narrative' of New Zealand's response to the pandemic. Although the pace and impact of slow violence have had different rhythms spatially and temporally globally and within New Zealand, no matter if pandemic wounds have been inflicted early or late in the process, the consequences are still felt and cause harm. Vannini (2020: 271) speaks, for example, of the loss of the rhythms of everyday life to lockdown, replaced by a sense of dis-ease as isolation became the primary atmospheric attunement; they describe isolation as a "geography of what doesn't happen: of cancelled events, of missed chances, of a shuttered consumer society, of shattered kinship".

We conceptualise New Zealand's pandemic journey as a polyrhythmic passage (Given, 2012: 2) subjecting to both normal rhythms of inequity of a pre-COVID life and disruptive rhythms of the pandemic that require different dealings at different pandemic stages. Pandemic rhythms are produced by a situatedness of socio-spatial practices that are relational and bring the inside and outside world together—both literally as inside and outside of the borders of New Zealand and metaphorically as the private and public sphere of COVID. In other words, pandemic slow violence has brought out different socio-spatial survival practices and coping strategies depending on the everyday context and stage of the pandemic. These practices build on and mobilise both pre-COVID and pandemic rhythms and change social relations based on expectations, discourses of non-conformity and stigmatisation, but they also bring out unexpected consequences both positive and negative. Violence "shapes, but does not wholly define" (McKittrick 2011: 947) people and the pace and practices of everyday life. In this chapter, we show how the diverse rhythms of pandemic slow violence affected specific communities and professions in New Zealand.

New Zealand's pandemic journey: from elimination to living with the virus

When COVID-19 emerged as a global pandemic in March 2020, some nations took the approach of "keeping COVID out" (Cousins, 2020). Such an approach required tight restrictions on the movement of people through a state's borders, mandatory quarantine and frequent testing of new arrivals in order to protect the national population and preserve the healthcare system from being overwhelmed (Jefferies et al., 2020).

New Zealand adopted a clearly structured four-tiered alert system which specified the public health and social measures to be taken to 'contain' COVID-19, for example, how many people can gather at each level in private and public spaces and what restrictions are in place for education providers or workplaces (e.g. working and studying from home). These four levels include the following, but at all levels, the border was firmly shut (Ministry of Health, 2022).

> **Alert level 1: prepare** (the virus is uncontrolled overseas, but the virus is contained within New Zealand with sporadic imported cases on the border, no restrictions on movement or gatherings within the country)

Alert level 2: reduce (the virus is contained, but the risk for community transmission exists and single cluster outbreaks might be occurring; travel locally and gatherings of people up to 100 indoors and outdoors)

Alert level 3: restrict (high risk, virus is not contained, cluster outbreaks which are controlled through testing; people stay home in their bubble and businesses can open if they can follow public health guidelines; gatherings of up to ten people are allowed but only for wedding services, funerals and *tangihanga* (mourning rites))

Alert level 4: lockdown (virus not contained and sustained and intensive community transmission occurring; people stay home in their bubble except for essential services)

The first officially recorded COVID case in New Zealand was reported on 28 February 2020 (see Figure 11.2). Public health experts lobbied the government to act with urgency to stop the spread of the virus and potentially eliminate it by implementing a strict nationwide lockdown. The "go hard—go early" approach taken by the Labour government of Prime Minister Jacinda Ardern resulted in a nationwide lockdown on 25 March 2020. Two days earlier, a text message sent to all cell phones in New Zealand informed the population about the temporal ending of 'normal' life; in these 48 hours, people needed to decide who would be part of their social 'bubble' and how to get ready for working and studying from home, stocking supplies and making any last minute arrangements for the unprecedented suspension of common activities. A section of the Health Act Order (2020) allowed the director-general of health to close all premises, including schools, universities and workplaces, as well as online, clothing and hardware stores, except those businesses deemed crucial for delivering essential and emergency activities to the population (e.g. supermarkets, health services and goods transport) (Kearns, 2021). New Zealanders remained at home and were required to stay within their 'bubble', often in their nuclear family or flatting constellation, and not to mingle with other 'bubbles' when exercising and playing outdoors locally for up to an hour per day. This first national state of emergency and associated lockdown restrictions, also known as alert level 4, was in place for almost two months until 13 May 2020.

New Zealand initially adopted an elimination strategy for the COVID virus, which led to one of the firmest public health measures globally, including, for example, the closure of the border except for returning citizens and residents. However, if people returned, it was mandatory they spend two weeks in a managed isolation and quarantine (MIQ) facility managed by the Ministry of Business, Innovation and Environment and the New Zealand Defence Force from 9 April 2020. From 11 August 2020, charges for some users were introduced to recover some of the costs of MIQ.[2] MIQ places were however limited, leaving many New Zealanders stranded overseas. As a consequence of this firmness, community transmission remained low, and the virus could be eliminated in the community again until August 2021 when the Delta variant arrived in New Zealand. The elimination strategy of the virus was achieved

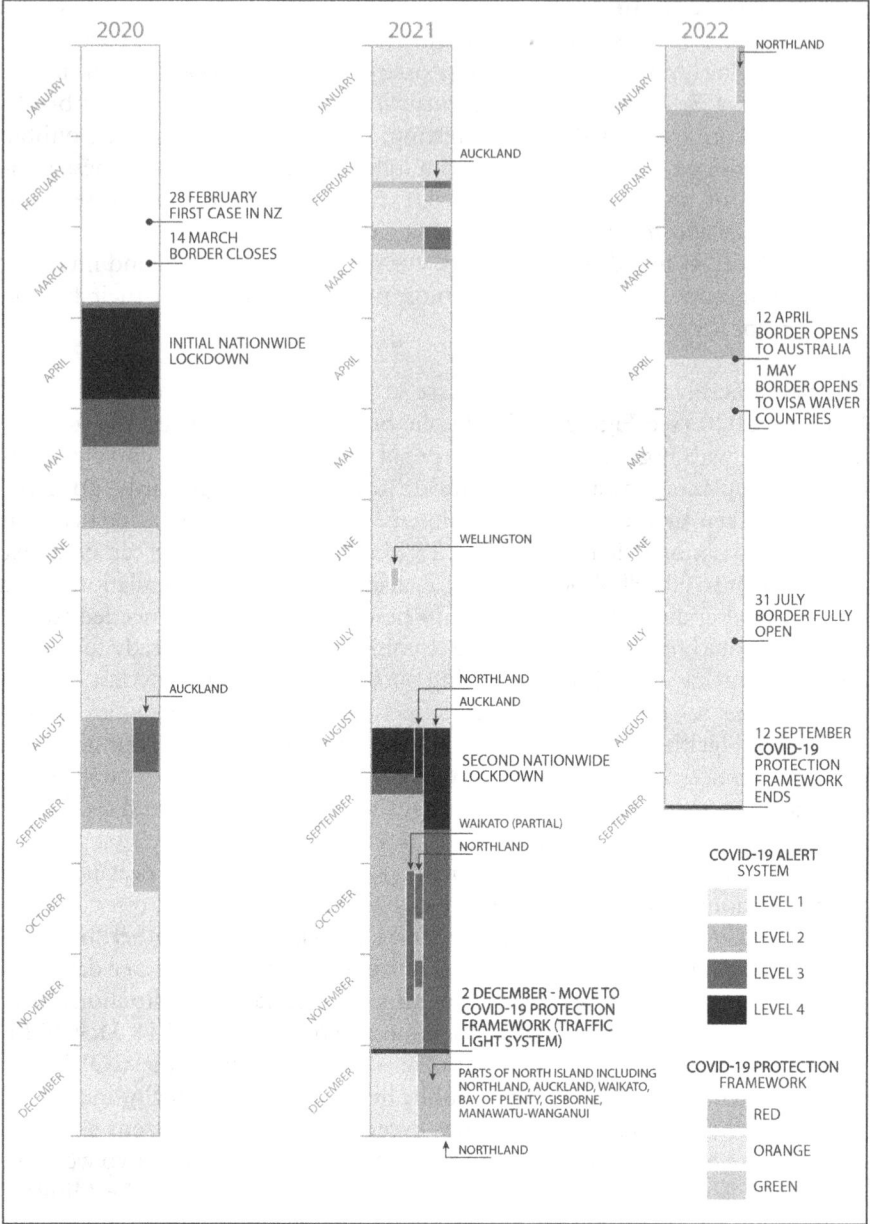

Figure 11.2 New Zealand's pandemic timeline.

Source: Figure created by Chris Garden, Geographical Information Systems, Otago University

with locally targeted shifts in the alert levels. For example, the city of Auckland moved for a few days to alert level 3, while the rest of the country moved to alert level 2 in August 2020 and February 2021 (for more details of changes in alert levels see Figure 11.2).

Until the abandonment of the alert level system in December 2021, New Zealand used QR code check-ins, but only to assist with contact tracing (O'Connor, Hopkins, and Johnston, 2021). Mobile apps were only an accessory to the COVID-19 policy of New Zealand's approach compared to some countries like Singapore and Taiwan, where data and location tracking through mobile phone apps were at the core of COVID-19 prevention strategies (Wang, Ng, and Brook, 2020). Instead, New Zealand, like many other states, continued to rely on a series of ancient methods that have been public health policy since antiquity to deal with a modern-day pandemic: selfisolation, quarantine, hand washing (Ergler et al., 2021); plus the compulsory wearing of face coverings on planes and medical facilities as the pandemic progressed.

The swift and strict implementation of the four-tiered alert level system resulted in very low infection rates, with just 1,504 cases and 22 deaths by 1 June 2020, virtually all of which were in March and April (Shaw, 2020). Exactly one year later, on 1 June 2021, there had been just 2,317 cases recorded, and only 13 active cases in managed isolation facilities (Ministry of Health, 2021a). Low-level infections remained until mid-August 2021, when the Delta variant of COVID emerged in NZ, linked to a traveller who had returned from Sydney, Australia (Al Jazeera 2021).

On 17 August 2021, the entire country moved into a second nationwide lockdown for almost four weeks, which continued on for Auckland and surrounding districts until December 2021. However, from 4 October 2021, the NZ government changed its pandemic management strategy from eliminating COVID to living with the virus (Ministry of Health, 2021b), which led to the abandonment of the alert level system and a move to a COVID-19 protection framework (traffic light system) on 2 December 2021.

A firm component of the new protection framework is a high vaccination rate among the eligible population that allows for a staggered five-step opening of the border with dependents of citizens and residents, work visa holders who still meet the visa conditions and Australian citizens or permanent resident visa holders. From 31 July 2022, all travellers, even unvaccinated travellers, can enter New Zealand.

New Zealand has so far been remarkably fortunate in avoiding the worst ravages of COVID. At the time of writing (early June 2022), the number of total COVID cases in NZ was 1,279,116 with 1,330 deaths. By any measure—for example, infections as a percentage of population, total cases, deaths—the case numbers in NZ are a fraction of those recorded in states in North America, Europe, Asia or Australia. Among OECD states with similar populations to NZ, Ireland has almost 5 million people and on 20 June 2022 had recorded 1,578,284 total COVID cases and 7,442 total deaths; Finland with 5.5 million people had recorded over 1,125,342 cases and 4,771 total deaths (Johns Hopkins 2022). Comparatively low numbers and deaths in NZ do not however diminish the social, economic, cultural and political consequences that were also felt and experienced in this country.

Social, economic, political and cultural consequences of New Zealand's pandemic journey

While many countries in Europe and North America were in lockdown, from mid-2020, life on the surface returned to the old 'normal' for many New Zealanders. People were encouraged to explore their 'own backyard' during the Christmas holidays to keep the struggling hospitality industry alive at a time when it was unclear when the border would open again (Frost, 2020). New Zealanders were able to roam freely within their country and did so, evidenced by the boom in motorhome purchases. However, not everything was rosy. House prices soared (The Economist, 2022). Many people struggled to pay their rent, mortgages, or to feed their families, even with the government's 'stay in job' subsidies (Prickett et al. 2020). The need for food parcels continued to grow even after the first lockdown when many businesses went into liquidation or closed and people lost their jobs. The government injected NZ$38.15 million into the country's food banks to mitigate the worst experiences and outcomes of the pandemic (Sepuloni, 2021).

For around 18 months, buy-in to the government's rhetoric of a "team of five million that stands together" remained strong. The discourse depicted a collective obligation to protect the health of the vulnerable while being 'kind' to each other, and it was reinforced by a relatively bleak international picture of successive lockdowns and pandemic 'waves'. Facing a pandemic election in October 2020, Jacinda Adern's Labour Party was returned with an increased majority and was able to form a government in its own right, unusual in New Zealand's Multi-Member Proportional (MMP) system.[3]

As 2021 progressed, cases of the Delta variant were detected in Auckland, and confidence in the country's elimination strategy began to waver. The country was plunged into a further lockdown in August 2021 that extended in Auckland for 107 days. Groups whose members reported feeling a sense of non-belonging to the 'team' became more vocal, criticising the government's elimination strategy and the social, political and economic consequences of NZ's border closures (Appelton et al. 2021; Ergler et al. 2021). Some questioned why families were separated, and they worried for the one million Kiwis stranded overseas since the pandemic commenced who were unable to obtain one of the limited spaces in quarantine, despite some no longer meeting the visa conditions of their host country (McClure 2021).

Opponents of the government's strict quarantine rules initially felt unable to speak up openly in public and censored themselves when among friends and colleagues, wary of being seen as unappreciative of their 'good fortune' (Ergler et al. 2021). Within the pandemic, disinformation and misinformation, as well as natural hesitancy, genuine questions and concern, have created vortexes of insiders and outsider labelling of the "team of five million" that denote who is accepted as part of the national polity. Many of those outside the 'mainstream' discourse lost social connections, but more broadly, the impact of lockdowns and alert level shifts on people's physical, social and mental well-being have not played a major role in the public discourse. For example, the impact of delays in routine check-ups (e.g. cancer prevention, ready for school), vaccination schedules and surgeries will only be able to be fully grasped in years to come (Quinn, 2022). The closest approximation to acknowledging any problem occurred during government "1pm Press conferences" with entreaties to 'be kind' to each other (Kearns 2021) until the occupation of Parliament grounds by people protesting against vaccine mandates and government ordinances in February 2022 (Thaker 2021; RNZ, 2022).

The social, cultural, economic and political consequences of and the wounds caused by the pandemic within New Zealand are manifold. Next, we discuss two examples that exemplify the rifts and slow violence that government ordinances (unintentionally) caused: COVID stigma and the forgotten pandemic children.

Example 1: COVID stigma in New Zealand

Age-old pandemic control methods such as quarantine and isolation seek to place physical boundaries around diseased persons and unsurprisingly are associated with similarly age-old social problems, notably, stigma. The word "stigma" originates from ancient Greece when persons with unwanted characteristics were physically tattooed, or *stitzo*, against their will in order to be easily identified in public (Bagcchi, 2020). The "casting out" of others is often constructed through stereotypes of otherness, and of persons being "out of place", a concept used by Cresswell (1992) that signifies how people structure their self-awareness of fitting into particular communities based on their own identity.

In medical terms, stigma is often cast at individuals who are thought to impose a health risk to the public good based on their actions rather than their identity, and hence the presence of such unwanted persons builds into social stigma (Ablon, 2002). The result is often the direct persecution of individuals or self-stigmatisation, which is when the potential to be targeted leads individuals to avoid public engagement for fear of stigma (Mahoudi et al., 2021). In the early days of the pandemic, social stigma emerged in many countries, New Zealand included, towards those who appeared to be of Asian descent (NZ Human Rights Commission, 2022). Disconnecting the association of disease to place can be a challenge for public health officials as popular media often seek out origin stories of illness along the lines of "where did it come from"? And, "Who is responsible" (Xue and White, 2021)? New Zealand's human rights commission recorded a significant increase in calls and complaints for public incidents discriminating against persons who appeared to be of Asian descent (NZ Human Rights Commission, 2022). Public ads and public education campaigns were commonplace in 2020 to discourage any sort of actions that could lead to stigmatisation of persons who appeared to be of Asian descent, and later to those of Pacific Islander (*Pasifika*) descent.

The experience of stigmatisation includes a reluctance to participate in public health initiatives or to engage with public health services for fear of being called out, blamed, humiliated or even attacked. Through the successful suppression of COVID-19 and the "hard and strong" public health response, the government created an environment ripe for stigmatisation of rare positive cases. For example, the August 2021 lockdown occurred, initially, on the basis of one positive case, with the media seeking intimate details of his movements, contacts and symptoms enabling the public to render his actions as deviant or conforming to the public health interests of the team of five million.

With each wave of the pandemic, stigma rolled onto other communities. Persons who returned to New Zealand from abroad were targeted. After the first wave of the pandemic, trust in the government-run quarantine services was high, and the popular perception grew that New Zealand would be protected from COVID-19 spreading within the community. Since many New Zealanders were under long and heavy lockdowns, the only associated risk popularly imagined in mid-2020 was that individuals with the ability to be mobile posed the greatest risk to the country (Power, 2021). Such "associated risk" extended to healthcare workers and essential workers. Despite their protective actions at work, many reported that they became disconnected from family, friends and community during the pandemic out of fear of association or contact (Bell et al., 2021). In particular, community cohesion and workplace well-being can be set back enormously. In New Zealand, such groups included, Pasifika communities, people with low incomes, gang members, sex workers and even MIQ workers, some of whom and their families reported losing rental contracts and being isolated from their social networks (Ergler et al., 2021). Partners and family members of MIQ workers in some cases quit their jobs or moved to work permanently at home rather than deal with the backlash of those who feared transmission. The impacts of stigma can have broad social impacts (Bayer 2008) and are fuelled by pre-COVID-19 structural inequities.

Stigma as a social consequence of the pandemic was not necessarily surprising, as it has occurred in past pandemics (Fischer, Mansergh, Lynch, and Santibanez, 2019). In contrast, with COVID, no particular group was singled out for the entirety of the pandemic, as groups affected by stigma changed over time, and in line with the global COVID-pandemic rhythms. What is particularly noteworthy in New Zealand's case is that early quarantine practices had limited success, in part due to short quarantine periods and variable notification of disease (Day, 1999). In March 2020, the government's pursuit of an elimination strategy informed by the Chinese response sought to identify and isolate all cases of COVID-19 (Baker et al., 2020). Rapidly, the language around New Zealand's use of self-isolation and quarantine became grounded in the spirit of the "team of 5 million", and keeping New Zealand COVID-free. With such lofty goals in place, those who were unwilling, or unable, to abide by these social measures were quick to fall to social stigma and self-stigmatisation.

Example 2: The forgotten population—children of the pandemic

Children and young people have been fairly invisible during New Zealand's pandemic journey, and so have their pandemic wounds. Children are often seen as a necessary corollary of the pandemic; their sacrifices are taken as a given without much further questioning (Freeman et al. 2022). They stayed at home during lockdowns, missing friends and extended family members while negotiating online learning, often without the much needed hardware or technological knowledge, and they were bored, as playgrounds were closed. Some were subjected to both verbal and physical abuse at home; some became wary of strangers, unsure when and with whom to interact in public and at home (Freeman et al. 2022; Children's Commissioner, 2020). Known practices were turned upside down.

Even when moving to lower alert levels, children suffered from cancelled or limited public social gatherings, such as the beloved Santa Parades, Midwinter Carnivals or big cultural festivals during the summer months; they lived with cancelled sporting and other extra-curricular activities. Implications of these profound changes on children's social, physical and mental well-being are often invisible and silenced in public. At the same time, their worries and need to comprehend ongoing events were, at best, dismissed. Children of the pandemic are again treated as "adults in the making" (Prout, 2005) rather than as social actors in their own right.

About 20% of New Zealand's population are children and young people, but their needs do not feature prominently in the public or government pandemic discourse (Freeman et al. 2022). If they feature in, for example, news outlets, they are often framed as an *at* or *as* risk population group. Children are *at* risk of getting sick, missing out on essential experiences and education and suffering from long COVID. Children also appear *as* a risk, their maskless school and social activities rendering them 'disease vectors' who endanger the life of older people. Rarely are they conceptualised as pandemic actors themselves who practice, shape, protect and live with the pandemic consequences (Smith et al. 2022; Spray and Hunleth, 2020). The struggles of being a pandemic child have been veiled by concerns about vaccination rates, inequities in access to technology, school dropouts and struggles of the economy as a result of border closures (Children's Convention Monitoring Group, 2021). In other words, their needs as children have been invisible to many public health experts and politicians, as they are not yet of voting age and are absorbed into a bigger family unit. Children were talked about, but talking *with* children rarely happened.

Speaking with children and taking them seriously reveals they care for the health of their immediate family members, older relatives, friends and strangers on the road or on TV. They remind parents to put on masks, follow public health hygiene, initiate neighbourhood support groups and put up with public health ordinances in solidarity with the greater good of the population (Freeman et al. 2022; Spray, 2020). Some children and young people worried about parents who are essential workers; others have witnessed their parents lose jobs and worry about family finances and friends and relatives overseas; others kept track and tried to make sense of the thousands of COVID-19 casualties globally. For others, wounds opened again or new ones were inflicted when moving back during lockdowns into a homophobic or transphobic home environment they were then unable to leave due to the dire economic situation; they were without any support from peers and an understanding wider support network (Murphy, 2020). This "stage-managed amnesia" (Kern, 2016) of children and young people's experiences and needs during the pandemic so far is surprising, especially as the prime minister was one of the few global leaders to hold a press conference in early 2020 just for children or to consider their concerns as to whether the Easter Bunny or the Tooth Fairy qualified as essential workers. But these rare acts of kindness hide a broader veiling of a fifth of the population's experiences, even when high-profile public figures call the government out on this oversight and for further fuelling the latent landscapes of inequity (Children's Monitoring Group, 2021). In October 2020, the Children's Commissioner presented a bleak outlook, especially for low-income families, as to the flow-on effects of children already living in poverty or falling into COVID-19-induced poverty, dealing with family violence caused by toxic stress and declining health due to a lack of affordable warm housing, and these concerns have only amplified further over time (Children's Monitoring Group, 2021). Thus, children's pandemic lives have been shaped by pre-COVID-19 structural violence, disruptive pandemic rhythms and the global stage, but not all experiences are so bleak.

Children reported enjoying the car-free environments during lockdowns, more time with family members and the joy of exploring their local environment (Children's Commissioner, 2020; Smith et al. 2022). Children created chalk hopscotch games on pavements, learned to ride bikes on empty roads, played board games in the evenings and explored new hobbies for which they had no time before lockdowns due to busy schedules and extra-curricula activities. They explored and got reattached to their neighbourhoods in a very different way than it was possible before the pandemic. Some of the joys of lockdowns have become a constant in their family life, while others remain a fond memory as their pandemic journey continues. Nonetheless, these positive experiences of a 'new normal' have not been translated into wide-reaching policies to ensure more family time through flexible work hours and places or low-speed neighbourhood zones.

Looking back and moving forward

The drive to protect the team of five million from COVID-19 through lockdowns and vaccinations has raised, and will likely continue to raise, social, economic and political concerns and consequences, especially as New Zealand's pandemic journey has been a polyrhythmic passage. Nonetheless, Prime Minister Jacinda Ardern's government was widely praised for handling the COVID-19 pandemic from the start to the present day, as we have outlined in this chapter. The first point of praise is given to the government for relying on all-source intelligence in the early days of the pandemic to effectively chart out a pandemic playbook that kept case counts to nearly nil during the onset of the pandemic and contributed to NZ having among the lowest rates of excess deaths in the OECD (OECD, 2021). The second point comes from the boasting rights to having over 95% of the population double vaccinated. Third, when the Omicron variant took hold of New Zealand in March 2022, because of the high vaccine rates, hospitalisations remained minimal, even though the country reported tens of thousands of cases daily, including the prime minister, who contracted COVID-19 in mid-May 2022.

While Jacinda Arden's government is widely respected for its COVID-19 strategy, both within the country and abroad, certain domestic challenges were put on the back burner during the pandemic. This violence of delayed destruction, as we have conceptualised in this chapter, may result in political consequences in the future; the political right-wing opponents are reinvigorating already. The shattered tourism industry, rising inflation and the cost of housing and energy all impact the daily lives of New Zealanders and can ultimately further social and economic inequalities. These are not challenges unique to New Zealand, but they are to be considered against a backdrop of two years of policy aimed at handling a common challenge for all. How New Zealand's post-COVID-19 recovery unfolds and handles specific challenges of social inequity that arose during the pandemic remains to be seen. However, in moving forward, the wounds inflicted through these processes need to be healed deeply, not just patched up with short-term band-aid solutions (Ergler et al. 2021); the furthered and deepening latent landscapes of violence beyond stigmatisation and unseen bodies of children need to be brought into the light to recognise and make visible the myriad pandemic experiences of New Zealand.

Notes

1 Microbiologist Siouxsie Wiles and cartoonist Toby Morris created for the online newspaper, the *Spinoff*, visual explainers of viral transmission, changing evidence and public health measures. Their work is for many New Zealanders part of the collective memory for making the complexity of the pandemic responses easily understandable and accessible https://thespinoff.co.nz/media/07-09-2021/the-great-toby-morris-siouxsie-wiles-covid-19-omnibus. (*The images have been released under a Creative Commons CC-BY-SA-4.0 licence. This means you are free to use them providing you give credit and share under the same conditions, so we could include one if we wanted.*)
2 In 2022, costs range between NZ$1,610 for an individual person with citizenship or residential status to NZ$2,760 for critical workers or temporary visa class holders. Additional adult family members and children sharing the same room needed to pay less depending on age, citizenship and visa status (NZ$230 for a child with citizenship—for an adult sharing the same room with an temporary visa class holder NZ$1,495) https://www.miq.govt.nz/charges-for-managed-isolation/.
3 New Zealand moved from first past the post to an MMP system for its general election in 1996. Under MMP, voters elect the candidate of their choice in regional electorates (72 seats), as well as voting nationally for the party list of their choice (48 seats). The unicameral chamber of 120 includes eight dedicated seats for Maori electors.

Bibliography

Ablon, J. (2002). The Nature of Stigma and Medical Conditions. *Epilepsy & Behavior*, *3*(6), 2–9.

Al Jazeera. (2021, September 17). 'New Zealand, Australia Travel Bubble Suspended as COVID Continues', https://www.aljazeera.com/news/2021/9/17/nz-australia-travel-bubble-suspension-stays-amid-delta-outbreaks.

Appleton R., Williams, J., Vera San Juan, N., Needle, J.J., Schlief, M., Jordan, H., Sheridan Rains, L., Goulding, L., Badhan, M., Roxburgh, E., Barnett, P., Spyridonidis, S., Tomaskova, M., Mo, J., Harju-Seppänen, J., Haime, Z., Casetta, C., Papamichail, A., Lloyd-Evans, B., Simpson, A., Sevdalis, N., Gaughran, F., and Johnson, S. (2021). 'Implementation, Adoption, and Perceptions of Telemental Health During the COVID-19 Pandemic: Systematic Review'. *Journal of Medical Internet Research*, 23(12), e31746, https://doi.org/10.2196/31746. PMID: 34709179. PMCID: 8664153.

Bagcchi, S. (2020). Stigma during the COVID-19 Pandemic. *The Lancet Infectious Diseases*, *20*(7), 782.

Baker, M. G., Kvalsvig, A., and Verrall, A. J. (2020). New Zealand's COVID-19 Elimination Strategy. *Medical Journal of Australia*, *213*(5), 198–200.e1. doi: 10.5694/mja2.50735

Bayer, R. (2008). Stigma and the Ethics of Public Health: Not Can We but Should We. *Social Science & Medicine*, *67*(3), 463–472.

Bell, C., Williman, J., Beaglehole, B., Stanley, J., Jenkins, M., Gendall, P., . . . Every-Palmer, S. (2021). Challenges Facing Essential Workers: A Cross-Sectional Survey of the Subjective Mental Health and Well-Being of New Zealand Healthcare and 'Other' Essential Workers during the COVID-19 Lockdown. *BMJ Open*, *11*, e048107. doi: 10.1136/bmjopen-2020-048107

Breen, C. and Gilliespie, A. (2021). Vaccine Mandates for NZ's Health and Education Workers Are Now in Force – but Has the Law Got the Balance Right? *The Conversation*. https://theconversation.com/vaccine-mandates-for-nzs-health-and-education-workers-are-now-in-force-but-has-the-law-got-the-balance-right-171392

Cahill, C. and Pain, R. (2019): Representing Slow Violence and Resistance: On Hiding and Seeing. *ACME An International Journal of Critical Geographies*, 18(5), 1054–1065.

Children's Commissioner. (2020). *Life in Lockdown*, https://www.occ.org.nz/publications/reports/life-in-lockdown/ [accessed 03.02.2022].

Children's Convention Monitoring Group. (2021). *Children's Rights in the Covid-19 Response*, https://www.occ.org.nz/publications/reports/childrens-rights-in-covid19/ [accessed 03.04.2022]

Cousins, S. (2020). New Zealand Eliminates Covid-19. *The Lancet*, *395*(10235), 1474.

Cresswell, T. (1992). *In Place/Out of Place: Geography, Ideology and Transgression*. Madison: The University of Wisconsin-Madison.

Day, A. (1999). Chastising Its People with Scorpians' Māori and the 1913 Smallpox Epidemic. *New Zealand Journal of History*, 33(2), 180–199.

Ergler, C., Huish, R., Georgeou, N., Simons, J., Eyles, O., Li, Y., . . . Tame, L. (2021). COVID-19 Stigma in New Zealand: Are We Really a 'Team' of Five Million? *New Zealand Geographer*, 77(3), 174–179.

Fischer, L., Mansergh, G., Lynch, J., and Santibanez, S. (2019). Addressing Disease-Related Stigma during Infectious Disease Outbreaks. *Disaster Medicine and Public Health Preparedness*, 13(5–6), 989–994.

Freeman, C., Ergler, C., Kearns, R., and Smith, M. (2022). Covid-19 in New Zealand and the Pacific: Implications for Children and Families. *Children's Geographies*, 20(4), 459–468, https://doi.org/10.1080/14733285.2021.1907312

Frost, N. (2020). Largely Free of the Virus, New Zealand Could Party Like It Was 2019, https://www.nytimes.com/2020/12/31/world/largely-free-of-the-virus-new-zealand-could-party-like-it-was-2019.html.

Given, L.M. (2012). Rhythmanalysis. In: *The Sage Encyclopedia of Qualitative Research Methods*. 794–797. https://methods.sagepub.com/reference/sage-encyc-qualitative-research-methods [accessed 02.06.2022]

Jefferies, S., French, N., Gilkison, C., Graham, G., Hope, V., Marshall, J., . . . Prassad, N. (2020). COVID-19 in New Zealand and the Impact of the National Response: A Descriptive Epidemiological Study. *The Lancet Public Health*, 5(11), e612–e623.

Johns, Hopkins (2022, June 20). 'What is the JHU CRC Now?' COVID Resource Centre, https://coronavirus.jhu.edu/.

Kearns, R. (2021). Narrative and Metaphors in New Zealand's Efforts to Eliminate COVID-19. *Geographical Research*, 59, 324–330.

Kern, L. (2016). Rhythms of Gentrification: Eventfulness and Slow Violence in a Happening Neighbourhood. *Cultural Geographies*, 23(3), 441–457.

Mahoudi, H., Saffari, M., Movahedi, M., Sanaeinsasab, H., Rashidi-Jahan, H., Pourgholami, M., and Pakpour, A. (2021). A Mediating Role for Mental Health in Associations between COVID-19-Related Self-Stigma, PTSD, Quality of Life, and Insomnia among Patients Recovered from COVID-19. *Brain and Behavior*, 11(5), e02138.

McClure, T. (2021, October 15). *New Zealand's Weird and Wonderful Vaccine Rollout*. Retrieved from The Guardian: https://www.theguardian.com/world/2021/oct/16/new-zealands-weird-and-wonderful-vaccine-rollout

McKittrick, K. (2011). On Plantations, Prisons, and a Black Sense of Place. *Social and Cultural Geography*, 12(8), 947–963.

Ministry of Health. (2021a, June 1). No New Community Cases; No New Cases of COVID-19 in Managed Isolation, https://www.health.govt.nz/news-media/media-releases/no-new-community-cases-no-new-cases-covid-19-managed-isolation-3.

Ministry of Health. (2021b, June 1). COVID-19: Protecting Aotearoa New Zealand. https://www.health.govt.nz/covid-19-novel-coronavirus/covid-19-response-planning/covid-19-protecting-aotearoa-new-zealand.

Ministry of Health. (2022). History of Covid-19 Alert System. https://covid19.govt.nz/about-our-covid-19-response/history-of-the-covid-19-alert-system/#alert-levels [accessed 03.06.2022]

Murphy. (2020). Concerns for LGBTQI People in Unsafe Homes during Covid-19 lockdown.https://www.rnz.co.nz/news/national/413386/concerns-for-lgbtqi-people-in-unsafe-homes-during-covid-19-lockdown 3 April 2020.

New Zealand Ministry of Health. (2022, June 1). *COVID-19: Vaccine Data*. Retrieved from Ministry of Health: https://www.health.govt.nz/covid-19-novel-coronavirus/covid-19-data-and-statistics/covid-19-vaccine-data

Nixon, R. (2013). *Slow Violence and the Environmentalism of the Poor*. Harvard University Press, Cambridge, MA and London, UK.

NZ Human Rights Commission. (2022, June 01). *Human Rights in Relation to COVID-19*. Retrieved from NZ Human Rights: https://www.hrc.co.nz/resources/human-rights-relation-covid-19/

O'Connor, H., Hopkins, W., and Johnston, D. (2021). For the Greater Good? Data and Disasters in a Post-COVID World. *Journal of the Royal Society of New Zealand*, 51(sup1), S214–S231.

OECD (2021). Health at a Glance, 2021. https://www.oecd.org/coronavirus/en/data-insights/excess-mortality-since-january-2020

Power, J. (2021, December 22). *No Way Home: Overseas New Zealanders Despair at Tightened Borders*. Retrieved from AlJazeera: https://www.aljazeera.com/economy/2021/12/22/no-way-home-overseas-new-zealanders-despair-at-border-rules

Prickett, Kate C., Fletcher, Michael, Chapple, Simon, Doan, Nyguen, and Smith, Conal. (2020). Life in Lockdown: The Economic and Social Effect of Lockdown during Alert Level 4 in New Zealand. *IGPS Working Paper*.

Prout, A. (2005). *The Future of Childhood*. Routledge, New York and London.

Quinn, R. (2022). Hospitals' Winter Illnesses Spell Long Waits for Heart and Cancer Surgeries. https://www.rnz.co.nz/news/national/471730/hospitals-winter-illnesses-spell-long-waits-for-heart-and-cancer-surgeries [28.07.2022]

RNZ. (2022). Parliament Protests – A Photo-Essay. https://www.rnz.co.nz/news/national/461421/photo-essay-parliament-grounds-occupation

Sepuloni, J. (2021). Additional Funding for Food Banks and Social Agencies. https://www.beehive.govt.nz/release/additional-funding-foodbanks-and-social-agencies [accessed 15.05.2022].

Shaw, R. (2020). 'New Zealand'. In N. Georgeou and C. Hawksley (eds.), *State Responses to COVID-19: A Global Snapshot at 1 June 2020*. Available at" https://researchdirect.westernsydney.edu.au/islandora/object/uws:56288/datastream/.

Smith, M., Donnellan, N., Zhao, J., Egli, V., Ma, C., and Clark, T. (2022). Children's Perceptions of Their Neighbourhoods during COVID-19 Lockdown in Aotearoa New Zealand. *Children's Geographies*, 1–15, https://doi.org/10.1080/14733285.2022.2026887.

Spray, J. (2020). Children and the Pandemic. Newsroom.

Spray, J. and Hunleth, J. (2020). Where Have All the Children Gone? Against Children's Invisibility in the COVID-19 Pandemic, *Anthropology Now*, *12*(2): 39–52, https://doi.org/10.1080/19428200.2020.1824856.

Thaker, J. (2021). The Persistence of Vaccine Hesitancy: COVID-19 Vaccination Intention in New Zealand. *Journal of Health Communication*, *26*(2), 104–111.

The Economist. (2022). New Zealand's Housing Crisis Is Worsening. https://www.economist.com/asia/2022/02/12/new-zealands-housing-crisis-is-worsening.

Vannini, P. (2020). 'COVID-19 as Atmospheric Dis-ease: Attuning into Ordinary Effects of Collective Quarantine and Isolation. *Space and Culture*, *23*(3): 269–273, https://doi.org/10.1177/1206331220938640.

Wang, C., Ng, C., and Brook, R. (2020). Response to COVID-19 in Taiwan: Big Data Analytics, New Technology, and Proactive Testing. *JAMA*, *323*(14), 1341–1342.

Ward, G. (2015). The Slow Violence of State Organized Race Crime. *Theoretical Criminology*, *19*(3), 299–314. https://doi.org/10.1177/1362480614550119

Xue, W. and White, A. (2021). COVID-19 and the Rebiologisation of Racial Difference. *The Lancet*, *10310*, 1479–1480.

12 Conclusion

Charles Hawksley and Nichole Georgeou

In this volume, we have presented a range of case studies that demonstrate the diversity of state responses to the COVID-19 pandemic in the Asia-Pacific as governments sought to protect their societies. These responses are all different, and some were more effective than others, but in the end, all states and all societies have had to learn to move from strategies of 'COVID elimination' to 'COVID suppression' to policies of adjusting to the omnipresent threat (including for those vaccinated) of infection with the COVID virus.

There may be more pandemics in the future, and more scrambles to discover effective vaccines, but for the generation who lived through the first two years of COVID-19, the memories of lockdowns, masks, restrictions, and the fear of infection will not quickly fade. In this very short conclusion, we reflect on some common themes that emerge from our case studies across the first two years of the pandemic (2020 and 2021) in the hope of sparking new areas of investigation around the effects of the COVID pandemic.

Making sense of state responses

The case studies in this volume have highlighted how in the first two years of COVID in Asia-Pacific states employed a variety of responses to combat the COVID pandemic, and no two states' responses were entirely the same. There can be parallels drawn between different states and their lockdowns, restrictions, masks, and vaccination, but there are a range of other factors that also affected individual state responses. These are not as consistent and can cover issues such as the relative wealth and level of economic development of the state, its capacity to implement and enforce effective restrictions; whether the state is unitary or federal, and the relevant powers of state and federal governments; and the quality of leadership.

A theoretical lens—biopolitics

So after a first seizure of power over the body in an individualizing mode, we have a second seizure of power that is not individualizing but, if you like, massifying, that is directed not at man-as-body but at man-as-species.

DOI: 10.4324/9781003311522-12

> After the anatomo-politics of the human body established in the course
> of the eighteenth century, we have, at the end of that century, the emer-
> gence of something that is no longer an anatomo-politics of the human
> body, but what I would call a "biopolitics" of the human race.
>
> Michel Foucault
"Society Must Be Defended"

The COVID pandemic perhaps confirms Foucault's (1976: 243), hypothesis
that modern society is regulated through biopolitics, or what is in effect the
'massification' of individual health needs by the state. In a situation of biopolitics the state governs by managing the health of the community as a whole,
making decisions on our welfare, supposedly driven by the public good. This
has various considerations including birth rates, death rates, and infections,
and information comes through records and censuses. Taking biopolitics as a
lens, the lockdowns, restrictions, masks, and vaccinations are all about ensuring that the mass of people are protected. The modern condition of biopolitics
also involves the collection of vast amounts of medical data on people that
enable the government to make decisions for the benefit of society. According
to Foucault, biopolitics further entrenches and reinforces pre-existing hierar-
chies of power in society. In this way pronouncements on infection rates from
Chief medical officers, based on statistics and expertise, serve as the basis of
public policy. A biopolitical approach to pandemic management is particularly
apparent when states moved to contain outbreaks in poorer neighbourhoods,
with extra vigilance and force deployed to curtail 'deviance', as if poorer people
required more discipline.

Biopolitics is not the only way to understand the COVID pandemic, but it
does suggest itself as a useful way of thinking about how states combatted
COVID.

Comparative levels of development

States that could afford to do so implemented social assistance packages, and
the level of expenditure was often truly massive. Japan's initial packages in
2020 were close to 20% of its gross domestic product, while Australia and
New Zealand also spent widely to prevent their economies from falling into
recession. This return of Keynesian pump priming in times of economic and
political crisis has not lasted, and the benefits were removed along with the
restrictions. The obsession with balanced budgets has however given way to an
acceptance that the costs of pandemic social support in payments and grants
will be present for decades to come. Politics in the Asia-Pacific has perhaps
become less ideological, although evidence from the rise of nationalist and
nativist parties in Europe and the Americas would indicate the divisions are
growing rather than reducing.

There has been however a recognition that states are not exactly like businesses and that they can survive a few years of unbalanced budgets if the re-
ceipts from taxation and other measures are strong. States like Indonesia, the

Philippines, Nepal, Bangladesh, Cambodia, and Vietnam did support their populations although less lavishly; all of them attempted some form of economic-social response to ameliorate the most severe effects of the COVID-19 lockdowns.

Far from being apart from the economy, the state remains as integral as ever—whether this be in making rules governing movement, prohibiting the eviction of renters from houses, raising income support, or deciding on where to allocate medical resources. The state was and remains essential to modern life, balancing public concerns with the realm of economic activity. As a mechanism for delivering resources, it is not perfect, but it is better than the market, as it is open to more influences than simply profit and it has more constituencies than just consumers.

Effective Implementation of controls—the state is still here

From the 1980s onwards, the push to globalisation saw states opening themselves to international capital, business, and people movements. COVID led to (in most cases) a retreat to attempting to police the borders of the basic territorial unit of the nation-state. The COVID pandemic has proved that border closures are indeed possible, but they are expensive and bad for trade. This was particularly apparent in the Pacific Islands where tourism basically stopped from 2020-2022 and there were significant falls in economic activity (Hawksley and Georgeou 2023).

Theoretically, the issue of state sovereignty is inextricably linked with notions of state power and state capacity, but sovereignty is essentially a legal term. Politically, sovereignty can mean effective control over borders, control over movement within the borders, having the power to make laws, and most importantly having the society obey the laws that are made. Even wealthy insular states such as New Zealand and Australia experienced several episodes of what might be termed civil disobedience by groups claiming to represent so-called sovereign citizens (i.e. those who did not accept the right of the state to make laws on their behalf).

There are limits to sovereignty: vaccination was not mandatory for citizens in any state covered in this book, but it was highly encouraged, and there were professions where a person could lose their job if they did not get vaccinated, so in some key industries (healthcare, transport, etc.), it was linked to workers continuing to be employed. Ostensibly, this was a requirement for the people being treated (the sick, the elderly). In the general public space, curfews and lockdowns were enforced (often differentially against the poor), and people were fined for disobeying the new rules and restrictions. All of this shows the state retains elements of what could be called 'sovereign power'. The pandemic quickly exposed the globalist line (see Ohmae 1991) that states since the late 1980s were becoming irrelevant. Pushed by neoliberals encouraging the free flow of capital and deregulation, this was always wishful thinking. In reality, states were the ones making their borders open, and they had the legal architecture to reverse this trend when required.

Unitary or federal state—what works better in a pandemic?

The legal formation of states is rarely considered when discussions of sovereignty ensue; however, when it came to the management of the pandemic, the power to make emergency laws at a national level appears to be an advantage in terms of consistency of regulation. Unitary states usually have the legal architecture for a "national state of emergency" (or something similar), and they could act before infections became acute within the community (New Zealand, Vietnam, Taiwan); however, this is not a cut-and-dried 'rule', as Japan, while a unitary state, did not have provision for emergency laws as a result of its post-war constitution, yet it managed its pandemic response rather effectively using social measures.

States that have been created as a result of a negotiation of legally equal parts and which decide to move into a federation (i.e. Australia), often have defined powers for the national government. These national powers do not always include the specific requirements for exercising emergency powers. As Australia found the individual states and territories (and their governments) ended up doing the day-to-day management of the pandemic, not the national state. The initial response was effective in that internal border controls did prevent the virus from spreading, but as restrictions lifted the national nature of the pandemic took over and the infections and deaths spiked. The same is however true for New Zealand, which is a unitary state. It had the lowest death rate of any of our case studies until it opted to lift restrictions.

Quality of leadership

Decisive leadership appears to have been a factor in pandemic management. In some states (Taiwan, New Zealand, Australia, and to an extent Japan), this is clear with early action preventing widespread infection. Less decisive leadership meant that life continued as the infection spread (Indonesia, Bangladesh, Nepal). For some jurisdictions, the pandemic was used as a political cudgel to silence dissent (Hun Sen in Cambodia), and in others, the pandemic response resembled a military operation (the government of Vietnam and Rodrigo Duterte's Philippines).

Political leadership is one of the great intangibles of political life. It can be linked to charisma in politics (some have it and some do not) and is generally more dependent on the individual human qualities of the leader than on the position of their party in the parliament. Jacinda Ardern in New Zealand did not enjoy a majority when the pandemic began and was rewarded at the ballot box by the electorate, which put her Labour Party into majority government. In Australia, Morrison's antics and overall mediocre performance led to his party's defeat in a federal election; however, the record for the state governments was mixed. In Victoria, Daniel Andrews was returned despite that state having the worst COVID death rates and the longest lockdowns, but Steve Marshall in South Australia was defeated despite an excellent overall COVID performance. Those who delayed taking action (Widowo in Indonesia, Hasina in Bangladesh, K. P. Oli in Nepal) found they were playing COVID catch-up and reacting to events. Decisive leadership appears to have been a factor, but like all matters that affect politics, its utility to explain everything is limited.

Conclusions

The experience of living through the COVID pandemic is not easily summarised. The chapters in this book have tried to do so, and have of course been partial in what they omitted and what they chose to include. The six areas discussed in this chapter suggest themselves for further research and exploration, whether for these same case studies or perhaps for states not included in this book. No state responded to the COVID pandemic entirely correctly. All had their problems and all could have done better in different ways. The years 2020–2021 were a collective learning experience, and as the COVID virus continues to evolve, there are doubtless lessons in these chapters about which measures work well, and which measures could be modified to be more effective when the next pandemic emerges.

References

Foucault, M. 1976. *"Society Must be Defenced": Lectures at the College de France 1975–1976*, [Translated D. Macey]. Picador, New York.
Hawksley and Georgeou September, 2023. 'Small States in the Pacific: Sovereignty, Vulnerability, and Regionalism', in T. Kolnberger and H. Koff (eds), *Agency, Security and Governance of Small States: A Global Perspective*. Routledge, London.
Ohmae. K. 1991. *The Borderless World*. HarperPerennial, New York.

Index

Pages in *italics* refer to figures and pages in **bold** refer to tables.

Abe, Shinzo 56, 59–60, 62–63
aged care (Australia) 136–161
AIDS 8, 14–15, *16*
Albanese, Anthony 142
anti-political ideology 13
Ardern, Jacinda 201, 205, 220
Argentina 4
army/armies/armed forces/defence
  forces 126–127, 140, 176
Asian Development Bank (ADB) 47, 93
Asian Infrastructure Investment Bank 93
Association of Southeast Asian Nations
  (ASEAN) 87, 97, 100
Auckland 206–208
Australia (case study) 136–161, *138–139*;
  other mentions 4, 6–9, 15, 20,
  38–39, 124, 168, 184, 207
Australian Federal Ministries/Ministers:
  Aged Care/Sport/Richard Colbeck
  145; Attorney General/Christian
  Porter 145; Finance/Matthias
  Corman 142; Health/Greg Hunt
  142; Treasury/Josh Frydenberg 143
Australian Labor Party (ALP) 140, 142,
  145, 149
Australian States/Premiers and
  Territories/Chief Ministers *144*;
  Australian Capital Territory/Andrew
  Barr 140, **149**; New South Wales/
  Dominic Perrottet 140, **149**, 152;
  New South Wales/Gladys Berejiklian
  140, **149**; Northern Territory/
  Michael Gunnar 140, **149**;
  Queensland/Anastasia Palaszczuk
  140, **149**; South Australia/Steve
  Marshall 140, **149**; Tasmania/Peter
  Gutwein 140, **149**; Victoria/Daniel

Andrews 140–143, **149**; Western
  Australia/Mark McGowan 140, **149**,
  152
Awami League 35

Baburam, Bhattari 127
Bangladesh (case study) 34–54, **36**, *39*;
  other mentions 6, 8, 20, 219–221
banks 39, 42, 45–48, 51, 93, 130, 154,
  183, 193–194
Beijing 125, 129, 172, 175
Bell, Virginia, Justice 142
Bhandari, Bidya Devi 127
Bhutan 130, 133
Bidyanondo Foundation 46
Bijukchhe, Narayan Man 124
Bin Duong 113, 115
Bloomfield, Dr Ashley 201
Bolsonaro, Jair 12
BRAC 43–44, 47
Brazil 4, 12
Brunei 39

Cambodia (case study) 182–200; other
  mentions 4, 6, 10, 219–220
Canberra 143, 156
Chang Sha 125
Chen Shui-bian 175, 177
children 2, 26–29, 43, 115, 117,
  188–189, 202–203, 209, 211–213
China 4, 7, 9–10, 15, 17, *21*, 38, 43, 62,
  88, 102, 107, 109, 112, 118,
  123–130, 140, 147, 154–155,
  163–165, 168–170, 172–177, 191
Chinese Communist Party (CCP) 170,
  172
Chinese Taipei (see Taiwan and) 175, 177

Chittagong 46
Chongqing 123
civil society 8, 12, 20, 25, 29, 154, 165, 176, 185, 187
contact tracing 23, 109–110, 136, 155, 165, 207
corruption 9, 49, 99, 122, 133, 140
COVID deaths 2–6, 25, 136, 145, 148, **149**, *150*, 156, 167; Asia Pacific comparative deaths **6**; global deaths 2–4, *3*
COVID strains 1; Delta 25, 38, 88, 108, 111, 115, 137, 147, 150, 162, 205, 207–208; Omicron 56, 88, 108, 137, 143, 152, 162, 184, 213
COVID vaccination 2, 4, 6, 8–9, 12, 17, 23, 25, 34, 41–42, 47, 50–51, 55–58, 88, *91*, 111–112, 122, 130, 137, 151–154, 156, 163, 167–168, 184, 188, 194, 207, 211–212, 218–219
COVID vaccines 7, 9, 13, 25, 29–30, 42, 45, 88, 107, 111–112, 118, 129–130, 132, 137, 140, 151–152, 156, 167–169, *170–171*, 178, 217; Abdala 112; AstraZeneca 42, 112, 129–130, 151–152, 167; Hayat-Vax 112; Jannsen 112, 130; Moderna 42, 112, 167; Pfizer (Comirnaty) 42, 88, 112, 129, 152, 167–168; Sinopharm 25, 130, 184; Sinovac 25, 88, 184; Sputnik V 42, 112; Vero Cell 112
Cruise ships 63, 136, 146–147; *Diamond Princess* 63; *Ruby Princess* 147
culture/cultural 69, 72, 109, 116, 202, 208–209, 211

Dahal, Pushpa Kamal 128
Deuba, Sher Bahadur 128
Dhaka 34, 39–40
disability 29, **98**, 150–151
Dong Nai 113, 115
Duterte, Rodrigo 9, 12, 82

education 1, 15, 28, 38, 43, 47, 49, 97, 109, 113, 122, 151, 154, 182–183, 188–190, 193–194, 204, 209, 211; online education 154, 189–190, 193–194, 211
Egypt 39
elderly/elder care 9, 25, 59, 112, 115–116, 130, 219
emergency powers/state of emergency 8–9, 55, 68–69, 73, 141, 145, 186–187, 193, 205, 220

federalism 140, 147
female/females 40–41, 43–44, 49–50
Ferdinand Marcos Jr 96
fines **64**, 67
Flemington Flats (Melbourne) 148–149
food banks 208
food security 133, 192
France 4, 182, 185

GAVI (The Vaccination Alliance) 130
GDP **36**, 38, 41, 44, 48, 93–96, *94*
gender-based violence 189
gender/gender imbalance 28–29, 40, 154, 189
Germany 35, 39
Ghebreyesus, Tedros Adhanom 169
Gonoshashatho Kendra 46
Guiyang 125

Hassina, Sheikh 35, 221
Health diplomacy 168
Health services 28–29, 46, 49, 92, 141, 154, 205, 210
HIV 8, 14–15, *16*
Ho Chi Minh City (HCMC) 113, 115
holidays and festivals 23, 44, 130, 141, 183, 208
Hong Kong 2, 164–165, 176
Hou Yanqi 124
Howard Springs Quarantine facility, Darwin 147–148
Humanitarian and Development Research Initiative (HADRI) 8–10
human rights 69, 87, 116–118, 123, 173, 182–188, 190–191, 193–194, 209
Hun Sen 184, 194, 220

India 4, 7, 9, 12, 20, 38, 41–42, 123–124, 128–130, 154
Indonesia (Case study) 12–33, *16*, *19*, *22*, *24*; other mentions 4, 6–8, 38, 87–88
inequality 29, 183, 193, 203
informal economy **98**, 113, 192, 194
International Labor Organisation (ILO) 47, 194
International Monetary Fund (IMF) 48, 182
International students 123, 147, 154, 172
Iran 4, 124–125, 147
Iraq 39
Italy 4, 15, 39, 43, 124, 147

Jakarta 13, *19*, 28
Japan (case study) 55–81, *61*; other
    mentions 4, 6, 8, 39, 124–125, 130,
    175, 184, 220
Job Keeper 153–154
Job Seeker 153
Johns Hopkins COVID Tracking Centre 2
Johnson, Boris 13
Jordan 39, *40*

Kathmandu 123, 128, 130, 132
Kingdom of Saudi Arabia (KSA) 35, 38,
    40, 42–44, 47
Kishida, Fumio 56, 69
Kuomintang (KMT) Taiwan 170, 176

Labour (New Zealand) 205, 208, 220
leadership 8, 11–12, 60, 82, 86, 107,
    137, 141, 148, 217, 220
Lebanon 39
Lee Teng-Hui 175
Liberal Democratic Party (LDP) (Japan)
    56
Liberal Party of Australia 137, 140, 143,
    145, **149**, 153
Libya 39
lockdown/lockdowns 2, 14, 40–41, 43,
    45, 50, 83–84, *85*, 87, 95, 107–109,
    113, 115
Long An 113, 115
long COVID 6, 211

Mahato, Rajendra 127
Malaysia 39
Manila 83, 86, 97
Mauritius 39
Melbourne 137, 145, 148, 150–153
mental health 29, 51, 113–115, 133
Mexico 4
migrant workers 8–9, 34, 38–44, *40*,
    46–51, 109, 130, 147, 167, 192;
    female migrant workers 44
migration 38, 43–44, 49, 113–115
militarisation 86
military 17–18, 20, 84–87, 100, 115,
    172, 220
Modi, Narendra 12, 128–129
moralised politics 8, 55, 73–75
Morrison, Scott 137, 140–143, 145,
    149, 151, 153–154

National disaster mitigation agency
    (Indonesia) *BNPB* 17
Nepal (Case study) 122–135; other
    mentions 6, 9, 219–221

Nepal Communist Party (Maoist) 123,
    128
Nepal Communist Party (NCP) 128, 130
New Zealand (case study) 201–216, *206*;
    other mentions 4, 6–9, 20, 147,
    218–220
1918 influenza 1–2, 11

Oli, K. P. Sharma 125–128
Oman 35, *40*

Pacific Islands 7, 151, 219; *Pasifika*
    peoples 210
Palmer, Clive 145
Parti Democrasi Indonesia–Perjuanjan
    (PDI-P) 15
Peru 4
Philippines (case study) 82–121, *87*;
    other mentions 4, 6, 8–9, 12, 17, 20,
    219–220
Phnom Penh 183
Poland 4, 35
police 20, 23, 41, 73–74, 84–87, 132,
    148–150, 152, 219
populism/populists 9, 12–13, 17, 82,
    100, 176
poverty 20, 26, 29, 35, 38, 41, 48, 93,
    126, 153, 183, 212
Probash Bondhu 47
Putin, Vladamir 12
Putranto, Tarawan Agus (Health
    Minister Indonesia) 13

Qatar 35, 38, *40*, 47
quarantine 43, 70, 82–84, *84*, 86,
    95–96, **98**, 99, 109–111, 113, 124,
    128, 130, 133, 136–137, 140,
    146–148, 164–165, 167, 204–205,
    207–210

Rajapaksa, Mahinda 12
recession 93, 182, 218
remittances 8, 30, 34, **36**, 38–39, *39*,
    42–44, 46
Royal Commission into COVID 146
rule of law 55, 69, 72–73, 75
Russia 4, 12, 48

schools 28–29, 35, 59, 108–109, 113,
    115, 117, 140, 151, 164, 166, **166**,
    170–171, 184, 188–190, 205, 209,
    211
securitisation 9, 18, 25, 82, 100
sexual abuse/sexual harassment 43, 49,
    189

sex workers 14, 154, 210
Shenzhen 125
Singapore 39, *40*, 43–44, 88, 207
slow violence 10, 150, 202–204, 209
South Africa 4, 12
South Asian Association for Regional Cooperation (SAARC) 129, 133
South Korea 39, 62, 124–125, 147
Spain 4, 35
stigma 15, 43, 47, 114, 150–151, 186, 209–210
stimulus packages 45–48, 50–51, **58**, 62, 67, 96, 136–137, 153–155
Sudan 39
Suga, Yoshihide 56, 63, 66
Suharto 12, 14
Sukarno 12
Sydney 137, 145, 147–148, 150, 207

Taipei 165, 172, 175
Taiwan (case study) 162–181; other mentions 4, 6, 10, 207, 220
Tokyo 56, 60, 66–68, 71; Tokyo Olympics 56, 60, 62, 66–67
tourism 10, 17, 60, 62, 97, 109, 125, 147–148, 172, 191–192, 213, 219
Trump, Donald/Trump Administration 12–13, 140, 163, 172
Turkey 4, 35, 125

Ukraine 4, 48, 51, 96
UNDP 47, 182, 192
unemployment 18, *19*, 43, 95, 153, 192
United Arab Emirates 35, *40*, 47

United Kingdom 4, 13, 35, 39, 66, 111, 116, 125, 152, 184
United Marxist Leninist (UML) Party 128
United Nations International Children's Emergency Fund (UNICEF) 25–26, 130, 189, 192
United States of America 35, 38–39, 96, 111, 113
universities 154, 190, 205

vaccine diplomacy 34
vaccine hesitancy 25, 88, 112, 152, 208
vaccine safety 88, 112
Vietnam (case study) 107–121; other mentions 6, 9, 88, 219–220
vigilantes/vigilantism 8, 73
volunteer(s)/voluntary sector 46, 129, 132

War on Drugs 9, 85–86, 100
Widodo, Joko ('Jokowi') 12–14
women 26, 28–29, **98**, 113, 117, 148, 191–192
World Health Organisation (WHO) 4, *5*, 18, 63, 88, 92, 107, 124, 130, 162, 165, 168–169, *170–171*, 173–176; WHO regions *5*
Wuhan, China 15, 17, 109, 123–124, 147, 164, 173

Xi Jingping 172

Zuma, Jacob 12

Taylor & Francis Group
an **informa** business

Taylor & Francis eBooks

www.taylorfrancis.com

A single destination for eBooks from Taylor & Francis
with increased functionality and an improved user
experience to meet the needs of our customers.

90,000+ eBooks of award-winning academic content in
Humanities, Social Science, Science, Technology, Engineering,
and Medical written by a global network of editors and authors.

TAYLOR & FRANCIS EBOOKS OFFERS:

A streamlined
experience for
our library
customers

A single point
of discovery
for all of our
eBook content

Improved
search and
discovery of
content at both
book and
chapter level

REQUEST A FREE TRIAL
support@taylorfrancis.com

Routledge
Taylor & Francis Group

CRC Press
Taylor & Francis Group